REVIEW
OF
PHARMACOLOGY

REVIEW OF PHARMACOLOGY

Sneha R. Ambwani
Professor, Pharmacology
Dr. S.N. Medical College
Jodhpur (Rajasthan) India

PEEPEE
PUBLISHERS AND DISTRIBUTORS (P) LTD.

Review of Pharmacology

Published by
Pawaninder P. Vij
Peepee Publishers and Distributors (P) Ltd.
Head Office:
160, Shakti Vihar, Pitam Pura, Delhi-110 034 (India)
Correspondence Address:
7/31, First Floor, Ansari Road, Daryaganj
New Delhi-110 002 (India)
Ph: 65195868, 23246245, 9811156083
e-mail: peepee160@yahoo.co.in
e-mail: peepee160@rediffmail.com
e-mail: peepee160@gmail.com
www.peepeepub.com

First Edition: 2012

ISBN: 978-81-8445-119-1

Dedicated to

My Guru

who has been a source of inspiration for me to work hard to write this book

To my mother and other family members for their unconditional support throughout writing this book

FOREWORD

In last few decades, significant advances have been made in pharmacology. A sound knowledge is essential to be a good practitioner, so students have to read and digest mammoth sized information from the large sized books. A comprehensive and simple book is always welcome all the time. This book has a unique combination and serves the dual purpose. In this book, the subject of pharmacology is divided into nine chapters. They are presented in outlined form from general principles of drug action to the minute pharmacology of the newer topics in a systematic and comprehensive manner. Each chapter is followed by multiple choice questions with answer and explanation arranged systematically to avoid repetition. This format is refreshing change from standard textbooks as in addition to MCQs and answers, a bird's eyeview of each topic has been presented in a good manner. As MCQs have become a standard tool of assessment of students at all levels, this book serve an excellent quick reference, not only for U.G. and P.G. students but also for different competitive examinations related to medical field. Drawing on the author, Dr Sneha Ambwani is having invaluable experience. As a teacher, she has provided the students, educators and practitioners with comprehensive text of pharmacology. This book should prove invaluable to some and useful to all. My blessings are to Dr. Sneha Ambwani with all the wishes for success in future.

Dr A. K. Mathur
Former Senior Professor and Head
Department of Pharmacology
Dr. S. N. Medical College
Jodhpur (Rajasthan)

Although, I gave my best efforts to prepare this book, yet, it is my humble request to my all readers and critics to kindly inform me about any deficiency and shortcoming [illegible] improve this book.

PREFACE

Review of Pharmacology presents the pharmacological basis for the students, who are preparing for the various entrance tests / qualifying examinations for the admission in different courses. All the scientific information given in this book is from different standard textbooks. The recent advances in the pharmacology also have been added.

Although, I gave my best efforts to prepare this book in concise pattern, yet, it is my humble request to my all readers and critics to kindly inform me about any deficiency and shortcomings and give me suggestions to improve this book.

Sneha R. Ambwani

ACKNOWLEDGEMENTS

I would like to express my sincere thanks to all my senior teachers, senior and junior colleagues and students who encouraged and supported me to write this book. I acknowledge the invaluable support, advice and guidance of Dr. A.K. Mathur, Former Senior Professor and Head, Department of Pharmacology, Dr. S.N. Medical College, Jodhpur, Rajasthan, in bringing the book to this shape.

I am also grateful to authors and publishers of the books which have been consulted for the preparation of the text and setting the MCQs and answers.

I give my sincere and deep thanks to the team of Peepee Publishers and Distributors (P) Ltd., for their efforts and suggestions in the timely publication of the book.

Sneha R. Ambwani

CONTENTS

REFERENCES

1. The Pharmacological Basis of the Therapeutics, Goodman and Gilman, 12th edition.
2. Essentials of Medical Pharmacology, KD Tripathi, 6th edition.
3. Multiple Choice Questions in Pharmacology, K.D. Tripathi, 4th edition.
4. Essentials of Pharmacotherapeutics, FSK Barar, 6th edition.
5. Pharmacology and Pharmacotherapeutics, Satoskar RS, Bhandarker SD, Rege NN, Revised 22nd edition.
6. Text Book of Pharmacology, Seth SD and Seth V, 3rd edition.
7. Principles of Pharmacology, HL Sharma and KK Sharma, 2nd edition.
8. Basic and Clinical Pharmacology, Katjung BG, 11th edition.
9. Pharmacology Examination and Board Review, Katjung and Trevors, 8th edition.
10. MCQs in Pharmacology and Drug Therapy, G Khilnani and S.K. Sharma.

1

GENERAL PHARMACOLOGY

INTRODUCTION
(Definitions, Nature and Sources of Drugs)

- **Pharmacology:** It is the science that deals with the effects of drugs on living system.
- **Drug:** WHO defines drug as a substance or product that is used or intended to be used to modify or explore physiological systems or pathological states for the benefit of the recipient.
- **Pharmacokinetics:** It is the study of movement of the drug within the body; it includes the processes of absorption (A), distribution (D), metabolism (M) and excretion (E). In short it means 'what the body does to the drug'.
- **Pharmacodynamics:** It is the study of mechanism of action, pharmacological actions and adverse effects of drugs. In short, it means 'what the drug does to the body'.
- **Pharmacy:** It is an art and science that deals with the collection, preparation, preservation, standardization, and compounding, dispensing and proper utilization of drugs.
- **Therapeutics:** It is the clinical aspect of medicine concerned with the treatment of diseases.
- **Chemotherapy:** It deals with the use of drugs for the treatment of infectious/parasitic diseases with chemical compounds that have relatively selective toxicity for the infecting organism without causing damage to the host cells (exception is chemotherapy of cancer).
- **Toxicology:** It is the study of poisons, their actions, detection, prevention and the treatment of poisoning.
- **Clinical Pharmacology:** It is the systematic study of a drug in human beings both in healthy volunteers and in patients. It includes the evaluation of pharmacokinetic and pharmacodynamic data, the safety, efficacy and adverse effects of a drug by comparative clinical trials.

- **Essential drugs:** According to WHO, essential drugs are those that satisfy the healthcare needs of the population; they should be available at all times in adequate amounts and in appropriate dosage forms.
- **Orphan drug:** Drugs or biological products that are used for the diagnosis, treatment or prevention of rare diseases, *e.g.*, digoxin antibody, erythropoietin fomepizole, chelating agents etc. They do not fetch much profit, thus neither manufacturer nor the chemists are interested in it.

Sources of Drugs

1. Natural Sources

a. *Plants:* (i) Alkaloids, *e.g.*, Morphine, Atropine, Quinine, Reserpine, Ephedrine (ii) Glycosides, *e.g.*, Digoxin, Digitoxin (iii) Oils, *e.g.*, clove oil, castor oil (iv) Gums, *e.g.*, gum acacia (v) Tannins, *e.g.*, tincture catechu (vi) Resins, *e.g.*, tincture benzoin.

b. *Animals:* Insulin, Thyroxine etc.

c. *Minerals:* Ferrous sulphate, Magnesium sulphate.

d. *Microorganisms:* Penicillin, Streptomycin, Griseofulvin, etc.

2. Synthetic Source

Most of the drugs used today are synthetic or semi-synthetic drugs, *e.g.*, Aspirin, Paracetamol, Cotrimoxazole and Chloroquine.

3. Genetic Engineering (DNA Recombinant Technology)

Human insulin, Human growth hormone, Hepatitis B vaccine.

ROUTES OF DRUG ADMINISTRATION

Drug and patient related factors determine the selection of routes for drug administration, *e.g.*

1. Characteristics of the drug (Physical or chemical properties).
2. Emergency / routine use.
3. Condition of the patient (unconscious, presence of vomiting, diarrhoea).
4. Age of the patient.
5. Associated diseases.
6. Sometimes patients and doctors choice.

Routes

- **Local**
  - **Topical**
  - **Deep tissue**
- **Systemic**
  - **Enteral**
    - Oral
    - Sublingual
    - Rectal
  - **Parenteral**
    - Inhalation
    - Injections
    - Transdermal

Local Route

Simplest mode of administration. Systemic side effects are minimal.

1. **Topical:** Drug is applied to the skin or mucous membrane for local action.
   a. *Oral cavity:* nystatin, clotrimazole.
   b. *GI tract:* neomycin.
   c. *Rectum and anal canal:*
      i. Evacuant enema, *e.g.* soap water enema.
      ii. Retention enema, *e.g.* methylprednisolone in ulcerative colitis.
      iii. As suppository, *e.g.* bisacodyl.
   d. *Eye, Ear and Nose:* as drops, ointments, sprays.
   e. *Bronchi:* as inhalation, *e.g.* salbutamol, ipratropium bromide.
   f. *Vagina:* as tablet, cream, pessary.
   g. *Urethra:* as jelly, *e.g.* lignocaine.
2. **Deep Tissue:** By using a syringe and needle, infiltration anaesthesia with local anaesthetics is given for local effect.

Systemic Route

Further divided into:

I. Enteral routes

It includes oral, sublingual and rectal route.

Oral route

It is the most common and acceptable route. Drugs are given as tablets, capsules, syrup, mixtures, etc.

Advantages

Safer, cheaper, painless, convenient for repeated and prolonged use and can be self-administered.

Disadvantages

Oral route has a slow onset of action, hence cannot be used in emergency. It is not suitable for unpalatable and highly irritant drugs, unabsorbable drugs (*e.g.* aminoglycosides) and drugs that are destroyed by digestive juices (*e.g.* penicillin G, insulin).

Enteric coated tablets and sustained or time release preparation are used for better compliance via oral route, *e.g.* Nifedipine (for hypertension), Pyridostigmine (for myasthenia gravis).

Sublingual route

The drug is absorbed through the buccal mucous membrane and enters into the systemic circulation directly, *e.g.* nitroglycerin for acute anginal attack and buprenorphine for myocardial infarction. Advantages of sublingual routes are:

- Quick onset of action.
- Action can be terminated by spitting out the tablet.
- Escapes the first pass metabolism, so smaller doses are required.
- Self administration is possible.

Rectal route

For systemic effects drugs are given as suppositories, *e.g.* indomethacin for rheumatoid arthritis, diazepam for status epilepticus (useful for irritant drugs).

II. Parenteral routes

Routes of administration of drugs other than enteral routes are called parenteral routes.

Advantages

1. It has a rapid onset of action, hence suitable for emergency.
2. It is useful in unconscious, uncooperative and unreliable patients and in presence of vomiting and diarrhoea.
3. It is suitable for drugs with high first pass metabolism, drugs not absorbed orally and drugs destroyed by digestive juices.

Disadvantages

It require sterilization and aseptic conditions. It is expensive, invasive and painful technique, cannot be self-administered, can cause local tissue injury to nerves, vessels, etc. and safe in skilled hands only.

Parenteral route is further divided into:

(A) Inhalation

Volatile liquids, gases and aerosols (salbutamol, beclomethasone) can be given by this route.

Advantages

Quick onset of action, dose required is very less, so systemic toxicity is minimized and amount of drug administered can be regulated.

Disadvantages

Local irritation may cause increased respiratory secretions and bronchospasm may occur.

(B) Injection

a. **Intradermal route:** Used for BCG vaccination, sensitivity tests.
b. **Subcutaneous route:** Used for adrenaline, insulin.
c. **Intramuscular route:** Drugs are injected into large muscles such as deltoid, gluteus maximus and lateral aspect of the thigh in children but the absorption is not always faster than oral route, *e.g.,* diazepam, digoxin, hydrocortisone etc.
d. **Intravenous route:** It can be given as:
   i. *Bolus:* Relatively large dose of a drug is injected rapidly or slowly as a single unit into a vein, *e.g.,* furosemide.
   ii. *Slow intravenous (I.V.) injection*: Given over 5-10 minutes, *e.g.,* morphine.
   iii. *Intravenous infusion:* It is given by adding the drug to a bottle containing dextrose/saline, *e.g.,* dopamine infusion in cardiogenic shock.
e. **Intra arterial route:** Used for angiography and for the administration of some anti-cancer drugs.
f. **Intrathecal route:** *e.g.,* Spinal anaesthesia (*e.g.,* lignocaine).
g. **Intra articular route:** *e.g.,* Hydrocortisone injection for rheumatoid arthritis.
h. **Intra peritoneal route:** Used for dialysis.

(C) Transdermal route (Adhesive patches)

The drug is administered in the form of patches that deliver the drug into the circulation for systemic effect, *e.g.,* scopolamine for motion sickness, nitroglycerine for angina, estrogen for hormone replacement therapy (HRT) and fentanyl for analgesia.

Other special drug delivery systems are:

1. *Occusert: e.g.* Pilocarpine in glaucoma for miosis.
2. *Progestasert:* As an intrauterine contraceptive.
3. *Liposomes:* They are minute vesicles made of phospholipids into which the drug is incorporated. It helps in targeted delivery of drugs, *e.g.* liposomal formulation of amphotericin B for fungal infections.
4. *Monoclonal antibodies:* They are immunoglobulin produced by cell culture, selected to react with a specific antigen. They are useful for targeted delivery of drugs, *e.g.* delivery of anti-cancer drug using monoclonal antibodies.

PHARMACOKINETICS

All biological membranes are made up of lipid bilayer. Drugs cross various biological membranes by the following mechanisms:

1. **Passive diffusion:** The drug molecules move from a region of higher concentration to lower concentration until equilibrium is attained. It does not require energy. This is most important mechanism of absorption for majority of drugs.
2. **Filtration:** Depends on the particle size and molecular weight of the drug. Free drug can pass through the pores in between the cells, *e.g.* urea, alcohol, glucose. Diffusion of drugs across capillaries is dependent on rate of blood flow.
3. **Specialized transport:**
   a. *Active transport:* The drug molecules move from a region of low concentration to high concentration against the concentration gradient. It requires energy.
   b. *Facilitated diffusion:* It is a type of carrier mediated transport and does not require energy, *e.g.* absorption of Vitamin B_{12} from the gut. It facilitates permeation of poorly diffusible substrate (from higher to lower concentration).
   c. *Pinocytosis:* It is the process of transport across the cell in particulate form (for proteins and other big molecules).

1. Drug Absorption

The movement of a drug from the site of administration into the circulation or passage of drugs across the biological membrane is known as absorption. Acidic drugs, *e.g.* salicylates, barbiturates are better absorbed in acidic medium of stomach while basic drugs, *e.g.* morphine and quinine are better absorbed in alkaline medium of intestine.

Factors influencing drug absorption:

1. Physicochemical properties of the drug:
   Physical state (Lipid soluble and unionized form are better absorbed).
   Particle size, Disintegration time, Dissolution time and formulations.
2. Route of drug administration.
3. pH and ionization.
4. Presence of other drugs and food.
5. Pharmacogenetic factors.
6. Area of the absorbing surface.
7. Gastrointestinal and other diseases.

Bioavailability

It is the fraction of a drug that reaches to the systemic circulation from a given dose in an unchanged form. Intravenous route of drug administration gives almost 100% bioavailability as it directly enters the circulation. The term bioavailability is used commonly for drugs given by oral route.

Measurement of Bioavailability

$$\text{Drug bioavailability (\%)} = \frac{\text{AUC (Oral)}}{\text{AUC (IV)}} \times 100$$

AUC = Area under curve

Factors Affecting Bioavailability

1. *First pass metabolism:* Certain drugs during their passage get metabolized in liver and are removed or inactivated before they reach to the systemic circulation. This process is known as first-pass effect. The net result is a decreased bioavailability of the drug and diminished therapeutic response.
2. Hepatic diseases.
3. Enterohepatic cycling.
4. Quality control by manufacturer.

Bio Equivalence

If two or more similar dosage forms of the same drug reach the blood circulation at the same relative rate and to the same relative extent, these are called bio equivalent.

Chemical Equivalence

If two or more dosage forms of the same drug contain the same labeled quantities of the drug as specified in pharmacopoeia are called chemically equivalent drugs.

2. Drug Distribution

Distribution is defined as the reversible transfer of drugs between various body fluid compartments.

Apparent Volume of Distribution

Apparent volume of distribution (aVd) is defined as the hypothetical volume of body fluid into which a drug is uniformly distributed at a concentration equal to that in plasma, assuming the body to be a single compartment.

$$aVd = \frac{\text{Total amount of drug in the body (mg/kg)}}{\text{Concentration of the drug in plasma (mg/L)}}$$

- Drugs with low volume of distribution confined to plasma (bind with plasma proteins).
- Drugs with high volume of distribution are widely distributed in various body fluids.

Factors affecting drug distribution (V_d)

1. Physicochemical properties of the drug.
2. Degree of plasma protein binding.
3. Tissue storage.
4. Disease states.
5. Fat – lean body mass ratio.

   Drugs extensively bound to plasma proteins are largely restricted to the vascular compartment and have low volume of distribution.

Redistribution

Highly lipid soluble drug such as thiopentone, on intravenous administration, immediately gets distributed to areas of high blood flow such as brain, and causes general anaesthesia. Immediately, it diffuses out of the blood brain barrier (BBB) and gets distributed into the blood and then to the less perfused tissues, such as muscle and adipose tissue which results in termination of drug action. This is called redistribution. Greater the lipid solubility, faster is redistribution of drug.

Protein Binding

Drugs usually bind to plasma and cellular protein. Most of the acidic drugs, *e.g.* warfarin, penicillins, aspirin etc. are bind to albumin, while most of the lipophilic basic drugs, *e.g.* quinidine, lidocaine etc. are bind to $alpha_1$ acid glycoprotein. Exceptions are steroids (bound to corticosteroid binding globulin transcortin), thyroxine (bound to alpha globulin) and antigen (bound to gamma globulins). Protein binding also act as drug reservoir.

Clinical importance of plasma protein binding:

1. Extensive protein binding reduces the intensity of drug action.
2. Drugs that are highly bound to plasma proteins have a low volume of distribution.
3. Plasma protein binding delays the metabolism of drugs and hence increases duration of action.
4. Bound form is not available for filtration at the glomeruli, hence delays its excretion. Also, they are difficult to remove by dialysis in case of poisoning.
5. Plasma protein binding can cause displacement interactions.

Drug Reservoirs or Tissue Storage

Some drugs are concentrated or accumulated in tissue or some organs, *e.g.* tetracyclines in bones, teeth; thiopentone and DDT in adipose tissue; chloroquine in liver and in retina; digoxin in heart, iodine in thyroid.

Blood Brain Barrier

The capillary boundary that is present between the blood and brain is called BBB. Only the lipid soluble and unionized drugs can pass through BBB and reaches to the brain, *e.g.* barbiturates, diazepam, volatile anaesthetics, amphetamine, morphine etc.

Pathological states like meningitis, encephalitis increase the permeability of the BBB and allow the normally impermeable substances to enter in the brain, *e.g.* penicillins, ampicillin etc.

Placental Barrier

The lipid membrane between the mother and foetus is called placental barrier.

Certain drugs when given during pregnancy may cross the placenta. Unionized and lipid soluble drugs can freely cross the placental barrier, *e.g.* anaesthetics, alcohol, morphine, etc. while polar or quaternary ammonium compounds (dTc), and substances with high molecular weight, *e.g.* insulin, cannot cross the placental barrier. Most effective biological barrier is sertoli cells.

3. Biotransformation (Drug Metabolism)

Chemical alteration of the drug in a living organism is called biotransformation. The metabolism of drug usually converts the lipid soluble and unionized compounds into water soluble and ionized compounds, so can be excreted easily.

Liver is the main site for drug metabolism. Other sites are GI tract, kidney, lungs, blood, skin, placenta, etc.

There are four ways by which the activity of a drug can be altered after its metabolism:

1. Active drug to inactive metabolite
   Phenobarbitone ⟶ Hydroxyphenobarbitone
   Phenytoin ⟶ p-Hydroxyphenytoin
2. Active drug to active metabolite
   Codeine ⟶ Morphine
   Diazepam ⟶ Oxazepam
3. Inactive drug to active metabolite (prodrug)
   L Dopa ⟶ Dopamine
   Prednisone ⟶ Prednisolone
4. Active drug to highly toxic metabolite
   Paracetamol ⟶ N-acetyl-p-benzoquinoneimine (NAPQI)

Drug get metabolized by:

1. **Microsomal enzymes:** They are mainly present in the endoplasmic reticulum of the cells.
2. **Non microsomal enzymes:** They are found in the cytoplasm, mitochondria of liver cells and in plasma.
3. **Hoffman elimination**.

Biotransformation reactions can be classified into:

a. *Non-synthetic / Phase I / Functionalization reactions:* A functional group is generated or exposed, metabolite may be active or inactive. They are mainly microsomal reaction.
b. *Synthetic / Phase II / Conjugation reactions:* Metabolite is inactive (except morphine). The metabolite from Phase I reaction may undergo Phase II reaction.

Phase I Reactions

Oxidation	*e.g.* Phenytoin, Phenobarbitone, Propranolol, Warfarin
Reduction	*e.g.* Chloramphenicol, Methadone, Cortisone, Chloral hydrate
Hydrolysis	*e.g.* Esters–Procaine, Succinylcholine (rarely microsomal)
	Amides–Lignocaine, Procainamide

Phase II Reactions — Always causes inactivation of drugs

Glucuronide conjugation	*e.g.* Morphine, Paracetamol, Diazepam, Sulfonamides
Acetylation	*e.g.* Isoniazid, Dapsone, PAS, Sulfonamides, Histamine, Procainamide
Glycine conjugation	*e.g.* Salicylic acid, Nicotinic acid (minor pathway)
Sulphate conjugation	*e.g.* Paracetamol, Sex steroids, Chloramphenicol
Glutathione conjugation	*e.g.* Paracetamol (minor pathway)
Methylation	*e.g.* Adrenaline, Dopamine (minor pathway)

Enzyme Induction

Repeated administration of certain drugs increases the synthesis of microsomal enzymes and thus increases the metabolism or drug itself and/or other drugs used. This is known as enzyme induction, *e.g.* rifampicin, phenytoin, barbiturates, carbamazepine, griseofulvin, etc.

Enzyme Inhibition

Certain drugs inhibit the activity of drug metabolizing enzymes and are known as enzyme inhibitors, *e.g.* chloramphenicol, ciprofloxacin, erythromycin, etc. (Enzyme inhibition is a rapid process as compared to enzyme induction).

Factors Affecting Drug Metabolism

1. *Age:* Neonates have low enzymatic activity.
2. *Diet:* Diet rich in proteins and low in carbohydrate enhance rate of metabolism.
3. *Presence of diseases, e.g.* hepatic diseases, thyroid diseases.
4. *Genetic factors (pharmacogenetics), e.g.*
   a. Slow acetylators and fast acetylators of isoniazid.
   b. Succinylcholine apnoea.
   c. Glucose-6-phosphate dehydrogenase deficiency (causes haemolytic anaemia).

Prodrug

It is an inactive form of a drug, which is converted to an active form after metabolism, *e.g.* L-dopa, prednisone, sulfasalazine, mercaptopurine, fluorouracil, cyclophosphamide, alpha methyldopa etc.

Uses of Prodrug

1. Improves the bioavailability of drug.
2. Prolong the duration of action.
3. Improves the taste/patient compliance.
4. Provide site specific drug delivery.

4. Drug Excretion

Removal of the drug and its metabolite from the body is known as drug excretion. The main channels of excretion of drugs are:

1. **Kidney**
   a. Glomerular filtration.
   b. Passive tubular reabsorption.
   c. Active tubular secretion.

   Rate of renal excretion =(Rate of filtration + Rate of secretion) – Rate of reabsorption
2. **Lungs:** Alcohol and volatile general anaesthetics such as ether, halothane, enflurane, isoflurane, etc. are excreted via lungs.
3. **Faeces:** Purgatives like senna, cascara, etc. excreted through faeces.
4. **Bile:** *e.g.* Erythromycin, phenolphthalein, tetracycline, ampicillin, rifampicin are excreted in bile. Some drugs are reabsorbed back and the cycle is repeated. This is known as enterohepatic circulation.
5. **Skin:** Metals, *e.g.* arsenic, mercury are excreted through skin.
6. **Saliva:** Rifmapicin.

7. **Milk:** Basic drugs taken by lactating women may appear in the milk, *e.g.*, tetracycline, chloramphenicol, morphine, diazepam, senna, metronidazole etc.

Plasma Half Life ($t_{½}$)

It is the time required for the plasma concentration of the drug to decrease by 50% of its original value. Plasma $t_{½}$ of lignocaine is 1 hour, and for aspirin it is 4 hours.

$$t_{½} = \frac{0.693}{K}$$

K is elimination constant.

Clinical Importance of Plasma Half Life

It helps to:

- Determine the duration of drug action.
- Determine the frequency of drug administration.
- Estimate the time required to reach the steady state. It takes approximately four to five half lives to reach the steady state during repeated administration of the drug. A drug is almost completely eliminated in four to five half lives after single administration.

Kinetics of Elimination

Clearance

The clearance (CL) of a drug is defined as the theoretical volume of the plasma from which the drug is removed in unit time.

$$\text{Clearance} = \frac{\text{Rate of elimination}}{\text{Plasma concentration of the drug (C)}}$$

1. **First order kinetics:** The important features are:
   a. A constant fraction of the drug in the body is eliminated per unit time.
   b. The rate of drug elimination is directly proportional to its plasma concentration.
   c. The $t_{½}$ of the drugs following first order kinetics will always remain constant.
   d. After a single dose 97% of the drug is eliminated at 4-5th half life time.

e. If a fixed dose is administered at every half life it, require 5 half life to achieve steady state, where the rate of absorption equals rate of elimination.
f. If the dose of the drug is doubled, duration of action is prolonged for one more half life.

2. **Zero order kinetics:**
   a. A constant amount of a drug in the body is eliminated per unit time.
   b. The rate of elimination is independent of plasma drug concentration, *e.g.* ethanol is eliminated from the body at the rate of about 10-15 ml /hours.
   c. The $t_{½}$ of the drug following zero order kinetics is never constant. Most of the drugs are eliminated by first order kinetics. Some drugs, *e.g.* phenytoin, digoxin, warfarin, tolbutamide show dose-dependent kinetic, where smaller dose are eliminated by first order kinetics but at higher plasma concentration, they follow zero-order kinetic.

Drug Dosage

1. *Loading dose:* Loading dose is the large dose of the drug to be given initially to provide the effective plasma concentration in short time.
2. *Maintenance dose:* This is needed to maintain the steady state plasma concentration.

Therapeutic Drug Monitoring (TDM)

Monitoring of drug therapy by measuring plasma concentration of a drug is known as TDM.

Indications

1. For drugs with narrow therapeutic index, *e.g.* lithium, digoxin, phenytoin, aminoglycosides, etc.
2. For drugs showing wide inter individual variations, *e.g.* tricyclic anti-depressants.
3. To ascertain patient compliance.
4. In patients with renal failure, *e.g.* aminoglycosides.
5. To check the bioavailability.
6. In patients who do not respond to therapy without any known reason.

TDM is not required in the following situations:

1. When clinical and biochemical parameters are available, *e.g.* blood pressure measurement for antihypertensive, blood sugar estimation for anti diabetic agents and prothrombin time, aPTT for anticoagulants.
2. For drugs producing tolerance, *e.g.* opioids.
3. For drugs whose effect persists longer than the drug itself, *e.g.* omeprazole (prodrug).

Fixed Dose Combination (FDC)

Combination of two different drugs in a single pharmaceutical formation is known as FDC.

Its examples are:

- Levodopa + Carbidopa: In Parkinsonism.
- Isoniazid + Rifampicin + Pyrazinamide: For Tuberculosis.
- Ferrous sulphate + Folic acid: For anaemia of pregnancy.
- Sulphamethoxozole + Trimethoprim (Cotrimoxazole) to broaden the spectrum.
- Amoxicillin + Clavulanic acid (Augmentin): To broaden the spectrum.
- Estrogen + Progesterone: As oral contraceptive.
- Aspirin + Codeine: As an analgesic.

Advantages

- Increased patient compliance.
- Synergistic effect.
- Increased efficacy.
- Reduce side effects.
- Reduced cost.
- Prevents development of microbial resistance.

Disadvantages

- The dose of any component drug cannot be adjusted independently, if desired.
- Unacceptable range of fluctuation may occur.
- Harmful or beneficial effects are difficult to identify.
- Inflexible fixed dose ratio.
- Increases the cost of therapy if patient not actually need all the drugs used in FDC.
- Discourages precise diagnosis.

Methods to Prolong the Duration of Drug Action

1. *For orally administered drugs:* By giving the drug in enteric coated form and sustained release preparations.
2. *For parenterally administered drugs:*
   a. By decreasing the vascularity of the absorbing surface, *e.g.* lignocaine and adrenaline.
   b. By decreasing the solubility.
   c. Injecting the drug in oily solution – Depot progesteron.
   d. Pellet implantation.
   e. By increasing the plasma protein binding of the drug, *e.g.* sulfonamides.
   f. By inhibiting drug metabolism, *e.g.* physostigmine/ neostigmine for ACh.
   g. By delaying renal excretion of the drug, *e.g.* penicillin and probenecid.

PHARMACODYNAMICS

It is the study of the biochemical and physiological effects of drug and their mode of action.

Types of Drug Action

The drug may act by/as:

1. **Stimulation:** By increasing the activity of specialized cells, *e.g.* catecholamine stimulates heart.
2. **Depression:** By decreasing the activity of specialized cells: barbiturates depresses CNS.
3. **Irritant and counter-irritant action:** Cause irritation of the skin, *e.g.* eucalyptus oil.
4. **Replacement:** Replaced by drugs, *e.g.* insulin in diabetes mellitus.
5. **Chemotherapeutic:** *e.g.* antibiotics, anti-cancer drugs.

Mechanism of Drug Action

Drug act either by:

A. Non receptor mediated mechanism

i. It is non-specific.
ii. Act at higher concentration.
iii. Donot act with specific receptors.

iv. Donot have specific antagonist.
v. Tend not to show structure activity relationship.

B. Receptor mediated mechanism

i. It is highly specific, act through specific receptors.
ii. Act at low concentration.
iii. Show structure activity relationship.
iv. Can be antagonized by specific antagonist.

Sites of Drug Action

The drug may act at:

1. Extracellular site, *e.g.* antacids, chelating agents, osmotic purgatives.
2. Cellular site, *e.g.* action of ACh on nicotinic receptors.
3. Intracellular, *e.g.* trimethoprim or sulfa drug acting by interfering synthesis of folic acid.

A. Non receptor mediated mechanisms

1. *By physical action*
   a. Osmosis – *e.g.* mannitol in cerebral edema.
   b. Absorption– *e.g.* kaolin.
   c. Demulcent– *e.g.* pectin.
   d. Radioactivity– *e.g.* barium sulphate.
2. *By chemical action*
   a. Neutralization – antacids.
   b. Chelation – Metals like iron, copper, mercury etc. are eliminated from the body with the help of chelating agents.
3. *Through enzymes*
   a. Drug action via enzyme inhibition
      (i) Angiotensin converting enzyme inhibitors, *e.g.* enalapril.
      (ii) Xanthine and hypoxanthine are oxidized to uric acid by xanthine oxidase enzyme. Allopurinol act by inhibiting xanthine oxidase enzyme.
   b. Drug action by activation of enzymes
      Cholinesterase reactivators in O.P.C. poisoning.
4. *Drug acting through antibody production:* Vaccines.
5. *Placebo effect:* Placebo is a pharmacodynamically inert and harmless substance, resembles with the actual medicament and when given to patient, cause relief in the subjective symptoms.

B. Receptor mediated mechanisms

Receptors are macromolecules, present either on the cell surface, cytoplasm or in the nucleus where the drug binds and interacts to produce cellular changes. They have specificity and selectivity. No drug is truly specific but many have a relatively selective action on one type of receptor. The basic functions of receptors are:

(a) Binding with appropriate regulatory ligands (neurotransmitter, hormones etc).
(b) Co-ordination of extracellular signals with intracellular activities.
(c) Transformation of such extracellular and intracellular reaction to generate an effect either directly or indirectly.

Affinity: The ability of the drug to get bound to the receptor is known as affinity.

Intrinsic activity: The ability of the drug to produce a pharmacological action after combining with the receptor is known as intrinsic activity of the drug.

Agonist: A drug that is capable of producing pharmacological action after binding to the receptor is called an agonist (have affinity and intrinsic activity both).

Antagonist: Drugs that bind to receptors but are not capable of producing pharmacological action are called antagonists. Antagonists have only affinity but no intrinsic activity. They cause receptor blockade.

Partial agonist: Drug that has affinity to the receptor but less intrinsic activity is called partial agonist.

Inverse agonist: It has full affinity towards the receptor but produces effect just opposite to that of an agonist, *e.g.* beta-carbolines (act on benzodiazepine receptor).

Receptor families (Transducer mechanism): They are:

1. Ligand gated ion channels (inotropic receptors).
2. G protein coupled receptors.
   G protein coupled receptors control cell function via.
   a. Adenylyl cyclase: cAMP system.
   b. Phospholipase C: Inositol phosphate system.
   c. Ion channel regulation (calcium).
3. Enzymatic receptors.
4. Receptor regulating gene expression (transcription factors) or the nuclear receptor.

Characteristics of various receptor families

	Ligand-gated ion channels	G-protein- coupled receptors	Enzymatic receptors	Nuclear receptors
Location	Membrane	Membrane	Membrane	Intracellular
Effector	Ion channel	Channel or enzyme	Enzyme	Gene transcription
Coupling	Direct	G-protein (Gs, Gi, Gq, etc.)	Direct	Via DNA
Examples	Nicotinic, $GABA_A$ receptors	Muscarinic, adrenergic receptors	Insulin, growth factor, cytokine receptors	Steroid, thyroid hormone receptors

Regulation of Receptors

Receptors are in a dynamic state. The density or the affinity of the receptors to drugs is not fixed. It alters according to the situation.

a. *Receptor down regulation:* Prolonged use of agonists, decreases number and sensitivity of receptors and decrease drug effect, *e.g.* chronic use of salbutamol down regulates the $beta_2$ adrenoceptors.

b. *Receptor up regulation:* Prolonged use of antagonists, increases receptor number and sensitivity of receptors and increase drug effect, *e.g.* withdrawal syndrome occurs with propranolol, when it is stopped after prolonged use.

Functions of Receptor

1. To propagate regulatory signals from outside to within the effector cell.
2. To amplify the signal.
3. To integrate various extracellular and intracellular signals.
4. To adopt short term and long term changes in the regulatory milieu and maintain homeostasis.

Therapeutic Index

Therapeutic index (T.I.) is an index of drug safety.

It is the ratio of median lethal dose to the median effective dose.

$$\text{T.I.} = \frac{\text{Median lethal dose } (LD_{50})}{\text{Median effective dose } (ED_{50})}$$

a. *LD_{50}*: It is the dose of a drug required to kill 50% of the unlimited animal population.

b. ED_{50}: It is the dose of the drug which produces desired effect in 50% of the population.

Wider the value of therapeutic index, safer is the drug. For example, penicillin has a high therapeutic index. Digitalis, lithium, phenytoin, etc. have narrow therapeutic index.

Drug potency: The quantity of a drug required to produce a desired response is potency of the drug.

Drug efficacy: It is the maximum effect of a drug.

Therapeutic Window

With certain drugs, therapeutic effect is seen only over a narrow range of plasma drug concentration. Both below and above this range, beneficial effects are less, *e.g.* tricyclic antidepressants, clonidine, lithium etc.

Combined Effect of Drugs

Increased Response (Synergism)

1. Additive effect – two drugs acting by the same mechanism, so, Effect of drugs A + B = Effect of drug A + Effect of drug B, *e.g.* Ibuprofen + Paracetamol.
2. Supra additive or potentiation – two drugs act by different mechanism, so,
   Effect of drugs A + B > Effect of drug A + Effect of drug B, *e.g.* trimethoprim + sulphamethoxozole.

Decreased Response (Drug Antagonism)

When combined effect of two drug is less. It may be:

1. *Physical antagonism: e.g.* activated charcoal adsorbs toxic substances in case of poisoning.
2. *Chemical antagonism: e.g.* antacids.
3. *Physiological (functional) antagonism: e.g.* insulin and glucagon.
4. *Receptor antagonism.*
   a. Competitive antagonism:
   For example,
   Acetylcholine (Agonist) → Muscarinic receptors ← Atropine (Antagonist).
   Morphine (Agonists) → Opioid receptors ← Naloxone (Antagonists).

The competitive antagonism can be overcome by increasing the concentration of the agonist.

b. **Non competitive antagonism:** The antagonist binds to a different site or to the same site with higher affinity, so that the agonist cannot displace it from the receptor. For example, phenoxybenzamine (antagonist) and noradrenaline bind to the same site on alpha adrenergic receptors.

Factors Modifying Drug Action

Variation in response to the same dose of a drug among individual is due to:

(A) Difference in pharmacokinetic handling of drug.
(B) Variation in number of receptors, coupling proteins.
(C) Variation in neurogenic/hormonal tone.

Various factors are:

Drug Factors

1. **Route of administration**
   a. *Quantitative variation:* Oral dose of the drugs are usually larger than intravenous dose.
   b. *Qualitative variation:* The drug may produce an entirely different response when administered by different routes. Magnesium sulphate orally produces purgative effect, on parenteral administration it causes CNS depression and locally reduces oedema in the inflamed area.
2. **Presence of other drugs.**
3. **Cumulation:** When elimination of a drug is slow.
4. **Placebo effect.**

Patient Factors

1. **Age:** In neonates, the metabolizing function of the liver and excretory function of the kidney is not fully developed. In the elderly, the renal and hepatic functions progressively decline. The incidence of adverse effect of drugs is also relatively more and so, drug doses have to be adjusted accordingly in both extremes of age.
2. **Body weight and body surface area.**

$$\text{Child's Dose} = \frac{\text{Body Weight (Kg)}}{70} \times \text{Average adult dose}$$

3. **Sex.**
4. **Environment.**
5. **Genetic factor.**
6. **Emotional factor/Psychological factor.**
7. **Pathological states:** *e.g.* GI disorders, liver diseases and renal failure.
8. **Tolerance:** Repeated administration of certain drugs can result in a decrease in their pharmacological effect. Hence, higher doses of such drugs are needed to produce a given response, *e.g.* ephedrine, organic nitrates, opioids, etc.

   Mechanism of development of tolerance
   i. Pharmacokinetic tolerance (Dispositional tolerance).
   ii. Pharmacodynamic tolerance (Functional tolerance).
   iii. Cross tolerance.
   iv. Tachyphylaxis.

ADVERSE DRUG REACTIONS

Adverse drug reaction (ADR) is defined as any undesirable or unwanted effect due to drug administration. ADRs could be either dose related or non dose related.

Dose Related ADR (Predictable)

1. *Side effects:* These are the unavoidable effects of a drug which are seen with therapeutic doses, *e.g.* atropine used in the treatment of heart block also produces dryness of mouth, blurring of vision, urinary retention, etc., they can be useful with some other conditions and proper adjustment of dose minimizes the symptoms. Drug withdrawal is usually not required.
2. *Unwanted or secondary effect:* They also develop with therapeutic dose but undesirable and if serious, may require withdrawal of drug, *e.g.* super infection by antibiotics, vomiting with morphine.
3. *Toxic effects:* These are the effects of a drug, which are either due to over dosage or chronic use, *e.g.* bleeding due to chronic or/over dosage of anticoagulants and nephrotoxicity with aminoglycosides especially in elderly patients.

Non Dose Related ADRs (Unpredictable)

(A) Hypersensitivity Reactions (Drug Allergy)

It is an abnormal response to a drug due to Ag:Ab reaction resulting in the release of various mediators, *e.g.*

- *Those associated with humoral antibodies:* Types I, II and III.
- *Those associated with cell mediated immunity:* Type IV (delayed hypersensitivity).

(B) Idiosyncrasy

It is usually a genetically determined adverse reaction to drugs, *e.g.* aplastic anaemia caused by chloramphenicol, succinylcholine apnoea, haemolytic anaemia seen with primaquine, sulphonamides, etc.

Other toxicities of drugs are:

- **Drug Dependence**
  1. Psychological dependence, *e.g.* cigarette smoking.
  2. Physical dependence, *e.g.* opioids, alcohol.
- **Iatrogenic Disease**—Parkinsonism due to metoclopramide.
- **Teratogenicity (Foetal abnormalities),** *e.g.* Warfarin, phyntoin, valproate.
- **Carcinogenicity and Mutagenicity,** *e.g.* Tobbaco, estrogens, radioisotopes.
- **Photosensitivity Reactions**—doxycycline, etc.
- **Hepatotoxicity,** *e.g.* Isoniazid, rifampicin, pyrazinamide, halothane, paracetamol, etc.
- **Nephrotoxicity,** *e.g.* Aminoglycosides, amphotericin B, cisplatin, cyclosporine, heavy metals, ACEI, NSAIDs etc.
- **Ototoxicity,** *e.g.* Aminoglycosides, loop diuretics, cisplatin, etc.
- **Ocular Toxicity,** *e.g.* Ethambutol, chloroquine, glucocorticoids, etc.
- **Haemopoietic,** *e.g.* sulfonamides, carbimazole, phenytoin, cytotoxic drugs.

CLINICAL EVALUATION

Drug development: It has following steps:

(A) *Drug discovery phase to find lead compound by*

a. Random screening

b. Serendipity (by chance)
c. Rational drug designing
It takes 3-5 years.

(B) *Preclinical trial:* To observe the effect of drug on animals:

a. Toxicological studies for
   i. Acute toxicity (up to 4 weeks)
   ii. Sub acute toxicity (4 weeks–12 weeks)
   iii. Chronic toxicity 1–2 years
   iv. Specific toxicity, *e.g.* reproductive, teratogenic, carcinogenic mutagenic, local toxicity etc.

b. Pharmacokinetic studies
c. Pharmacodynamic studies
d. To find safety index LD_{50}, ED_{50} and TI

(C) *Clinical trials.*

CLINICAL TRIALS

Clinical trial is the evaluation of pharmacological properties of the drug including drug toxicity both in healthy volunteers and diseased persons in a recognized hospital centre where all the infrastructural facilities of medical care are available.

Phase I trial

Phase I trial is conducted on a small number (25-50) of healthy volunteers to determine the safety and tolerability of a drug and to study the pharmacokinetic parameters. It is open label trials/non blind trial in which both the volunteer and the investigator know the identity of the drug.

Phase II trial

In phase II trial, the drug effects are studied in patients with the known disease for which the trial is meant to determine the efficacy of the drug.

a. *Early phase:* Number of subjects up to 200 and is single blind (subject does not know the identity of drug).

b. *Late phase:* Number of subjects 200-400 patients double blind (both investigator and subject do not know the identity of drug and the third person hold the code). The duration of the trial is about six weeks.

Phase III trial

Conducted on several hundreds of patients and are conducted at multiple centers (multi-centric study), double blind crossover studies. Phase III studies are based on specific clinical end points and secondary end points which lasts for about six months or more. All the three phases takes 5-6 years and then at the end of the study statistical analysis done.

If the results of phase III meet the requirements of the study, permission is granted by the regulatory authorities to market the product and promote the same, using a brand name.

Phase IV trial

The post-market surveillance is mainly aimed to know the profile of the adverse drug effects or to know the safety of drug.

Pharmacovigilance means continuous monitoring for unwanted effect and other safety related aspects of marketed drugs.

MULTIPLE CHOICE QUESTIONS

Q. 1 According to WHO drug is substance that is:

(A) Used therapeutically only
(B) Modify physiological system
(C) Always safe to used in human being
(D) Used as diagnostic agent

Q. 2 Which agent is derived from animal source?

(A) Insulin (B) Digoxin
(C) Chloroquine (D) Ferrous sulphate

Q. 3 High first pass metabolism is seen with which of the following route of drug administration?

(A) Oral (B) Subcutaneous
(C) Sublingual (D) Intravenous

Q. 4 Which of the following route of administration show slow but sustained release of the drug for several days?

(A) Transcutaneous (B) Transdermal
(C) Sublingual (D) Subcutaneous

Q. 5 All of the drugs can be given by intravenous route only *except:*

(A) Heparin (B) Dopamine
(C) Pancuronium (D) Diazepam

Q. 6 All statements are true regarding the sublingual route of drug administration *except:*

(A) It has quick and rapid onset of action
(B) The drug passes directly into the systemic circulation
(C) Drug absorbed through buccal mucosa
(D) It is very useful route for the drugs having high molecular weight

Q. 7 Which of the following route of administration of drug is free from 1st pass effect?

(A) Oral (B) Subcutaneous
(C) Intra arterial (D) Intravenous

---

1 (B) 2 (A) 3 (A) 4 (B) 5 (D) 6 (D) 7 (C)

Q. 8 All of the following drugs will be absorbed from stomach *except:*

(A) Aspirin (B) Phenytoin
(C) Phenobarbitone (D) Morphine

Q. 9 Duration of action of I.V. administered drug depends on:

(A) Clearance (B) Volume of distribution
(C) Lipid solubility (D) Half life

Q. 10 Majority of drugs cross biological membrane primarily by:

(A) Passive diffusion (B) Facilitated diffusion
(C) Active transport (D) Pinocytosis

Q. 11 All are important factors governing absorption of the drug through passive diffusion *except:*

(A) Ionization (B) Lipid solubility
(C) pH (D) Carrier transport or energy

Q. 12 Which of the following statement is not correct?

(A) pKa of a drug is the pH at which the drug is 50% ionized and 50% unionized
(B) Strongly acidic or strongly basic drugs remain predominantly unionized at all pH
(C) Small changes of pH near the pKa value of a weak acidic drug affect the degree of ionization
(D) Knowledge of pKa of a drug is useful in predicting its behavior in various body fluids

Q. 13 Which of the following drug is not bound to plasma proteins?

(A) Sulphadiazine
(B) Ketoconazole
(C) Penicillin
(D) Lithium carbonate

Q. 14 A drug which is more protein bound may show:

(A) Longer duration of action
(B) Shorter duration of action
(C) Decreased absorption
(D) Increased renal excretion

---

8 (D) 9 (D) 10 (A) 11 (D) 12 (B) 13 (D) 14 (A)

Q. 15 All of following drug interactions are due to displacement of drug from its binding site *except:*

(A) Phenylbutazone and tolbutamide
(B) Salicylate and methotrexate
(C) Sulfonamides and bilirubin
(D) Phenytoin and isoniazid

Q. 16 Which of the following statement is not true for the effect of pregnancy on drug disposition?

(A) Drug absorption may be delayed
(B) Clearance is decreased
(C) Half life may be prolonged
(D) Hepatic drug metabolism is increased

Q. 17 Which is the incorrect statement regarding volume of distribution?

(A) Non-ionized, lipid soluble drugs have large volume of distribution
(B) Drugs which are highly plasma protein bound have high volume of distribution
(C) Drugs sequestrated in other tissue may have large volume of distribution
(D) Pathological states can alter the volume of distribution

Q. 18 Redistribution is a feature of:

(A) Highly plasma protein bound drugs
(B) Depot preparations
(C) Poorly lipid soluble drugs
(D) Highly lipid soluble drugs

Q. 19 All drugs which show significant entero hepatic recycling *except:*

(A) Indomethacin
(B) Phenolphalthalein
(C) Digitoxin
(D) Penicillin

---

15 (D) 16 (B) 17 (B) 18 (D) 19 (D)

Q. 20 All statements are true about glucuronide conjugation reaction *except:*

(A) It is the microsomal conjugation reaction
(B) Metabolites of phase I reactions contain phenolic group undergoes conjugate reaction
(C) It forms inactive and readily excreted products
(D) It is non-microsomal conjugation reaction

Q. 21 The false statement regarding biotransformation of drugs is:

(A) Formation of inactive metabolite from active drug
(B) Formation of active metabolite from inactive drug
(C) Formation of active metabolite from equally active drug
(D) Convert of non lipid soluble drugs to lipid soluble drugs

Q. 22 The true statement regarding a drug given in presence of hepatic dysfunction is:

(A) In the presence of hepatic dysfunction, protein binding of acidic drugs increased
(B) Bioavailability of drugs having high first pass metabolism is increased
(C) Morphine is more rapidly metabolized by the liver
(D) Solubility of the drug is affected in the presence of hepatic damage

Q. 23 Which sub family of Cytochrome P-450 is responsible for the highest fraction of clinically important drug interactions resulting from metabolism?

(A) CYP1A (B) CYP2A
(C) CYP3A (D) CYP4A

Q. 24 The most important factor which governs filtration of drugs across capillaries other than those in the brain is:

(A) Blood flow through the capillary
(B) Lipid solubility of the drug
(C) pKa value of the drug
(D) pH of the medium

---

20 (D) 21 (D) 22 (B) 23 (C) 24 (A)

Q. 25 Chronic long term administration of the prodrug with increase in cytochrome P450 expression will cause:

(A) Decrease in potency
(B) Increase in potency
(C) Decrease in efficacy
(D) Increase in efficacy

Q. 26 A 17 years old male epileptic patient was given carbamazepine to control seizure. After some time he was prescribed macrolide for control his asthmatic attack of URI. After few days the patient again develops seizures. The reason for the new seizure activity is:

(A) Inhibition of the cytochrome P-450 mono-oxygenase system
(B) Induction of the cytochrome P-450 mono-oxygenase system
(C) Impairment of renal excretion of the carbamazepine
(D) Induction of glucuronyl transferase activity in the liver

Q. 27 Which of the following is a prodrug?

(A) Captopril (B) Clonidine
(C) Hydralazine (D) Sulfasalazine

Q. 28 The most commonly occurring conjugation reaction for drugs and their metabolite is:

(A) Glucuronide conjugation (B) Acetylation
(C) Methylation (D) Glutathione conjugation

Q. 29 Which of the following drug metabolism reaction is entirely non microsomal?

(A) Glucuronide conjugation (B) Hydrolysis
(C) Acetylation (D) Oxidation

Q. 30 Induction of drug metabolizing enzymes involves:

(A) Conformational changes in enzyme protein
(B) Expression of enzyme molecules on the surface of hepatocytes
(C) Enhanced transport of substance molecule
(D) Increased synthesis of enzyme proteins and enzymatic activity

---

25 (B) 26 (B) 27 (D) 28 (A) 29 (C) 30 (D)

Q. 31 Microsomal enzyme induction can be a cause of:

(A) Tolerance
(B) Physical dependence
(C) Psychological dependence
(D) Idiosyncrasy

Q. 32 In toxic doses paracetamol undergoes:

(A) Acetylation (B) Dealkylation
(C) N-methylation (D) N-hydroxylation

Q. 33 Microsomal oxidative pathway involves the participation of enzyme:

(A) Dehydrogenase (B) Cytochrome oxidase
(C) Xanthine oxidase (D) Mono amine oxidase

Q. 34 Drug which is excreted largely unchanged without being metabolized?

(A) Morphine (B) Paracetamol
(C) Alcohol (D) Streptomycin

Q. 35 Acetylation is a major pathway of metabolism of all drugs *except:*

(A) Isoniazid (B) Procainamide
(C) Hydralazine (D) Lorazepam

Q. 36 For a drug obeying first order kinetic the time taken to achieve steady state plasma concentration equals:

(A) 8 half lives (B) 2 half lives
(C) 4 half lives (D) Six half lives

Q. 37 Which of the following correctly describes the formula for a loading dose?

(A) Loading dose = desired plasma concentration of drugs × clearance
(B) Loading dose = 0.693 × volume of distribution / clearance
(C) Loading dose = amount of drug administered / initial plasma concentration
(D) Loading dose = desired plasma concentration of the drug × volume of distribution

---

31 (A) 32 (D) 33 (B) 34 (D) 35 (D) 36 (C) 37 (D)

Q. 38 The rational of frequent dosing schedule for the drugs having short half-life is:

(A) To achieve the steady-state plasma concentration of the drug
(B) To avoid the toxicity of the drug
(C) To aid more complete distribution of the drug
(D) To inhibit the first-pass metabolism

Q. 39 Following IV administration, the initial rates of the drug distribution to different tissues depend primarily on which of the following?

(A) Blood flow to the tissue
(B) Fat content of the tissue
(C) Degree of ionization of the drug in the tissue
(D) Specific organ clearances

Q. 40 If the oral dosing rate of a drug is held constant what will be the effect of increasing the bioavailability of the preparation?

(A) Increase the half-life for the first-order elimination
(B) Decrease the first order elimination rate constant
(C) Increase the steady-state plasma concentration
(D) Decrease the total body clearance

Q. 41 True statement regarding therapeutic drug monitoring is:

(A) Dose of the drug is adjusted according to plasma concentration
(B) It is done for the drugs having wide variation in pharmacokinetics
(C) It is done for the drugs having wide therapeutic index
(D) It is done for the drugs whose effect can be easily measured

Q. 42 Which of the following is not true about fixed-dose combination?

(A) It has better patient compliance
(B) It minimizes adverse effects
(C) It enhances the effect
(D) Dose of the individual drug can be adjusted

Q. 43 All of the following drugs have both direct and immunological mediated hepatic toxicity *except:*

(A) Alpha methyldopa (B) Isoniazid
(C) Chlorpromazine (D) Paracetamol

---

38 (A) 39 (A) 40 (C) 41 (B) 42 (D) 43 (D)

Q. 44 An undesirable effect of a drug that occurs at therapeutic doses and can be predicted from its pharmacological action is called:

(A) Side effect (B) Toxic effect
(C) Allergic reaction (D) Idiosyncrasy

Q. 45 Pharmacogenetics is associated with:

(A) Variability of enzyme action
(B) Environmental influence
(C) Individual variability in oral absorption
(D) Different dose response curve in different individual

Q. 46 Adaptive neuro physiological changes produced by repeated administration of a drug which results in withdrawal symptom on discontinuation is called:

(A) Drug addiction (B) Drug abuse
(C) Psychological dependence (D) Physical dependence

Q. 47 Glomerular filtration of a drug is affected by its:

(A) Lipid solubility (B) Plasma protein binding
(C) Degree of ionization (D) Rate of tabular secretion

Q. 48 The plasma half life of penicillin G is longer in the newborn because their:

(A) Plasma protein level is low
(B) Drug metabolizing enzymes are immature
(C) Glomerular filtration rate is low
(D) Tubular transport mechanism is not well developed

Q. 49 All are true regarding a drug eliminated by first order kinetic *except:*

(A) A constant amount of drug will be eliminated per unit time
(B) Its clearance value will remain constant
(C) Its elimination half life is not affected by dose
(D) It will be completely eliminated from the body in 4-5 life period

Q. 50 The loading dose of a drug is governed by its:

(A) Renal clearance (B) Plasma half life
(C) Volume of distribution (D) Elimination rate constant

---

44 (A) 45 (A) 46 (D) 47 (B) 48 (D) 49 (A) 50 (C)

Q. 51 Characteristics of zero order (non linear) kinetic is:

(A) The time required to eliminate 50% of a dose increases with increasing dose
(B) Doubling the dose of drug doubles the plasma concentration
(C) The proportion of excretion of drug in urine is not dependent on dose and route of administration of drug
(D) There is exponential decline in drug concentration after parenteral dose

Q. 52 Which of the following drugs do not require dose adjustment in renal impairment?

(A) Sulfadoxine (B) Digitoxin
(C) Doxycycline (D) Morphine

Q. 53 All are correct statements regarding half life ($t_{½}$) *except:*

(A) It is a useful kinetic indicator of time required by drug to attain steady state
(B) It is not a good parameter of studying kinetics of elimination/distribution
(C) It reflects drug clearance
(D) It is a good indicator of estimation of dosing interval

Q. 54 A decrease in which of the following parameters explain higher than anticipated plasma drug concentration?

(A) Bioavailability (B) Volume of distribution
(C) Clearance (D) Half life

Q. 55 The rational behind using loading dose regimen is:

(A) Drug is administered in loading dose to achieve the desired plasma concentration rapidly
(B) Loading dose of the drug does not depend on the volume of distribution
(C) Loading dose does not depend on the clearance
(D) It is useful for drugs having short $t_{½}$

Q. 56 Alkalinization of urine increases the excretion of:

(A) Weakly acidic drugs (B) Weakly basic drugs
(C) Strong electrolytes (D) Non polar drugs

---

51 (A) 52 (C) 53 (C) 54 (C) 55 (A) 56 (A)

Q. 57 All statements regarding inverse agonist are false *except:*

(A) It binds to receptor and cause intended action
(B) It binds to receptors and cause opposite action
(C) It binds to receptor and cause no action
(D) It binds to receptor and cause submaximal action

Q. 58 Which of the following is a G-coupled receptor?

(A) Muscarinic cholinergic receptors
(B) Nicotinic cholinergic receptors
(C) Glucocorticoid receptors
(D) Androgen receptors

Q. 59 Which of the following parameters is used to indicate the ability of a drug to produce the desired therapeutic effect relative to a toxic effect?

(A) Potency (B) Therapeutic index
(C) Efficacy (D) Bioavailability

Q. 60 Which of the following factors will determine the number of drug-receptor complexes formed?

(A) Efficacy of the drug
(B) Receptor affinity for the drug
(C) Therapeutic index of the drug
(D) Half-life of the drug

Q. 61 Action of alpha subunit of G protein is:

(A) Binding of agonist
(B) Conversion of GDP to GTP
(C) Breakdown of GTP to GDP
(D) Internalization of receptors

Q. 62 All are second messenger *except:*

(A) Cyclic AMP (B) Guanylyl cyclase
(C) DAG (D) IP_3

Q. 63 Short half life of thiopentone is due to:

(A) Excretion (B) Metabolism
(C) Spontaneous degradation (D) Redistribution

---

57 (B) 58 (A) 59 (B) 60 (B) 61 (C) 62 (B) 63 (D)

Q. 64 All of the following agents act by intracellular receptors *except:*

(A) Thyroid hormones (B) Vitamin D
(C) Insulin (D) Steroid

Q. 65 All of the following statements regarding bioavailability of a drug are true *except:*

(A) It is a fraction of administered drug that reaches the systemic circulation in unchanged form
(B) Bioavailability of an orally administered drug can be calculated by comparing the area under curve after oral and intravenous administration
(C) Low oral availability always and necessarily means poor absorption
(D) Bioavailability can be determined from plasma concentration or urinary excretion data

Q. 66 All of the following drugs can cross placenta *except:*

(A) Phenytoin
(B) Diazepam
(C) Morphine
(D) Heparin

Q. 67 All are the reasons for alteration of drug dosage in the elderly *except:*

(A) They have decreasing renal function with age
(B) They are lean and their body mass is less
(C) They have increased baro receptor sensitivity
(D) Body water is decreased

Q. 68 Which of the following statement is true?

(A) As the concentration of the drug increases over the therapeutic range, the bound form of the drug increases
(B) The bound form is not available for metabolism but is available for excretion
(C) Acidic drugs binds to α_1–acid glycoprotein and basic drugs bind to albumin
(D) Binding sites are non-specific and one drug can displace the other

---

64 (C) 65 (C) 66 (D) 67 (C) 68 (D)

Q. 69 Which of the drug should not be given in hepatic failure?

(A) Diazepam
(B) Theophylline
(C) Streptomycin
(D) Penicillin

Q. 70 True about tachyphylaxis is:

(A) Direct sympathomimetics are involved
(B) Mechanism of action is clearly understood
(C) It is an anaphylactic reaction
(D) Indirect sympathomimetics are involved

Q. 71 Fastest acting receptor/ transduction mechanism is:

(A) Adenylyl cyclase – cyclic AMP pathway
(B) Phospholipase C–IP_3:DAG pathway
(C) Intrinsic ion channel operation
(D) Nuclear receptor

Q. 72 Which of the following drug act through heptahelical (serpentine) receptors?

(A) Insulin
(B) Estrogen
(C) Local anaesthesia
(D) Salbutamol

Q. 73 A drug which produces qualitatively different actions when administered through different route is:

(A) Phenytoin sodium
(B) Hydralazine
(C) Magnesium sulphate
(D) Nitroglycerine

Q. 74 Tolerance is generally not acquired to following effect of drug:

(A) Anti secretory action of atropine
(B) Emetic action of L-dopa
(C) Euphoria due to morphine
(D) Vasodilator action of nitrates

Q. 75 Which of the following is an idiosyncratic adverse drug reaction?

(A) Muscle dystonia caused by triflupromazine
(B) Insomnia after pentobarbitone
(C) Precipitation of asthma by morphine
(D) Gum hyperplasia caused by phenytoin

---

69 (A) 70 (D) 71 (C) 72 (D) 73 (C) 74 (A) 75 (B)

Q. 76 In which phase (period) of pregnancy, foetal malformation occur due to any drug?

(A) During 18-55 days of gestation (organogenesis)
(B) During 56-84 days of gestation
(C) During second trimester
(D) 36 weeks onwards

Q. 77 If the effect of combination of two drugs is equal to the sum of their individual effect, the two drugs are exhibiting:

(A) Potentiation of action
(B) Additive effect
(C) Cross tolerance
(D) Antagonism

Q. 78 Which of the following statement about spare receptors is most correct?

(A) Spare receptors in the absence of drug are sequestered in the cytoplasm
(B) Spare receptors may be detected by finding that the drug receptors interaction lasts longer than the intracellular effect
(C) Spare receptors influence the maximal efficacy of the drug receptor system
(D) Spare receptors may be detected by the finding that the EC_{50} is smaller than the Kd for the agonist

Q. 79 What is the true in relation to drug receptors?

(A) All drugs act through specific receptors
(B) All drug receptors are located on the surface of the target cells
(C) Agonist induce a conformational changes in the receptor
(D) Partial agonists have low affinity for the receptor

Q. 80 Drug acting through receptor exhibit all of the following features *except:*

(A) Structural specificity
(B) High potency
(C) Competitive antagonism
(D) Dependence of action on lipophilicity

76 (A) 77 (B) 78 (D) 79 (C) 80 (D)

Q. 81 Down regulation of receptor can occur as a consequence of:

(A) Continuous use of agonists
(B) Continuous use of antagonists
(C) Chronic use of CNS depressants
(D) Denervation

Q. 82 A drug which is administered without the need for dose individualization is:

(A) Insulin (B) Digoxin
(C) Mebendazole (D) Prednisolone

Q. 83 True statement about competitive antagonist is:

(A) Dissociate from receptors faster than their respective agonist
(B) Alters the shape of the log dose response curve of an agonist
(C) Have low dissociation rate constant
(D) Initiate the opposite cellular response to receptor occupancy to that obtained by the agonist

Q. 84 Which of the following is an action of a non-competitive antagonist?

(A) Alters the mechanism of action of an agonist
(B) Shifts the dose-response curve of an agonist to the right
(C) Decrease the maximum response to an agonist
(D) Binds to the same site on the receptor as the agonist

Q. 85 Find correct statement regarding a placebo:

(A) It is not always an inert substance
(B) It is an indispensable element in routine clinical practice
(C) It produces subjective improvement in symptoms
(D) It is not an integral part of a good trial

Q. 86 Single blind study is a feature of:

(A) Phase I trial (B) Phase II trial
(C) Phase III trial (D) Phase IV trial

Q. 87 In which phase of clinical trial approval of ethical committee is not required?

(A) Phase I (B) Phase II
(C) Phase III (D) Phase IV

---

81 (A) 82 (C) 83 (C) 84 (C) 85 (C) 86 (B) 87 (D)

ANSWERS

Ans. 1 **(B)** WHO define the drug as any substance or product that is used or intended to be used to modify or explore the physiological system or pathological state in the benefit of the recipient. It can be used for the treatment, cure (antimicrobial agents), preventions (vaccines) symptomatic relief (analgesic) or for the diagnostic purposes (radio-opaque dye).

Ans. 2 **(A)** The various sources of obtaining drugs are plants (morphine, atropine, digoxin, various oils) animals (insulin, vitamins, vaccines, sera) microbiological sources (penicillins, aminoglycosides, antifungal drug griseofulvin,) minerals (ferrous sulphate, antacids, kaolin) and by genetic engineering (human insulin). But nowadays majority of drugs are obtained synthetically and semi-synthetically.

Ans. 3 **(A)** The main disadvantage/demerit of oral route of administration is metabolism of many drugs in liver during first pass before reaching to systemic circulation, *e.g.* morphine, propranolol etc.

Ans. 4 **(B)** Transdermal route of administration produce smooth and non fluctuating plasma concentration, avoid hepatic first pass metabolism. It minimizes inter individual variations in the achieved plasma drug concentration of the drug and produce slow sustained plasma concentration of the drug.

Ans. 5 **(D)** The drugs which can be given only by IV routes are GDW, GNS, aminophylline, pancuronium (SMR) and dopamine (IV infusion). Other drugs çan be given by IV route (*e.g.* Diazepam, furosemide antibiotic, hydrocortisone etc.) to get maximum bioavailability or in emergency, but they can be given by other (oral/parenteral) route also.

Ans. 6 **(D)** In sublingual route of drug administration, drug is kept under tongue. It directly reaches to systemic circulation through buccal mucosa bypassing the portal circulation. Thus have good bioavailability and rapid onset of action. The drugs having high molecular weight do not absorbed well by this route.

Ans. 7 (C) First pass effect or first pass metabolism or pre systemic metabolism means the drug metabolism occurring before it enters the systemic circulation. This leads to decrease in bioavailability and ultimately decrease in the therapeutic response. When a drug is given orally it passes through GIT and then to portal system before reaching to systemic circulation. By parenteral administration (*i.e.* subcutaneous, and even intravenous) some drugs get inactivated during passage in the lungs but in intra arterial injection, drug directly injected into the lumen of desired artery and the first pass and cleansing effect of the lungs are not available.

Ans. 8 (D) Weakly acidic drugs like phenytoin, barbiturates, aspirin remain predominantly non-ionized in acidic media and are better absorbed from acidic media of stomach, while morphine, diazepam and amphetamine are weakly basic drugs and remain unionized predominantly at alkaline pH and thus are better absorbed from intestine.

Ans. 9 (D) When a drug having first order elimination is given I.V. and when we plot a graph as shown in graph, it has two slopes (i) initially rapidly declining alpha-phase due to distribution and (ii) later less declined beta-phase due to elimination. Only the $t_{½}$ calculated over the therapeutic plasma concentration range is clinically relevant.

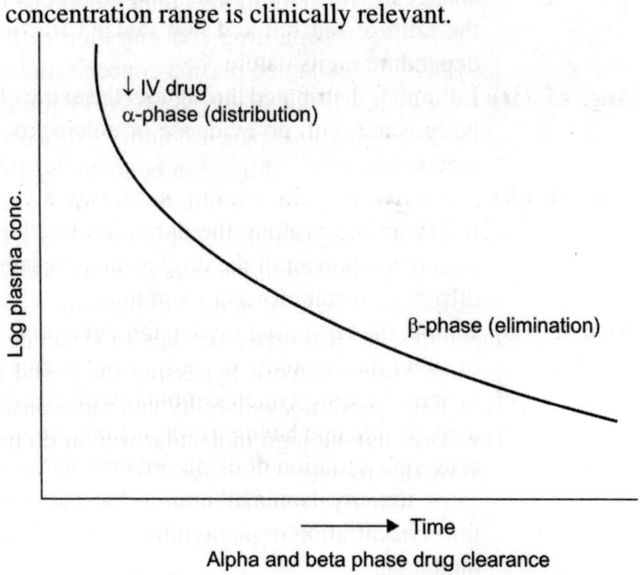

Alpha and beta phase drug clearance

Ans. 10 (A) Most biological membranes are relatively permeable to water. The transport of water carried water soluble substance of small molecular weight. In such passive diffusion, bidirectional movement of the concerned molecule occur against the concentration gradient (from higher to lower concentration) without input of energy and this is the most important mechanism for most of the drugs.

Ans. 11 (D) Absorption of drug depends on the ionization, lipid solubility and the pH. Weak acids are largely unionized at gastric pH so better absorbed from acidic media of stomach while weak base are unionized in alkaline pH so better absorbed in the alkaline pH of intestine. Lipid soluble drugs diffuse by dissolving in the lipoidal matrix of the membrane and attain higher concentration quickly regardless of the pH of the medium.

Ans. 12 (B) Strongly acidic/ basic drugs and quaternary compounds remain predominantly ionized at all pH and are therefore poorly absorbed, while weakly acidic drugs, *e.g.* aspirin, phenytoin, barbiturates remain predominantly non ionized in acidic media and are better absorbed. The stronger the acid, the lower will be its pKa value. Thus the slightest change in pKa value by changing pH, decreases or increases the ratio of ionized and non ionized fraction of the drug depending on its nature.

Ans. 13 (D) Lithium is distributed throughout the extracellular fluid and body water with no evidence of either protein binding or metabolism.

Ans. 14 (A) Extensive protein binding serves as a circulating drug reservoir and prolong the duration of action. The protein bound component of the drug is not accessible to capillary diffusion, metabolism or excretion.

Ans. 15 (D) If more than one drug bind to the same protein binding site of albumin (protein) it causes displacement interaction. Wherein a drug which is bound with higher affinity will displace the one having lower affinity, to increase the free drug concentration of displaced drug and have potential to cause toxicity. Isoniazid inhibits the enzyme and increases the concentration of phenytoin and toxicity due to enzyme inhibition.

Ans. 16 (B) In pregnancy apparent volume of distribution and plasma half life is increased but clearance remains unaltered or increased due to increase in renal blood flow which makes the elimination of polar drugs faster.

Ans. 17 (B) Non ionized, lipid soluble drugs readily crosses the membrane and distributed throughout the body and have large volume of distribution (*e.g.* thiopental sodium) while those drug with high protein binding largely restricted to the vascular compartment and have low volume of distribution (*e.g.* warfarin, phenylbutazone). Drugs sequestrated in other tissue may have volume of distribution much more than total body water or even body mass, *e.g.* digoxin, propranolol, morphine, and such drugs are difficult to be removed by haemodialysis, if toxicity occurs.

Ans. 18 (D) Redistribution is a feature of highly lipid soluble drugs, *e.g.* thiopentone. These drugs, enter the brain very rapidly causing general anaesthesia but also diffuses out of the brain through blood circulation and are then redistributed in the muscle, lean tissue and fat and their action gets terminated (have short duration of action).

Ans. 19 (D) Liver cells transfer various drugs and endogenous substances from plasma to bile. These are then subsequently eliminated through bile. Some drugs are secreted through bile but after being delivery to intestine are reabsorbed back and cycle is repeated. This is known as enterohepatic circulation. The net result of enterohepatic circulation is the prolongation of drug action as the drug serves as a small circulating reservoir (see text).

Ans. 20 (D) Glucuronide conjugation reaction is the sole example of microsomal conjugation reaction. Parent drug or metabolite of phase I reactions having phenolic, alcoholic, carboxylic, amino or mercapto group can undergo conjugate reaction. They usually yield polar, readily excreted and inactive substances.

Ans. 21 (D) Biotransformation of drugs make / convert lipid soluble drugs to water soluble drugs hence not reabsorbed from the renal tubules and thus finally excreted.

Ans. 22 (B) In the presence of liver dysfunction, bioavailability of drugs having first pass metabolism is increased, while protein binding of acidic drugs is reduced due to hypoalbuminaemia. Metabolism of morphine slows down in presence of hepatic dysfunction. Solubility of drugs has nothing to do with hepatic damage.

Ans. 23 (C) The CYP3A subfamily is responsible for roughly 50% of the total cytochrome P-450 activity present in the liver and is estimated to be responsible for most of the clinically important untoward drug interactions resulting from metabolism.

Ans. 24 (A) Filtration is passage of drugs through aqueous pores in the membrane or through para cellular spaces. Majority of cells have very small pores (4A°) and drugs with M.W. > 100-200 are not able to penetrate. However, capillaries (except those in brain) have large para cellular space (40A°) and most drugs (even albumin) can filter through these, and the filtration is dependent on rate of blood flow through them rather than on lipid solubility of the drug or pH of the medium.

Ans. 25 (B) The induction of the cytochrome P450 following chronic administration will increase the conversion of the inactive prodrug to the active form. This will shift the dose response curve to the left without changing its efficacy.

Ans. 26 (B) Both carbamazepine and macrolide antibiotics are enzyme inducer of the cytochrome P450 enzyme system. Though reversible, it leads to an enhanced microsomal enzyme activity and accelerated metabolism and consequently decreased pharmacological response of carbamazepine.

Ans. 27 (D) Few drugs are inactive as such and need conversion in the body to one or more active metabolites. Such a drug is called a prodrug, *e.g.* L-dopa, enalapril, sulfasalazine, alpha methyl dopa etc.

Ans. 28 (A) Glucuronide conjugation is the most important synthetic reaction carried out by a group of UDP glucuronyl transferases (UGTs). Compounds with a hydroxyl or carboxylic acid group are easily conjugated with glucuronic acid, *e.g.* chloramphenicol, aspirin, paracetamol etc.

Ans. 29 (C) Non microsomal enzymes are present in the cytoplasm and mitochondria of hepatic cell as well as in other tissues including plasma. Some oxidation and reduction, many hydrolytic and all conjugation reaction (except glucuronidation) undergoes entirely by non-microsomal enzymes. Non-microsomal enzymes are non inducible but show genetic polymorphism. Acetylation reactions are entirely non-microsomal reactions.

Ans. 30 (D) Many drugs on repeated administration stimulate or induce the growth of smooth endoplasmic reticulation and leads to an enhanced synthesis of microsomal enzyme protein and enzyme activity. This results in accelerated metabolism of inducing drug itself and /or other drugs utilizing the same enzymatic pathway and decrease the response of the drugs, *e.g.* phenobarbitone, phenytoin, carbamazepine, rifampicin insecticides, omeprazole etc.

Ans. 31 (A) Microsomal enzyme induction may leads to decrease action of drugs (oral contraceptive pill failure) increase intensity of action/ toxicity (paracetamol toxicity due to its metabolite) tolerance, (carbamazepine) and precipitation of acute porphyria.

Ans. 32 (D) Normally paracetamol is metabolized by glucuronide and sulfate conjugation (major pathway) while a litter amount of metabolite, *e.g.* N-acetyl P-benzoquinone imine, which is highly toxic is metabolized by glutathione conjugation. With toxic doses it is not detoxified through glutathione conjugation and increasing amounts undergo CYP mediated N-hydroxylation to form NAPQI which is eliminated rapidly.

Ans. 33 (B) Oxidative reactions are mostly carried out by a group of mono oxygenase in the liver which in the final step involves a cytochrome P450 haemoprotein, NADPH, cytochrome P-450 reductase.

Ans. 34 (D) Most hydrophilic drugs, *e.g.* streptomycin, neostigmine, pancuronium etc. are little biotransformed and are largely excreted unchanged. Penicillin is also secreted by renal tubules. Its action can be enhanced by using probenecid which inhibits its secretion.

Ans. 35 (D) Compounds having amino or hydralazine residues are conjugated with the help of acetyl CoA, *e.g.* sulfonamides isoniazid, PAS, hydralazine, clonazepam, procainamide. Rate of acetylation show genetic polymorphism. Lorazepam on the other hand is metabolized by glucuronide conjugation.

Ans. 36 (C) In first order kinetic of elimination, a constant fraction of the drug is eliminated at a constant interval of time and the rate of elimination is directly proportional to the plasma concentration and the plasma half life remains constant irrespective of the dose. So it requires 4-5 half lives to achieve steady state when a drug is given repeatedly.

Ans. 37 (D) Drugs having longer half life have a high volume of distribution, slow rate of clearance and are cumulative in nature. Since 4-5 half lives are needed to reach the steady state, when there is a clinical emergency and such a delay is bound to be fatal for the patient, an initial loading dose is given to reduce the time needed to reach the steady state plasma concentration.

Ans. 38 (A) Dosing schedule of the drugs is adjusted according to their half-life to achieve steady state plasma concentration. Attempting to avoid the toxicity of the drug because of its low therapeutic index one would reduce the dosing schedule. Neither distribution of the drug nor first-pass metabolism is affected by the dosing schedule.

Ans. 39 (A) The initial rate of distribution of a drug to a tissue depends primarily on the rate of blood flow to the tissue. At longer times, a drug may undergo redistribution among various tissues, *e.g.* a very lipophilic drug may become concentrated in adipose tissue with time.

Ans. 40 (C) If the oral dosing rate is constant but bioavailability increases, the fraction of the administered dose that reaches the general circulation unaltered increases. This in turn, will increase the steady state plasma concentration.

Ans. 41 (B) TDM is done for those drugs that have low therapeutic index (*e.g.* lithium, theophylline anti-epileptics etc.) and for those drugs that show wide variation in pharmacokinetics. It is not done for those drugs whose effect can be measured easily (*e.g.* antihypertensive) and which are activated in the body or produce active metabolite.

Ans. 42 (D) In FDC, two different drugs which are having same pharmacokinetics are combined in a single preparation for convenience and better patients compliance. It enhances the efficacy and may produce the synergistic effect. So the dose of individual drug can be reduced and minimize the incidence of adverse effects, *e.g.* Co-trimaxazole (sulphamethoxozole + trimethoprim) and combination of L-dopa and carbidopa. As they are available in a combination of fixed doses, we cannot adjust the individual component, if required.

Ans. 43 (D) Drugs can damage liver by its direct action (either themselves or through metabolite). Such toxicity is predictable. Some drugs render a constituent of the liver antigenic (immunologic) which is unpredictable. In case of methyl dopa, isoniazid and chlorpromazine both the mechanism can operate while paracetamol causes direct hepatic toxicity due to its metabolite N-acetyl -p-benzoquinone imine.

Ans. 44 (A) Side effects are undesirable but unavoidable, predictable effects. Toxic effects are predictable effects due to over dosage or prolong use of the drug. Allergic and idiosyncrasy are not drugs known effect (unpredictable). They are less common but generally serious and require withdrawal of the drug.

Ans. 45 (A) Variation in response of a drug is mainly because of different rates of drug metabolism due to different enzyme levels contributed by genetic factors, *e.g.* slow and fast acetylators for isoniazid, prolongation of apnea with succinylcholine due to deficiency of pseudo cholinesterase enzyme.

Ans. 46 (D) **Drug addiction** is a pattern of compulsive drug use (*e.g.* amphetamine, LSD etc). **Drug abuse** refers to use of a drug by self medication in a manner and amount that deviates from the approved medical and social pattern. **Drug dependence** is a state in which use of drug for personal satisfaction is a higher priority. In psychological dependence feeling of well being or euphoria is there while in **physical dependence** neuroadaptation is there in nervous system and discontinuation of drugs leads to characteristic withdrawal symptoms.

Ans. 47 (B) Several factors influence the renal excretion by glomerular filtration, *e.g.* molecular size (small molecules filters readily), plasma protein binding (only free drug can be filtered) and renal blood flow (greater the perfusion faster the drug removal).

Ans. 48 (D) Penicillin is mainly excreted through tubular secretion. Tubular transport mechanism is not well developed in newborn.

Ans. 49 (A) In first order kinetics, constant fraction of drug is eliminated at a constant interval of time and its plasma $t_{½}$ remains same irrespective of the dose (see text also).

Ans. 50 (C) A loading dose of a drug is given initially to provide the effective plasma concentration rapidly. For the drugs having long $t_{½}$ show high volume of distribution, slow rate of clearance and are cumulative in nature, *e.g.* digoxin (~40 hours), diazepam (40 hours) etc. Since five half lives are needed to reach the steady state plasma concentration, several days are required to achieve steady state (effective plasma concentration), so when there is clinical emergency, *e.g.* CHF, an initial loading dose followed by maintenance dose is prescribed (also see Ans. 37).

Ans. 51 (A) Very few drugs obey zero order kinetic, *e.g.* ethyl alcohol, in which a constant or fixed quantity of the drug is eliminated per unit time at fixed rate. Thus increase in dose does not result in a proportional rise in rate of elimination. So half life of these drugs is never constant.

Ans. 52 (C) Doxycyclin is a broad spectrum antibiotic (tetracycline group) having long half life and lack of renal toxicity so dose adjustment is not required and it is preferred in patients with pre existing renal disease. Long acting sulfonamides causes crystalluria and renal toxicity especially in presence of renal dysfunction due to its acetylated metabolite. The conjugated metabolites of morphine require adequate renal function for their excretion. Digoxin is mainly excreted unchanged in urine so digitoxin is usually preferred in these patients and digoxin is preferred in patients with hepatic insufficiency.

Ans. 53 (C) The half life ($t_{½}$) is the time taken for the plasma concentration or the amount of drug in the body to be reduced by 50% of its original concentration. It is a poor index of drug elimination, it does provide a good indication of the time required to reach steady state after a dosage regimen is initiated, the time for a drug to be removed from the body and a means to estimate the appropriate dosing schedule but not reflects clearance.

Ans. 54 (C) Steady state plasma concentration of drug = dose rate / clearance. Thus a decrease in clearance will increase in the plasma concentration, whereas an increase in any of the other three parameters will decrease the steady state plasma concentration.

Ans. 55 (A) The loading dose depends on the volume of distribution, whereas maintenance dose depends on the clearance of the drug (also see Ans. 50).

Ans. 56 (A) Renal tubular reabsorption of the drugs depends on lipid solubility, ionization constant and pH of the urine. Hence when pH of the urine is acidic all acidic drugs (barbiturates, salicylic acid, sulfonamides) remain non ionized and reabsorbed back. When pH of the urine is alkaline (by giving sodium bicarbonate or citrate) the ionization of the acidic drug increase and reabsorption is decreased rather excretion is facilitated. So alkalinization of urine is a part of therapeutic regimen for poisoning of acidic drugs.

Ans. 57 (B) Inverse agonist binds to the receptor and produce opposite action as that of agonist, *e.g.* Beta carboline, which bind to benzodiazepine receptors and have opposite effect, *e.g.* insomnia. There is no clinical utility of these drugs but they are used experimentally. They differ from competitive antagonist, in the sense; they show effect even in absence of agonist so they also called negative antagonists. They have full affinity but the efficacy ranges from 0 to minus one.

Ans. 58 (A) Muscarinic cholinergic receptors are both Gi (inhibitory - M_2 subtype) and Gq (M_1 subtype), coupled receptors while nicotinic receptors are ion channel receptors. Glucocorticoid and androgen both are cytosolic receptors.

Ans. 59 (B) Potency of the drug is the amount of drug needed to produce a given response. Efficacy of the drug is the maximum drug effect that can be achieved in a patient under a given set of condition. Bioavailability of the drug is the fraction of the drug that reaches the blood stream unaltered. Lithium is an example of drug with a very low therapeutic index, which requires frequent monitoring of the plasma level to achieve the balance between the desired effect and untoward effects (Toxic effect).

Ans. 60 (B) Receptor affinity for the drug will determine the number of drug-receptor complexes formed. Efficacy is the ability of the drug to activate the receptor after binding has occurred. Therapeutic index is related to safety of the drug. Half-life is the property of elimination and do not influence formation of drug receptor complex.

Ans. 61 (C) Alpha subunit of G-protein contains GTP activity and thus dissociated GTP to form GDP.

Ans. 62 (B) Guanylyl cyclase is an enzyme and not a second messenger (cGMP is a second messenger).

Ans. 63 (D) Due to high lipid solubility, thiopentone is quickly redistributed and thus is short acting.

Ans. 64 (C) Receptors may be (A) Intracellular (B) Membranous. **Intracellular** receptors are (a) **Nuclear**, *e.g.* T_3, T_4, Vitamin A, PPAR estrogen, testosterone progesterone (b) **cytoplasmic**: Glucocorticoid, mineralocorticoids, Vitamin D. **Membranous receptor** are tyrosine kinase (insulin, GH, prolactin) IP3/DAG/Ca2+ ADH, oxytocin and cAMP. Insulin is a membranous receptor.

Ans. 65 (C) Low oral bioavailability can also be due to high first pass metabolism.

Ans. 66 (D) Placental membrane is lipoidal and allows the transfer of non polar lipid soluble substance mainly by passive diffusion. Thus lipid soluble non ionize drugs like hypnotics, narcotics, general anaesthetics, cardiac glycosides, alcohol, neuroleptics and certain antibiotics can readily cross placental barrier, while polar substances and quaternary ammonium compounds, *e.g.* (dTc) and substances with high molecular weight (heparin, dextran) cannot cross placental barrier.

Ans. 67 (C) Action of drugs in elderly is decrease as age declines. Total body water, lean body mass, and body fats are reduced which reduces distribution of drugs, while decrease in hepatic and renal function, metabolism and excretion of drug is decreased, which leads to toxicity. Slow absorption due to reduced motility, blood flow, less plasma protein binding, decrease responsiveness to the receptors are all responsible for the altered response in elderly.

Ans. 68 (D) Acidic drug bind to albumin while basic drugs bind to alpha$_1$ acid glycoprotein. It is the free form of the drug that is increased as concentration of drug is increased, or get metabolized or excreted. Bound form is not available for either metabolism or excretion. Binding sites are non specific and many drugs can bind to same plasma protein binding site resulting in the displacement reaction.

Ans. 69 (A) Diazepam is contraindicated in hepatic failure. Other drugs contraindicated in hepatic failure are narcotics, salicylates, benzodiazepine (except lorazepam, oxazepam triazolam and estazolam) and diuretics.

Ans. 70 (D) Indirect sympathomimetics, *e.g.* ephedrine, amphetamines etc show tachyphylaxis. It is defined as rapid development of tolerance when the drug is given repeatedly in short duration. It may be due to depletion of stored neurotransmitter in the vesicle.

Ans. 71 (C) Intrinsic ion channel opening are the fastest channels. Drugs acting via inotropic receptors are fastest acting whereas acting through nuclear receptors is slowest in action.

Ans. 72 (D) Salbutamol acts through G-protein coupled receptors (GPCR) which are serpentine or hepta helical. They act through beta$_2$ G protein coupled receptors.

Ans. 73 (C) Magnesium sulphate act as osmotic purgative, antacids and anti arrhythmic drug when given by rectal, oral and intravenous route respectively.

Ans. 74 (A) Significant tolerance does not develop with anti secretory effect (dryness of mouth) to atropine. While tolerance develop to all other drugs, *e.g.* with nitrates efficacy is reduced by using the drug for prolonged period, chances of vomiting reduces with L-dopa, euphoric effect with morphine is also decreased.

Ans. 75 (B) Idiosyncrasy is a genetically determined abnormal reactivity to a chemical. Certain uncharacteristic or bizarre drug effects due to peculiarities of an individual may occur, *e.g.* normally barbiturates (pentobarbitone, phenobarbitone etc) cause sedation but may cause excitement and mental confusion in some. All other three reactions occur as a common adverse effect due to some alteration or changes in physiological function.

Ans. 76 (A) The drug can affect the foetus at the stages of organogenesis (18-55 days of gestation) while from 56 days onwards growth and developmental abnormalities can occur when given during pregnancy.

Ans. 77 (B) When the action of one drug is facilitated or increased by other drug they are said to be synergistic. If the effect of two drugs is simply add, it is known as additive (A+B=effect of + effect of B), *e.g.* Aspirin and Paracetamol. If the effect of combination is greater than it is known as super additive (potentiation) A+B=effect is more than A+B, *e.g.* ACh and neostigmine, sulfonamide+trimethoprim.

Ans. 78 (D) Spare receptors may be defined as those which are not needed for binding drug to achieve the maximum effect. Spare receptors influence the sensitivity of the system to an agonist because the statistical probability of a drug receptor interaction increases with the total number of receptors. They do not alter the maximal efficacy. If they do not bind an agonist molecule, spare receptors do not activate an effector molecule. EC50 less than Kd is an indication of the presence of spare receptors.

Ans. 79 (C) Large number of drugs bind directly to the receptor and act through receptors, but few drugs does bind with enzymes, channels, transporters, structural proteins etc. Receptors are defined as macromolecules located on the surface or inside the effector cells. Agonist activates the receptor to produce similar effect. Partial agonist activates a receptor to produce sub-maximal response but can antagonizes the action of full agonist (have high affinity).

Ans. 80 (D) Action of drug through receptor is not dependent on lipophilicity (expl. as with text).

Ans. 81 (A) Continue intense receptor stimulation by agonist causes desensitization and may cause decrease synthesis or increased destruction of the receptor. This is known as down regulation. In contrast, prolonged deprivation of agonist or continuous use of antagonist results in super sensitivity or proliferation of receptor occurs. This is known as up regulation of receptors.

Ans. 82 (C) Standard dose is the same dose which is appropriate for most of the patients because individual variation is minor or the drug has a wide safety margin, *e.g.* oral contraceptive, mebendazole, chloroquine. In regulated dose the dose modification is done by regulating body function measure (anti hypertensive, hypoglycemic). Titrated dose is given for those drugs which have intolerable adverse effects, *e.g.* anti-cancer drugs.

Ans. 83 (C) Competitive antagonist binds to the receptor with strong covalent bond or dissociate from it very slowly. The have affinity but not intrinsic activity, so no response is produced and the log DRC of the agonist is shifted to right (no change in shape) with no suppression of maximal response.

Ans. 84 (C) A non-competitive antagonist decreases the magnitude of the response to an agonist but does not alter the agonist's mechanism of action and potency. A competitive type of agonist interacts at the agonist binding site.

Ans. 85 (C) Placebo is a pharmacodynamically inert and harmless substance, which resembles with actual medicament and causes improvement in subjective symptom only but not in objective response. It is necessary when a trial is to be conducted on healthy volunteers but have no place in the trials of a new drug in the patients suffering from a disease.

Ans. 86 (B) In phase II trial, the drug is studied in patients with target disease, to determine its efficacy. In early phase a small number (20-200) patients are studied and is a single blind design where the subject does not know whether he is taking an inert placebo or a drug. In late phase of II trial it is conducted in double blind manner where investigator is also ignorant, about what he is prescribing.

Ans. 87 (D) Clinical trial phase IV, is a post licensing surveillance phase which has no fixed duration and is started after complete satisfaction from phase III regarding the efficacy and safety of drug.

2

AUTONOMIC NERVOUS SYSTEM (ANS)

GENERAL CONSIDERATION

There are two systems in our body, one is **Central Nervous System (CNS)** and another is **Peripheral Nervous System** or **Autonomic Nervous System (ANS)**. The ANS controls the functioning of viscera and innervates almost all the tissues of the body except the voluntary muscles. The ANS thus regulates the vital functions in the body including respiratory system, blood pressure, body temperature, water balance, urination, digestion and many metabolic functions. The ANS comprises three major subdivisions: Sympathetic, Parasympathetic and Enteric Nervous System (ENS).

Acetylcholine (ACh) is the neurotransmitter at all sympathetic and parasympathetic ganglion synapse (autonomic ganglia), post ganglionic parasympathetic fibers (except apocrine sweat gland). So, all somatic motor neurons to skeletal muscle (NMJ), all pre ganglionic parasympathetic and sympathetic fibers (including adrenal medulla), postganglionic parasympathetic fibers of neuro effector junction (NEJ) and post ganglionic fibers to sweat glands of palm and sole are cholinergic in character which act through cholinergic receptors.

All postganglionic sympathetic fibers release norepinephrine at NEJ except of sweat gland, fibers supplying to arteriole of skeletal muscles and some postganglionic sympathetic neurons of splanchnic and renal blood vessels. They act through adrenergic receptors.

Receptor Characteristics

The major receptor systems in the ANS include:

A. Cholinergic receptors: Cholinergic receptors are subdivided as follows: (Table 2.1)

a. *Muscarinic receptors:* As their name suggests, these receptors respond to muscarine as well as to acetylcholine. The effects of

Table 2.1: Some characteristics of cholinergic receptors in the ANS

	Location	Agonist	Antagonist	Mechanism	Major function
Muscarinic (M_1)	Autonomic ganglia, CNS, GIT	Oxotremorine	Atropine, Pirenzepine, Telenzepine	G_q-coupled	Increase IP_3, DAG cascade
Muscarinic (M_2)	Heart S.A. node Atrium, AV node Ventricles Smooth muscles	Methacholine	Methoetramine Tripitramine	G_i-coupled	Decrease cAMP, activates K^+ channels
Muscarinic (M_3)	Smooth muscles secretory glands	Bethanecol	Hexa-hydrosila fenidol Darifenacin Tolterodine	G_q-coupled	Increase IP_3, DAG cascade
Nicotinic (Nm) Muscle	Neuromuscular junction	Nicotine, PTMA Succinyl choline	d-Tubocurarine	Intrinsic Ion channel	Depolarizes, evokes action potential Contraction of skeletal muscle
(Nn) Neuronal	Autonomic ganglia Adrenal medulla	DMPP, nicotine	Hexamethonium Trimetharphan	Ion channel	Depolarizes, evokes action potential, secretion of NE and E

DMPP - Dimethyl phenyl piperizinium
PTMA - Phenyl trimethyl ammonium

activation of these receptors resemble those of postganglionic parasympathetic nerve stimulation. Muscarinic receptors are located primarily on autonomic effector cells (including heart, vascular endothelium, smooth muscle, pre synaptic nerve terminals and exocrine glands). They are of 5 subtypes, of which 3 appear to be important in peripheral autonomic transmission.

b. *Nicotinic receptors:* These receptors are parts of ion channels and respond to acetylcholine and nicotine, but not to muscarine. The two major nicotinic subtypes are located in ganglia and in skeletal muscle end plates (Nn and Nm type respectively).

B. Adrenergic receptors: They are divided into two subtypes: (Table 2.2)

Table 2.2 Characteristics of some important adrenoceptors in the ANS

Receptor type	Location	G protein	Second messenger	Major functions	Agonist	Antagonist
Alpha$_1$ (post-junctional on effector organs)	Vascular, GIT Genitourinary, smooth muscles Heart	G_q	Increase IP_3 DAG	Increase Ca^{2+} causes contraction of smooth muscles increase secretion	Adr. NA, Iso Phenylephrine Methoxamine	Prazosin
alpha$_2$ (pre junctional on nerve endings)–(α2A) to also post-junctional in brain	Pancreatic beta cells, Platelets, Nerve terminals, Vascular smooth muscles	G_i	Decrease cAMP activate K^+ channels	Decrease transmitter release, causes vaso-contraction decrease insulin	Adr, NA Iso	Yohimbine
Beta$_1$	Heart and JG cells	G_s	Increase cAMP	Increase heart rate, increase force, increase renin release	Iso, Adr, NA Dobutamine	Metoprolol-Atenolol
Beta$_2$	Bronchial, vascular, GIT, smooth muscles	G_s	Increase cAMP	Relax smooth muscle; increase glycogenolysis; increase heart rate and force of contraction	Iso, Adr, NA	α-methyl propranolol Butoxamine
Beta$_3$	Adipose tissue	G_s	Increase cAMP	Increase lipolysis Thermogenesis	Iso, NA	ICI 48537
Dopamine (D$_1$)	Smooth muscles of renal, coronary vascular bed and myocardium	G_s	Increase cAMP	Relax renal vascular smooth muscle	Fenol dapam	SCH 23390
Dopamine (D$_2$)	Mainly in the CNS, renal and vascular bed	G_i	Decrease cAMP, increase K^+ conductance	Decrease NE release, modulate DA release	Bromo-criptine	Sulpride

a. *Alpha receptors:* These are located on vascular smooth muscle, pre synaptic nerve terminals, blood platelets, fat cells, and neurons in the brain. Alpha receptors are further divided into two major types, alpha$_1$ and alpha$_2$.

b. *Beta receptors:* These receptors are located on most types of smooth muscle, cardiac muscle, some pre synaptic nerve terminals, and lipocytes as well as in the brain. Beta receptors are divided into three major sub-types, beta$_1$, beta$_2$ and beta$_3$.

C. Dopamine receptors: Dopamine (DA) receptors are a subclass of adrenergic receptors but with different distribution and function. Dopamine receptors are especially important in the renal and splanchnic vessels and in the brain. Although at least 5 subtypes exist, but the D_1, subtype appears to be the most important peripheral effector cell dopamine receptor. D_2 receptors are found on presynaptic nerve terminals. D_1, D_2 and other types of dopamine receptors also occur in the CNS.

Non-adrenergic non-cholinergic transmission (NANC): Some nerve fibers in autonomic effector tissues do not show the histochemical characteristics of either cholinergic or adrenergic fibers. Some of these are motor fibers that cause the release of ATP and other purines related to it. Purine evoked responses have been identified in the bronchi, gastrointestinal tract and urinary tract. Other motor fibers release peptides as the primary transmitters. These peptides are potent agonist in many autonomic effector tissues.

CHOLINERGIC DRUGS
(Parasympathomimetic Drugs)

Acetylcholine (ACh) an ester of choline, is the neurotransmitter of the parasympathetic system. The nerves that synthesize, store and release ACh are called 'cholinergic nerves'. Acetylcholine is synthesized from acetyl CoA and choline and released into the synaptic cleft. This ACh binds to and activates the cholinergic receptor on the postsynaptic membrane leading to the depolarization of the membrane.

ACh released into the synaptic cleft is rapidly destroyed by the enzyme acetylcholinesterase (AChE). There are two types of AChE present:

1. **True cholinesterase:** It present at neurons, ganglia and neuromuscular junction.
2. **Pseudo cholinesterase:** It present in plasma, liver and intestine.

Cholinergic drugs may be classified as:

1. *Esters of choline*: Acetylcholine, Methacholine, Carbachol, Bethanechol.
2. *Cholinomimetic alkaloids*: Pilocarpine, Muscarine, Arecoline.
3. *Anticholinesterases*:
   a. *Reversible:* Physostigmine, Neostigmine, Pyridostigmine, Donepezil, Edrophonium, Ambenonium, Demecarium, Rivastigmine.
   b. *Irreversible:* **Organophosphates,** *e.g.* Echothiophate, Malathion, Sumithion, Diazinon. **Carbamates,** *e.g.* Carbaryl (SEVIN), Propoxure (BAYGON), Aldicarb (TEMIK), Toxic nerve gases (Sarin, Tabun).

Actions of Acetylcholine

Muscarinic Actions

1. **Heart:** It depresses the SA node and thereby reduces the heart rate and force of contraction, decreases rate of diastolic depolarization and increase refractory period (through M_2 receptors).
2. **Blood Vessels:** ACh relax the vascular smooth muscles and dilate the blood vessels of the skin and mucous membrane. The BP falls due to a fall in total peripheral resistance and reflex tachycardia (arteries have no parasympathetic innervations, but have M_3 receptors which release EDRF).
3. **Smooth Muscle:** ACh increases the tone of all other (nonvascular) smooth muscles.
   a. *Intestinal:* Peristalsis is enhanced, sphincters are relaxed, resulting in rapid forward propulsion of intestinal contents (M_1 and M_3 receptors).
   b. *Urinary bladder:* detrusor contracts and trigonal sphincter relaxes thus promotes voiding of urine (M_3 receptors).
   c. *Bronchial smooth muscle:* contraction of bronchial muscles resulting in bronchospasm (M_3 receptors).
4. **Secretory Glands:** Acetylcholine enhances the secretions of all glands; salivary, lacrimal, nasopharyngeal, tracheobronchial, gastric (M_1 receptor) and intestinal secretions (M_3 receptors).
5. **Eye:** Acetylcholine brings about constriction of pupil (miosis) by contracting the circular muscles of the iris. Drainage of aqueous humor is facilitated and intraocular pressure falls. Ciliary muscle contracts resulting in spasm of accommodation.
6. **Male Sex Organ:** Erection of penis (M_3 receptors).

Nicotinic Actions

1. **Neuromuscular junction (NMJ):** Contraction of skeletal muscles by stimulating Nm receptors present in the neuromuscular junction. Large doses cause paralysis.
2. **Autonomic ganglia:** Acetylcholine stimulates both sympathetic and parasympathetic ganglia and the adrenal medulla and causes rise in BP.
3. **CNS:** IV injection of ACh does not penetrate BBB and no central effect are seen but direct injection into brain produce stimulation followed by depression.

Actions of Acetylcholine

CVS	Decrease HR, decrease BP
Non-vascular smooth muscle	Contraction, increase gut peristalsis, promotes urine voiding, bronchospasm
Glands	Increase secretion
Eye	Miosis, spasm of accommodation, decrease IOP
Ganglia	Stimulation
NMJ	Muscle contraction

Uses

Acetylcholine is not used therapeutically.

Carbachol and **bethanechol** are resistant to both pseudo and true cholinesterases and have a longer duration of action. Carbachol is sometimes used in glaucoma.

Bethanechol is used to:

a. Reverse post-operative atony of bladder.
b. GIT atony (without obstruction).
c. Xerostomia as an alternative to pilocarpine. Sevimeline is a new drug used now-a-days. It is long acting and less toxic to pilocarpine.
d. Alzheimer's disease (by intracerebroventricular injection).

Contraindications of Choline Esters

1. Hyperthyroidism
2. Bronchial asthma
3. Peptic ulcer
4. Myocardial infarction

Cholinomimetic Alkaloids

Pilocarpine: Its muscarinic actions are prominent (M_3 receptor), with mild action at Nn receptor. It is too toxic for systemic use. Main therapeutic uses are:

1. Open angle glaucoma (ocusert).
2. Pilocarpine is also used alternately with mydriatics like homatropine to break the adhesions between the iris and the lens.
3. It is used to counter dryness of mouth that is seen following radiation of head and neck and after laryngeal surgery.

Anti Cholinesterases

Anti cholinesterases (anti ChEs) or cholinesterase inhibitors are drugs which inhibit the enzyme cholinesterase. As their structure resembles that of ACh, they bind to acetyl cholinesterases and inactivate them. Thus ACh is not hydrolyzed and it accumulates. The actions of all these drugs are due to this accumulated ACh. Hence the actions are similar to cholinergic agonists.

They may be:

(A) Reversible

They bear the structural resemblance to AChE and combined with anionic and the esteratic sites of AChE, which hydrolyze slowly and causes temporary inhibition.

(a) *Physostigmine:* It is a tertiary ammonium compound, has better penetration into tissues and also cross the BBB. It is used in glaucoma and in atropine poisoning.

(b) *Neostigmine:* is a synthetic quaternary ammonium compound, poorly absorbed from the gut and it does not cross the BBB. It is used in myasthenia gravis. The mechanism to improve muscle power in myasthenia gravis is:
  (i) Its anti ChE activity (accumulate ACh at motor end plate).
  (ii) Increase the amount of ACh released during each nerve impulse.
  (iii) Directly stimulate cholinoceptive receptor sites on motor end plate, so act as partial agonist.

(c) *Edrophonium:* is rapid and short acting (as it binds with anionic site only). It is used for the diagnosis of the myasthenia gravis and in snake bite and in curare poisoning (intravenously).

Uses of Reversible Anti Cholinesterases

1. As a miotic (in glaucoma).
2. Myasthenia gravis.
3. Alzheimer's disease.
4. Poisoning due to anticholinergic drugs, TCA.
5. Curare poisoning.
6. Postoperative paralytic ileus and urinary retention.
7. Cobra bite (with atropine) .
8. Post operative decurarization.
9. Paroxysmal atrial and supra ventricular tachycardia (now-a-days CCBs are preferred).

TREATMENT OF GLAUCOMA, MYASTHENIA GRAVIS AND ALZHEIMER'S DISEASE

Treatment of Glaucoma

Beta blockers are the first line drugs. They reduce aqueous humor formation by blocking $beta_2$ receptors in the ciliary body. **Adrenergic agonist** reduces aqueous humor formation ($alpha_2$ receptor) present on ciliary epithelium. **Miotics** improve drainage of aqueous humor by constricting the pupil and opening the iridocorneal angle, contraction of ciliary muscle and thus increase drainage of aqueous humor.

Latanoprost is a prostaglandin analogue. It increases the outflow of aqueous humor probably by relaxing the ciliary muscle. It can be used as an adjuvant to other drugs.

Drugs used in glaucoma are summarized in Table 2.3.

Table 2.3: Drug used in glaucoma

Drug	Adverse effects	Comments
Beta blockers – Timolol, betaxolol carteolol, levobunolol	Conjunctival irritation, redness and discomfort	First line drug, no miosis hence no headache or brow ache
Cholinergics – pilocarpine, carbachol, physostigmine, echothiophate	Corneal edema, spasm of accommodation, brow ache, myopia, retinal detachment	Used with beta blockers
Adrenergic agonists–dipivefrine, adrenaline Apraclonidine brimonidine	Conjunctival redness, photosensitivity allergic reactions	2nd line drug adjuvant
Carbonic anhydrase inhibitors (acetazolamide), dorzolamide	Hypokalemia, anorexia, drowsiness	2nd line drugs — given orally Given topically

Treatment of Myasthenia Gravis

Myasthenia gravis is an acquired auto-immune disorder causing skeletal muscle fatigability and weakness, which worsen after exercise.

Drug used are:

(a) Anti cholinesterase (Reversible)–Neostigmine, Pyridostigmine, Ambenonium (with atropine to minimize muscarinic adverse effects).

(b) Glucocorticoids–Prednisolone which may inhibit antibodies production.

(c) Immunosuppressants–Azathioprine, Cyclosporine.

(d) Thymectomy.

(e) Plasmapheresis – To remove antibodies.

Drugs which aggravate myasthenia gravis are aminoglycosides, morphine, procainamide, quinidine dTc, lithium etc.

Treatment of Alzheimer's Disease

It is a neuro-degenerative disorder characterized by progressive loss of memory (dementia). Drug used are:

a. *Tacrine:* Long acting anti ChE. This facilitate release of Ach, NA, DA and 5HT and inhibits MAO, GABA release, may cause hepatotoxicity.
b. *Donepezil, Rivastigmine, Galantamine* are the other drugs nowadays preferred.
c. *Vitamin E,* Vitamin A, Zn, Acetyl-L-carnitine, DHEA (dehydro-epi androsterone).

(B) Irreversible Anticholinesterases

Organophosphorus (OP) compounds are powerful inhibitors of AChE enzyme, they bind only to the esteratic site (except echothiophate, which bound with anionic site) and the enzyme is phosphorylated. This phosphorylated complex hydrolyses very slowly or sometimes does not hydrolyze. So recovery takes very long time. Organophosphates are highly lipid soluble and hence are absorbed from all routes including intact skin. Since they are very toxic, so they are not used.

Acute Organophosphorus Compound Poisoning

Treatment

1. Remove/Termination of further exposure.
2. Gastric lavage.
3. Purgative (sodium sulphate/magnesium sulphate).
4. Maintain BP and patent airway.
5. Specific Therapy.
   a. Atropine: IV, high doses.
   b. Cholinesterase reactivators (Pralidoxime, Obidoxime, Diacetylmonoxime). These oxime compounds combine with cholinesterase enzyme by attaching themselves on anionic site and form complex with phosphate group which is soluble. Thus set free the binding and AChE enzyme. Thus they reactivate the cholinesterase enzyme. They should be given within minutes after poisoning preferably immediately,

because the complex undergoes 'aging' (strengthening of phosphate enzyme) and the enzyme cannot be released. They are ineffective in carbamate poisoning. Only diacetyl monoxime crosses BBB.

ANTI-CHOLINERGIC DRUGS

Anti-cholinergic drugs are agents which block the effects of acetylcholine on cholinergic receptors (anti muscarinic). Drugs that block the nicotinic receptors are ganglionic blockers and neuromuscular blockers.

Classification

1. *Natural alkaloids:* Atropine, Hyoscine (scopolamine).
2. *Semisynthetic derivatives:* Homatropine, Ipratropium bromide, Tiotroprium bromide.
3. *Synthetic derivatives:* Glycopyrrolate, Dicyclomine, Oxybutynin, Pirenzepine, Tropicamide etc.

Actions

The actions of atropine and scopolamine are similar except that atropine is a CNS stimulant while scopolamine is a CNS depressant and causes sedation.

1. **CVS:** Brief bradycarida (M_1) followed by increases heart rate (M_2), vasodilatation and hypotension occurs (due to histamine releases in toxic doses).
2. **Secretions:** Atropine reduces all secretions (except milk and bile) results in dry mouth and difficulty in swallowing. It is an antisialogogue. Sweating is also reduced.
3. **Smooth muscle:**
   a. *GIT:* Decrease tone and motility, sphincters are closed may result in constipation.
   b. *Biliary tract:* Biliary spasm is relieved (less marked).
   c. *Bronchi:* Broncho-dilatation, reduce airway resistance.
   d. *Urinary bladder:* Relaxes ureter (useful in uretric colic), tone of fundus is reduced, while that of sphincter is increased, so may cause urinary retention.
4. **Eye:** Atropine produces mydriasis by blocking the muscarinic receptors in the sphincter pupillae. The ciliary muscle is paralyzed

resulting in cycloplegia or paralysis of accommodation. It block the drainage of aqueous humor, thus IOP increases and may precipitate glaucoma in some patients.

5. **CNS:** In higher doses atropine stimulates the CNS resulting in restlessness, disorientation, hallucinations and delirium. In contrast, scopolamine produces sedation and drowsiness.

Pharmacokinetics: Atropine and hyoscine are well absorbed from gut, widely distributed, cross the BBB and metabolized in the liver. About 50% of atropine is excreted unchanged.

Adverse effects are common but not serious and include blurring of vision, dry mouth, dysphagia, dry skin, fever, constipation and urinary retention. High doses cause palpitation, flushing, restlessness, delirium, hallucinations, psychosis, convulsions and coma.

Uses of Anti-Cholinergic Drugs

1. As anti-secretary
   a. Pre anaesthetic medication
   b. Peptic ulcer
   c. Pulmonary diseases
   d. Parkinsonism.
2. As anti-spasmodic in renal colic, biliary colic, spastic constipation.
3. As mydriatric and cycloplegic.
4. In organophosphorus poisoning.
5. In bronchial asthma (ipratropium bromide is used).
6. Motion sickness: Hyoscine given 30 minutes before the journey.

Contraindications

1. Narrow angle glaucoma.
2. Patients with enlarged prostate.
3. COPD.
4. CCF with tachycardia.

Atropine Substitues

Atropine substitutes and their uses

	Indications	Derivatives
1	On the eye – mydriatics and cycloplegia	Homatropine, Eucatropine Cyclopentolate, Tropicamide
2	As antispasmodics	Propantheline, Methantheline, Dicyclomine, Flavoxate hydrochloride, Oxybutynin chloride, Oxyphenonium, Glycopyrrolate, Clidinum
3	Peptic ulcer	Pirenzepine, Telenzepine
4	Bronchial asthma	Ipratropium, Tiotropium
5	Pre anaesthetic medication	Glycopyrrolate
6	Urinary disorders	Oxybutynin, Tolterodine, Propiverine, Dicyclomine
7	Antiparkinsonian drugs	Benzhexol, Benztropine
8	Motion sickness	Scopolamine

Adrenergic System

The prime function of the adrenergic or sympathetic nervous system is to help the human being to adjust to stress and prepare the body for fight or flight reactions.

Neurotransmitters of the sympathetic system are norepinephrine (nor adrenaline NA) and dopamine (DA). Epinephrine (Adrenaline) is the major hormone secreted by the adrenal medulla.

The stimulation of alpha receptors mainly produces excitatory effects (exception GIT); beta stimulation causes mainly inhibitory effects (exception heart).

ADRENERGIC AND ANTI- ADRENERGIC DRUGS

Adrenergic Drugs (Sympathomimetics)

Sympathomimetics are drugs that produce actions which mimic that of sympathetic stimulation by activating alpha and/or beta receptors, directly or indirectly.

Classification

1. **Chemical classification**
   a. *Catecholamines:* Norepinephrine (NE), Epinephrine (E), Dopamine (DA), Isoprenaline (Synthetic).

b. *Non-catecholamine:* Ephedrine, Amphetamine and other vasopressor as well as smooth muscle relaxants.

2. **Depending on the mode of action**
   a. *Directly acting sympathomimetics* (by interacting with adrenergic receptors): Norepinephrine (NE), Epinephrine, Dopamine, Isoprenaline.
   b. *Indirectly acting sympathomimetics* (by releasing NE from nerve terminals or from storage): Amphetamine, Tyramine.
   c. *Mixed action amines* (both direct and indirect actions): Ephedrine, Methoxamine.
3. **Therapeutic or clinical classification**
   a. *Vasopressors:* Norepinephrine, Dopamine, Methoxamine, Metaraminol, Phenylephrine.
   b. *Cardiac stimulants and inotropic:* Epinephrine, Dopamine, Dobutamine, Isoprenaline, Ephedrine.
   c. *CNS stimulants:* Amphetamine, Ephedrine.
   d. *Bronchodilators:* $Beta_2$ agonist, *e.g.* Albuterol (Salbutamol), Salmeterol, etc.
   e. *Nasal decongestants:* Ephedrine, Pseudoephedrine, Phenylpropanolamine, Phenylephrine, Oxymetazoline, Xylometazoline.
   f. *Appetite suppressants (Anorectics):* Fenfluramine, Dexfenfluramine, Phenteramine, Sibutramine.
   g. *Uterine relaxants:* Salbutamol, Terbutaline, Isosxuprine, Ritodrine.
   h. *Used for allergic reaction (anaphylaxis):* Epinephrine (Adrenaline) Ephedrine.

Pharmacological Actions of Catecholamines

1. **Cardiovascular System**
   a. *Heart:* Epinephrine (Adrenaline) is a powerful cardiac stimulant. Acting through $beta_1$ receptors, it increases the heart rate, force of contraction, cardiac output and conduction velocity. It abolishes reflex vagal bradycardia in response to carotid sinus compression, so causes tachycardia.
   b. *Blood vessels and BP:* Blood vessels of the skin and mucous membrane are constricted (alpha) and that of the skeletal muscles are dilated ($beta_2$) by epinephrine. So, epinephrine raises SBP by cardiac action and fall in DBP by peripheral action. Rapid increase

in BP followed by a fall (a biphasic response) is observed with epinephrine. When alpha receptors are blocked (with ergot alkaloids which is an alpha blocker), epinephrine produces only a fall in BP and this is named as Dale's vasomotor reversal.

Norepinephrine is mainly an alpha agonist and brings about a rise in BP with bradycardia due to ++ of cardiac baro- receptors.

Other vascular beds: It causes renal, pulmonary and mesenteric vasoconstriction. Cerebral and coronary blood flow is enhanced.

2. **Smooth Muscles**
   a. *Bronchi:* It causes bronchodilatation.
   b. *Uterus:* Non pregnant uterus contracts.
   Pregnant: Last month of pregnancy relaxes.
   c. *Gut:* Smooth muscles relaxed (alpha and beta effect).
   d. *Bladder:* Detrusor is relaxed (beta receptors) while trigon is contracted (alpha effect).
   e. *Others:* Splenic capsule contracts, pilomotor muscles contract.
3. **Eye:** Mydriasis due to contraction of the radial muscles of the iris ($alpha_1$); reduces intraocular pressure.
4. **Metabolic Effects:** Increases the blood sugar level ($beta_2$ and $alpha_1$ action) by increasing glycogenolysis and by inhibiting insulin release ($alpha_2$), increases free fatty acids ($beta_3$ and alpha receptors), increase BMR and increase body temperature ($beta_3$ effect).
5. **Skeletal Muscles:** Catecholamines facilitate neuromuscular transmission by action on both alpha and beta receptors.
6. **CNS:** Do not cross BBB.
7. **Respiration:** Epinephrine is a weak stimulant of respiration and induces apnea.

Pharmacokinetics: As catecholamines are rapidly inactivated in the gut and the liver, so not given orally. Epinephrine and NE are metabolized by COMT and MAO and converted into VMA.

Adverse reactions: Anxiety, palpitation, weakness, tremors, pallor, dizziness, restlessness and throbbing headache may (occur). NE infusion should be controlled carefully.

Uses

1. Anaphylactic shock.
2. Cardiac arrest.
3. Control of haemorrhage.
4. With local anaesthetics.

5. Acute bronchial asthma (used rarely nowadays).
6. Glaucoma (alpha-adrenergic).
7. **Isoprenaline** is used in heart block and shock for its cardiac stimulant actions.

Contraindications

They are contraindicated in angina pectoris, hypertension and hyperthyroidism and in patients on beta blockers and digitalis, with halothane.

Dopamine is the precursor of NE. It acts on dopaminergic and adrenergic receptors.

1. In low doses (2.5 μg/kg/min) it stimulate vascular D_1 receptors and increases renal blood flow and thereby GFR and excretion of sodium.
2. In moderate doses (5-10 μg/kg/min) it causes cardiac stimulation through $beta_1$, receptors and increases force of contraction, cardiac output and B.P.
3. In high doses (more than 10 μg/kg/min) $alpha_1$ receptors are activated resulting in vasoconstriction and increase BP and nullify the beneficial effects.

Dobutamine is a recemic mixture of dopamine and is a selective $beta_1$ agonist. In therapeutic doses, increase in the force of contraction, without a significant increase in the heart rate is observed. The l-form of dobutamine is potent $alpha_1$ agonist while d-form is having $alpha_1$ antagonist and beta agonist action. So the net results are $beta_1$ agonist action.

Dopexamine is a synthetic analog of dopamine acting on D_1, D_2 and $beta_2$ receptors and have beneficial effects in CCF.

Fenoldopam is a selective D_1 agonist (no alpha or beta receptor agonist action) which dilates coronary, renal and mesenteric arteries. It is used as an IV infusion in severe hypertension to rapidly reduce the BP (short term use).

Non-catecholamines

They are effective orally, have longer duration of action and may cross BBB and have CNS effect.

Ephedrine: It acts by direct stimulation of alpha and beta receptors and indirectly through release of NE from sympathetic neurons. It causes increases in force of contraction; increase BP, relaxations of smooth muscles and CNS effects. Mydriasis and increase BMR is also observed.

Uses

Its use declined due to lack of selectivity and low efficacy.

1. Bronchial asthma.
2. Nasal decongestion.
3. Mydriasis.
4. Hypotension.
5. Narcolepsy – Amphetamine is preferred.
6. Nocturnal enuresis.
7. Stokes Adam's syndrome (isoprenaline is preferred).

Amphetamine: CNS stimulant and decreases appetite but not used because of its drug abuse liability and other toxic effect.

Uses

1. Attention deficit hyperactivity disorder – in children.
2. Narcolepsy.
3. Obesity.
4. Epilepsy.

Vasopressors (NE, DA, Phenylephrine, Metaraminol etc.)

They increase the BP by increasing total peripheral resistance (TPR) or cardiac output (CO) or both. They are given parenterally with constant monitoring of BP. Tachyphylaxis may develop with these agents. Vasopressors are used to raise the BP in hypotension as seen in cardiogenic or neurogenic shock and during spinal anaesthesia. Mephenteramine is preferred to treat or to prevent hypotension due to spinal anaesthesia and surgical procedure.

Nasal Decongestants (Xyelometazoline, Oxymetazoline, Nephazoline)

Nasal decongestants are $alpha_2$ agonists. They bring about vasoconstriction of the nasal mucosa, resulting in its shrinkage and they decrease the volume of the mucous and used as nasal drops (0.05-1% solution).

Disadvantages of these agents, as a result from long term use, are atrophy of the nasal mucosa and loss of efficacy or tolerance due to desensitization.

Selective $Beta_2$ Stimulants

They are used in bronchial asthma and details discuss with respiratory system and with tocolytic drugs (Uterine relaxants).

Anorectic Agents (Anorexiants)

Though amphetamine suppresses appetite, it is not recommended for the treatment of obesity due to its central stimulant effects. Fenfluramine, dexfenfluramine, mazindol, phenylpropanolamine (now banned), penmetrazine and others are used.

Sibutramine: It inhibits the uptake of NA and 5 HT.

Adrenergic Antagonists

Alpha Adrenergic Blocking Agents (Alpha-receptor Antagonist)

Alpha receptor antagonists block the adrenergic responses mediated through alpha adrenergic receptors. Some of them have selectivity for $alpha_1$ or $alpha_2$ receptors.

Classification

1. **Non-selective**
   a. *Non-competitive blocker (Irreversible):* Phenoxybenzamine.
   b. *Competitive blockers (Reversible):* Tolazoline, Phentolamine.
2. **Selective**
   a. *$Alpha_1$ blockers:* Prazosin, Terazosin, Doxazosin, Tamsulosin, Alfuzosin, Bunazosin, Silodosin.
   b. *$Alpha_2$ blocker:* Yohimbine, Idazoxan.
3. **Miscellaneous:** Ergot alkaloid, Chlorpromazine.

Non Selective Alpha Blockers

Phenoxybenzamine binds covalently to both $alpha_1$ and $alpha_2$ receptors causing irreversible blockade. It can be used orally in the treatment of pheochromocytoma.

Phentolamine and tolazoline, in addition, also block 5 HT receptors; stimulate gut motility and increase gastric secretion, causes nasal stiffness, miosis, improved urine flow and impotence.

Selective Alpha Blockers

$Alpha_1$ blockade inhibits vasoconstriction leading to vasodilatation and thereby decrease BP. This fall in BP is opposed by the baroreceptor reflexes (++) which tend to increase heart rate and cardiac output.

$Alpha_2$ blockade Enhances release of NE which stimulates beta receptors (alpha are already blocked) – $beta_1$, stimulation in heart results in tachycardia and increased cardiac output.

Selective Alpha$_1$ Blockers

Selective alpha$_1$ blockade results in hypotension without significant tachycardia.

Prazosin: It is a potent, highly selective, alpha$_1$ blocker. Arterioles and venules are dilated, resulting in decreased peripheral vascular resistance and cardiac output (CO falls because of venodilation and leads to decreased preload). There is no significant tachycardia (alpha$_2$ receptors are spared there is no increase in NE release). It may decrease central sympathetic outflow. Prazosin also inhibits phosphodiesterase enzyme, resulting in increase cAMP which also contributes to vasodilatation. It also decrease LDL and triglycerides and increase HDL cholesterol and relax the urinary bladder neck and the prostatic capsule. Prazosin is orally effective, extensively bound to plasma proteins and is metabolized in the liver.

Adverse effects marked postural hypotension, impotence, nasal congestion GIT upset, retention of water and Na^+ is observed with prazosin.

Prazosin congeners (Terazosin, Doxazosin, Tamsulosin etc.)

- These congeners are longer acting and can be given once daily.
- They are highly selective for alpha$_1$ receptors.
- Postural hypotension is milder than with prazosin with these agents.
- No significant effect on cardiac function is observed.
- They decrease LDL and increase HDL cholesterol.
- Tamsulosin has selective activity on alpha$_{1A}$ receptors in the bladder and prostate while hypotension (mediated by alpha$_{1B}$) is mild. So used in BPH.
- Alfuzosin is useful in BPH but have short duration of action.
- Terazosin and doxazosin are used in hypertension.
- Urapidil is useful in BPH with hypertension.

Selective Alpha$_2$ Blockers

Yohimbine is a relatively selective alpha$_2$ blocker which increases BP and heart rate due to increase NE release. It is used to treat psychogenic impotence.

Ergot alkaloids blockade is of short duration. Cause contraction of the uterus and increase BP due to vasoconstriction.

Adverse Effects of Alpha Blockers

Postural hypotension, palpitation, nasal stuffiness, miosis, impaired ejaculation and impotence.

Uses of Alpha Blocker

1. Hypertension.
2. Pheochromocytoma.
3. Peripheral vascular diseases.
4. Congestive cardiac failure.
5. Benign prostatic hypertrophy (BPH).

Beta Adrenergic Blocking Agents

Classification

1. *Non-selective (beta$_1$ and beta$_2$ blocker)*
   a. Without intrinsic sympathomimetic activity (ISA), *e.g.* Propranolol, Nadolol Timolol, Sotalol).
   b. With both ISA and membrane stabilizing activity, *e.g.* Pindolol, Oxyprenolol, Alprenolol.
2. *Selective (Cardioselective beta$_1$ blocker):* Metoprolol, Atenolol, Acebutolol, Esmolol, Betaxolol, Bisoprolol, Nebivolol.
3. *Partial agonists:* Pindolol, Oxprenolol, Carteolol, Bopindolol, Penbutotol.
4. *With additional alpha blocking property:* Labetalol, Carvedilol.
5. *Beta$_1$ blocker, beta$_2$ agonist:* Celiprolol.

Pharmacological Actions

1. *CVS:* Beta blockers decrease heart rate, force of contraction and cardiac output. So, decrease cardiac work and O_2 consumption.
2. *Blood pressure:* They causes fall in BP (the effect is more pronounced in presence of increased sympathetic tone than in a normal situation), decrease plasma renin activity (propranolol) and decrease sympathetic outflow.
3. *Respiratory tract:* They increases airway resistance and may precipitate acute attack of asthma.
4. *Eye:* Beta blockers (Timolol) reduce intraocular pressure by decreasing secretion and formation of aqueous humor.
5. *Metabolic:* They block lipolysis and glycogenolysis (beta$_2$ mediated) thus, decrease FFA and insulin release. Plasma LDL and triglycerides may increase and HDL levels decrease in some patients.
6. *CNS:* Sedation, lethargy, disturbed sleep.
7. *Skeletal muscle:* Propranolol inhibits adrenergically provoked tremors during anxiety.

8. *Propranolol have local anaesthetic activity* but not used due to its irritant effect.

Pharmacokinetics: Beta blockers are well absorbed on oral administration, propranolol undergo extensive first pass metabolism and has low bioavailability. Marked individual variation is seen.

Adverse Reactions

1. Bradycardia and hypotension.
2. *CCF:* may exacerbate heart failure in patients with compensatory heart.
3. Cold extremities.
4. Beta blockers precipitate acute asthmatic attack.
5. CNS insomnia, depression and rarely hallucinations.
6. Fatigue due to decreased blood flow.
7. Abrupt withdrawal of beta blockers after prolonged use can cause rebound hypertension and attack of angina.
8. Beta blockers can also cause dizziness.
9. *Hypoglycemia:* They mask the symptoms of hypoglycemia and delay recovery.
10. Altered lipid profile.

Contraindications

They are contraindicated in bradycardia, heart block, asthmatics, in chronic obstructive pulmonary disease, variant angina, diabetes and with other cardio depressant drugs (Verapamil).

Drug Interactions

1. Propranolol + insulin: Beta blockade masks tachycardia which is the first warning signal of hypoglycemia.
2. Propranolol + verapamil causes myocardial depression.

Cardioselective Beta Blockers

These drugs:

- Selectively block $beta_1$ receptors; $beta_2$ receptor blocking action is weak.
- Bronchospasm is less/negligible.
- Inhibition of glycogenolysis is less–hence safer in diabetics.
- Exercise performance is impaired to a lesser degree.
- Lesser chances of peripheral vascular disease.
- No/less deleterious effects on lipid profile.

Disadvantages

1. Rebound hypertension occurs on abrupt withdrawl.
2. Ineffective in controlling tremors.

Uses of Beta Blockers

1. CVS: Hypertension, Angina pectoris, Cardiac arrhythmias, Myocardial infarction, Congestive cardiac failure, Obstructive cardiomyopathy.
2. Pheochromocytoma.
3. Thyrotoxicosis.
4. Glaucoma.
5. Prophylaxis of migraine.
6. Anxiety.
7. Oseophageal varies.

Mixed Alpha and Beta Antagonist

a. **Labetalol** blocks both $alpha_1$ and beta ($beta_1$ and $beta_2$) receptors. It decrease heart rate, contractility, AV conduction and fall in BP. Vasodilatation ($alpha_1$ and $beta_1$ blockade) and reduced C.O.P. contribute to antihypertensive effect. Blood flow to the limbs increases. Labetalol is used in hypertensive emergencies and in pheochromocytoma.

b. Carvedilol is more cardio protective, inhibits vascular smooth muscle mitogensis, inhibit free radical induced peroxidation.

SKELETAL MUSCLE RELAXANTS (SMR)

Skeletal muscle relaxants (SMR) are drugs that reduce the muscle tone either by acting peripherally at the neuromuscular junction or centrally in the cerebrospinal axis or directly by acting on the contractile mechanism. They reduce the spasticity in a variety of neurological conditions and are also useful in surgeries to obtain relaxation of skeletal muscles.

Classification

1. Drugs acting peripherally at the NMJ

a. *Non-depolarizing agents (Competitive blockers)*
d Tubocurarine, Pancuronium, Alcuronium, Atracurium, Mivacurium*, Rocuronium, Doxacurium, Pipecuronium, Vecuronium, Rapacuronium*, Gallamine* (*short acting).

b. *Depolarizing blockers (Persistent depolarizers)*
Succinylcholine, Decamethonium.

2. **Drugs acting centrally:** Diazepam, Baclofen, Mephenesin derivatives (Carisoprodol, Methocarbamol, Chlorzoxazone), Tizanidine.
3. **Drugs acting directly on the muscle:** Dantrolene.

Peripherally Acting Skeletal Muscle Relaxants

Competitive Neuromuscular Blockers

All these are quaternary ammonium compounds because of which they are not well absorbed orally and are quickly excreted. d tubocurarine (dTc) is the dextrorotatory quaternary ammonium alkaloid.

Mechanism of Action: Non depolarizing blockers bind to nicotinic receptors (Nm) on the motor end plate and block the actions of acetylcholine by competitive blockade action. They do not interfere with the release of ACh. So no depolarization occurs, thus, contraction does not occur by impulse.

Pharmacological Actions

Skeletal muscle: On parenteral administration, tubocurarine initially causes muscular weakness followed by flaccid paralysis. Small muscles of the eyes and fingers are the first to be affected, followed by those of the limbs, neck and trunk. Later the inter costal muscles and finally the diaphragm are paralyzed and respiration stops. Consciousness is not affected throughout. Recovery occurs in the reverse order; the effect lasts for 30-60 minutes.

Autonomic ganglia: In high doses tubocurarine can block autonomic ganglia and adrenal medulla resulting in hypotension.

Histamine release: Tubocurarine can cause histamine release from the mast cells leading to bronchospasm, increased tracheobronchial and gastric secretions. Histamine release also contributes to hypotension. It also reduces venous return and increase HR. Being a quaternary ammonium compound they do not cross BBB.

Pharmacokinetic: They are well absorbed on IM/IV injection, widely distributed, redistribution to non-muscular tissues play an important role in termination of action.

Adverse Reactions

1. Respiratory paralysis and prolonged apnea.
2. Hypotension.
3. Flushing and bronchospasm.

d-Tubocurarine is not used now. The synthetic compounds are preferred.

Synthetic Competitive Blockers

They have the following advantages over d-tubocurarine:

- Less/no histamine releases.
- Do not block autonomic ganglia hence cause less hypotension.
- Spontaneous recovery takes place with most of these drugs.
- Some are more potent than tubocurarine.
- Rapacuronium and rocuronium—have a rapid onset of action.
- Rocuronium does not cause hypotension, tachycardia and is fast acting.
- Atracurium can be safely used in patients with renal impairment because it is degraded by plasma esterase and does not depend on the kidney for elimination.
- No pharmacogenetic variation in metabolism/response.

Reversal of blockade: Neostigmine and pyridostigmine are used which increases ACh availability in synaptic cleft.

Depolarizing Blockers

Succinylcholine (SCh, Suxamethonium) is a quaternary ammonium compound with the structure resembling two molecules of acetylcholine joined together.

Mechanism of Action: SCh reacts with the nicotinic receptors and depolarizes the skeletal muscle membrane. But, unlike ACh, it is destroyed very slowly by pseudo cholinesterase. Thus continued presence of the drug causes persistent depolarization resulting in flaccid paralysis. This is phase I block. In high doses SCh produces a dual block, initial depolarizing block is followed by non-depolarizing block. The membrane gets slowly repolarized but cannot be depolarized again.

Pharmacological Actions

Skeletal muscle: On intravenous administration onset of action is very rapid (within 1 minute). Initial transient muscular fasciculation and twitching, mostly in the chest and abdominal regions are followed by skeletal muscle paralysis. SCh is rapidly hydrolyzed by pseudo cholinesterase and is shortacting muscle relaxant.

CVS: Initially hypotension and bradycardia may result from stimulation of vagus. This is followed by hypertension and tachycardia due to stimulation of sympathetic ganglia. Higher doses can cause cardiac arrhythmias. SCh can also cause histamine release.

Adverse Reactions

Postoperative muscle pain due to the damage to muscle fibers that occurs during initial fasciculation, hyperkalemia, cardiac arrhythmias, malignant hyperthermia, increased intragastric pressure, prolonged apnea, rise in IOT, masseter muscle rigidity are common adverse effects.

Uses of Peripherally Acting Skeletal Muscle Relaxants

1. Adjuvant to anaesthesia.
2. In electroconvulsive therapy to prevent trauma.
3. In spastic disorders.
4. To control ventilation.

Centrally Acting Muscle Relaxants

Centrally acting muscle relaxants depress the spinal polysynaptic reflexes. These reflexes maintain the muscle tone, *e.g.* Diazepam, Baclofen, Mephenesin, Tizanidine, Riluzole, Gabapentin and Progabide.

Tizanidine is a central alpha$_2$ agonist and alter neuronal activity in the spinal cord, in doses which hardly have any effect on blood pressure.

Uses

1. Musculoskeletal disorders.
2. Spastic neurological disorders (to relieve painful spasticity in multiple sclerosis but not of very useful in cerebral palsy).
3. Tetanus.

Directly Acting Muscle Relaxants

Dantrolene directly affects the skeletal muscle contractile mechanism. It inhibits the muscle contraction by preventing the calcium release from the sarcoplasmic reticulum and interferes with excitation contraction coupling.

Dantrolene is used in spastic disorders of upper motor neuron like hemiplegia, paraplegia, spinal injuries, multiple sclerosis and cerebral palsy. Dantrolene is the drug of choice in malignant hyperthermia.

MULTIPLE CHOICE QUESTIONS

Q. 1 All are endogenous catecholamines *except:*

(A) Epinephrine (B) Norepinephrine
(C) Dopamine (D) Doubtamine

Q. 2 Metabolic degradation of catecholamines involves:

(A) COMT (B) MAO
(C) COMT and MAO (D) None of the above

Q. 3 Major pathway of termination of action of the catecholamine is:

(A) Reuptake into nerve terminals
(B) Reuptake into extraneuronal effector cells
(C) Inactivation by MAO enzyme
(D) Hepatic inactivation

Q. 4 The location of the alpha$_1$ adrenoceptor (peripheral) is predominantly:

(A) Pre junctional on nerve ending
(B) Sympathetic adrenergic nerve terminals
(C) Post synaptic neurons
(D) None of the above

Q. 5 Beta$_2$ adrenergic receptors are found in all of the following *except:*

(A) Coronary vessels (B) Uterine smooth muscles
(C) SA node (D) Myocardium

Q. 6 All of the following are molecular mechanisms involved in mediating the response to catecholamines *except:*

(A) Activation of Gs protein receptors
(B) Activation of Gi protein receptors
(C) Inhibition of phospholipase-C
(D) Opening of receptor operated calcium channel

Q. 7 What intracellular effect does a beta agonist produce?

(A) Allows passage of sodium through a ligand gated ion channel
(B) Activates Gs-protein, resulting in stimulation of adenylyl cyclase
(C) Activates Gq-protein, resulting in increase of phosphatidylinositol and calcium
(D) Activate Gi-protein, resulting in inhibition of adenylyl cyclase

1 (D) 2 (C) 3 (A) 4 (B) 5 (C) 6 (C) 7 (B)

Q. 8 Activation of beta$_3$ receptors results in:

(A) Tachycardia
(B) Lipolysis
(C) Bronchodilatation
(D) Uterine relaxation

Q. 9 Activation of muscarinic receptors results in all of the following *except:*

(A) Activation of IP_3-DAG cascade
(B) Inhibition of adenylyl cyclase activity
(C) Increased cellular concentration of cyclic GMP
(D) Opening of potassium channel

Q. 10 Activation of nicotinic receptor results in:

(A) Stimulation of adenylyl cyclase activity
(B) Opening of cation selective ion channels
(C) Increased concentration of diacylglycerol
(D) Increased concentration of cyclic AMP and cyclic GMP

Q. 11 The drug used as a marker for nicotine receptor is:

(A) Latrotoxin (B) Alpha bungarotoxin
(C) Capsaicin (D) Conotoxin

Q. 12 Which of the following is a G-coupled receptor?

(A) Muscarinic cholinergic receptors
(B) Nicotinic cholinergic receptors
(C) Glucocorticoid receptors
(D) Androgen receptors

Q. 13 Botulinum toxin causes paralysis by:

(A) Inhibiting choline acetyl transferase
(B) Blocking transport of choline into neurons
(C) Blocking release of acetyl choline from storage vesicles
(D) Inhibiting acetyl cholinesterase

Q. 14 Which of the following neurotransmitter interacts with guanethidine?

(A) Epinephrine (B) Dopamine
(C) Norepinephrine (D) Serotonin

---

8 (B) 9 (D) 10 (B) 11 (B) 12 (A) 13 (C) 14 (C)

Q. 15 Full activation of the sympathetic nervous system as in maximal exercise, can produce all of the following *except:*

(A) Bronchodilation
(B) Decreased intestinal motility
(C) Increased renal flow
(D) Mydriasis

Q. 16 Epinephrine causes decrease in:

(A) cAMP in heart muscle (B) Glucose in blood
(C) Triglyceride in fat cells (D) Free fatty acids

Q. 17 Which of the following effects of epinephrine would be blocked by phentolamine but not by metoprolol?

(A) Cardiac stimulation
(B) Relaxation of the uterus
(C) Contraction of radial muscles
(D) Relaxation of bronchial smooth muscles

Q. 18 Epinephrine (adrenaline) is not combined with local anaesthetic agent used for finger (phalanges or digital) surgery because:

(A) Epinephrine causes increased blood loss during delicate surgery
(B) Epinephrine causes swelling of the tissue
(C) Epinephrine is contraindicated in emergency surgery
(D) Epinephrine causes vasoconstriction, which can lead to vascular ischemia in digits

Q. 19 Epinephrine acts on which of these receptors to contract arteriolar smooth muscle?

(A) $Alpha_1$ adrenoceptors (B) $Beta_1$ adrenoceptors
(C) $Alpha_2$ adrenoceptors (D) $Beta_2$ adrenoceptors

Q. 20 The beta action of epinephrine includes:

(A) Constriction of bronchioles
(B) Increase in the force of cardiac contraction
(C) Decrease in the force of cardiac contraction
(D) Constriction of arterioles in the skin

15 (C) 16 (C) 17 (C) 18 (D) 19 (A) 20 (B)

Q. 21 Rational of using amphetamine in assumed attention hyperactivity disorder in children is:

(A) It inhibits epinephrine reuptake
(B) It indirectly act on norepinephrine receptors
(C) It blocks effect of norepinephrine
(D) It inhibits serotonin reuptake

Q. 22 All of the following agents are therapeutically used as nasal decongestants *except:*

(A) Ephedrine (B) Fenfluramine
(C) Pseudoephedrine (D) Phenylephrine

Q. 23 Epinephrine is drug of choice in the management of all *except:*

(A) Acute attack of bronchial asthma
(B) Anaphylactic shock
(C) Cardiac arrest (cardiac asystole)
(D) Cardiogenic shock

Q. 24 Which of the following presser agent produces both vasoconstriction and cardiac stimulation?

(A) Phenylephrine (B) Methoxamine
(C) Meteraminol (D) Mephenteramine

Q. 25 Which of the following medication is used to prevent premature labor?

(A) Tamsulosin (B) Cevimeline
(C) Tolterodine (D) Ritodrine

Q. 26 Clonidine is:

(A) $Alpha_1$ selective agonist
(B) $Alpha_2$ selective antagonist
(C) $Alpha_1$ selective antagonist
(D) $Alpha_2$ selective agonist

Q. 27 Mechanism of action of clonidine in opioid withdrawal is:

(A) Beta-blocking effect
(B) Inhibition of opioid receptors
(C) Action of $alpha_2$ pre synaptic nerve ending situated centrally
(D) Postsynaptic action

---

21 (B) 22 (B) 23 (D) 24 (D) 25 (D) 26 (D) 27 (C)

Q. 28 A drug that act at pre junctional alpha$_2$ adrenoceptors and is used to treat hypertension is:

(A) Clonidine (B) Methoxamine
(C) Metaproterenol (D) Dobutamine

Q. 29 The direct cardiac effects of dobutamine would be blocked by which one of the following agent?

(A) Prazosin (B) Metoprolol
(C) Clonidine (D) Isoproterenol

Q. 30 Which of the following is true regarding dobutamine?

(A) It acts on dopamine receptors
(B) It activates alpha receptors
(C) It activates cyclic AMP (cAMP)-related pathways
(D) It produces bradycardia

Q. 31 All of the following may be associated with beta$_2$ agonist treatment *except:*

(A) Hyperkalemia
(B) Hyperglycemia
(C) Detrusor relaxation
(D) Relaxation of gut and bronchial muscles

Q. 32 All of the following are non-selective beta blockers with additional alpha action *except:*

(A) Carvedilol (B) Betaxolol
(C) Carteolol (D) Labetalol

Q. 33 Which statement is true about sotalol?

(A) It is a selective beta blocker
(B) It prolongs action potential duration throughout the heart
(C) It is excreted through bile
(D) Bradycardia is a common side effect

Q. 34 All of the following are selective beta$_1$(β_1) blockers *except:*

(A) Atenolol (B) Esmolol
(C) Bisprolol (D) Celeprolol

28 (A) 29 (B) 30 (C) 31 (A) 32 (B) 33 (B) 34 (D)

Q. 35 Beta blocker which cannot be used in renal failure:

(A) Propranolol (B) Pindolol
(C) Sotalol (D) Metoprolol

Q. 36 Beta blocker with peripheral vasodilator action is:

(A) Carvedilol (B) Propranolol
(C) Atenolol (D) Acebutolol

Q. 37 Anti-adrenergic drug which does not cross blood brain barrier (BBB) is:

(A) Propranolol
(B) Atenolol
(C) Alprenolol
(D) Oxprenolol

Q. 38 Propranolol is used in all of the following *except:*

(A) Thyrotoxicosis
(B) Variant angina
(C) Migraine
(D) Hypertension

Q. 39 Timolol can be used in all *except:*

(A) Myocardial infarction
(B) Hypertension
(C) Bronchial asthma
(D) Migraine

Q. 40 Which of the following drug is not used topically for the treatment of open angle glaucoma?

(A) Latanoprost
(B) Brinzolamide
(C) Acetazolamide
(D) Dorzolamide

Q. 41 Pretreatment with propranolol will block which one of the following?

(A) Methacholine induced tachycardia
(B) Nicotine induced hypertension
(C) Norepinepherine induced bradycardia
(D) Phenylephrine induced mydriasis

35 (C) 36 (A) 37 (B) 38 (B) 39 (C) 40 (C) 41 (A)

Q. 42 Topical application of timolol causes:

(A) Miosis
(B) Mydriasis
(C) Increased formation of aqueous humor
(D) Decreased formation of aqueous humor

Q. 43 Beta blockers alone are not indicated in the treatment of hypertension due to:

(A) Renal disease
(B) Pheochromocytoma
(C) Thyrotoxicosis
(D) Atherosclerosis

Q. 44 Adrenergic beta receptor stimulation mediated metabolic response includes all *except:*

(A) Gluconeogenesis
(B) Hypokalemia
(C) Lipolysis
(D) Decreased insulin secretion

Q. 45 Beta-receptor blocking agent which have an effect on plasma renin activity is:

(A) Atenolol
(B) Pindolol
(C) Nodalol
(D) Propranolol

Q. 46 The mechanism of action of propranolol in hyperthyroidism involves:

(A) Blockade of release of thyroxine from the thyroid gland
(B) Beta receptor blockade
(C) Beta receptor blockade and inhibition of conversion of T_4 to T_3
(D) Beta receptor blockade and inhibition of release of thyroxine from the gland

Q. 47 Which of the following drug abolishes the antihypertensive action of propranolol?

(A) Cimetidine
(B) Indomethacin
(C) Chlorpromazine
(D) Imipramine

Q. 48 Adrenergic $beta_1$ selective blockers offers the following advantages *except:*

(A) Lower propensity to cause bronchospasm
(B) Less prove to produce cold hands and feet as side effect
(C) Withdrawal is less likely to exacerbate angina pectoris
(D) Less liable to impair exercise capacity

42 (D) 43 (B) 44 (D) 45 (D) 46 (C) 47 (B) 48 (C)

Q. 49 In a patient of myocardial infarction, beta adrenergic blockers are used with the following objects:

(A) To reduce the incidence of reinfarction
(B) To prevent cardiac arrhythmias
(C) Myocardial salvage
(D) All of the above

Q. 50 Beta adrenergic antagonist are useful antihypertensive agent in all *except:*

(A) Young patients with high renin levels
(B) Patients with associated conditions like migraine
(C) Patients receiving vasodilators to counteract tachycardia
(D) Patients on oral hypoglycemic agents

Q. 51 In contrast to propranolol, metoprolol:

(A) Is used for the management of hypertension
(B) Has greater selectivity for $beta_2$ adrenoceptors
(C) May be beneficial for the acute attack of migraine headache
(D) Is less likely to precipitate bronchoconstriction in patients with asthma

Q. 52 Timolol is preferred for local use in the eye because of all of the following *except:*

(A) It has no partial agonistic activity
(B) It has no local anaesthetic activity
(C) It is a selective blocking agent
(D) It has longer duration of action

Q. 53 All are true about beta blockers *except:*

(A) Atenolol is longer acting than metoprolol
(B) Labetalol has both alpha and beta blocking action
(C) Carvedilol has alpha agonistic and selective beta blocking action
(D) Nadalol has longest half life

Q. 54 Which is a selective $alpha_{1A}$ blocker?

(A) Prazosin (B) Terazosin
(C) Tamsulosin (D) Indoramine

49 (D) 50 (D) 51 (D) 52 (C) 53 (C) 54 (C)

Q. 55 All are true regarding prazosin *except:*

(A) It is an $alpha_2$ presynaptic blocker
(B) It is effective orally
(C) It is metabolized in liver
(D) First dose effect may occur

Q. 56 Postural hypotension is common side effect of:

(A) Prazosin (B) Nifedipine
(C) Atenolol (D) ACE inhibitors

Q. 57 The common side effect of terazosin is:

(A) Bronchospasm (B) Postural hypotension
(C) Sedation (D) Heart failure

Q. 58 The tachycardia induced by non-selective alpha-receptor blocking agent is due to:

(A) Direct stimulation of beta-receptors in the heart
(B) Release of adrenaline from adrenal medulla
(C) Reflex in nature due to postural hypotension
(D) Postural hypotension and blockade of presynaptic $alpha_2$ receptors

Q. 59 The drug which have $alpha_1$ receptor antagonist with a weak $alpha_2$ agonist and weak $beta_1$ antagonistic action is:

(A) Indoramine (B) Urapidil
(C) Labetalol (D) Terazosin

Q. 60 The drug occasionally used to treat drug induced sexual dysfunction is:

(A) Phentolamine (B) Phenylephrine
(C) Yohimbine (D) Papaverine

Q. 61 The drug which produce vasoconstriction despite being an alpha adrenergic blocker is:

(A) Phenoxybenzamine
(B) Ergotamine
(C) Dihydroergotoxine
(D) Tolazoline

55 (A) 56 (A) 57 (B) 58 (D) 59 (B) 60 (C) 61 (B)

Q. 62 Which of the following is true of sildenafil?

(A) It enhances sexual enjoyment in normal men
(B) It delays ejaculation
(C) It is indicated only for the treatment of erectile dysfunction
(D) It blocks cavernosal $alpha_2$ adrenoceptors

Q. 63 Labetalol has:

(A) More potent beta-adrenergic blocking than alpha blocking activity
(B) More potent alpha adrenergic blocking than beta blocking activity
(C) Equal alpha and beta blocking activity
(D) $Beta_1$ agonistic activity in addition to alpha and beta adrenergic blockade

Q. 64 In the comparison of bethanechol and pilocarpine which one of the following is correct?

(A) Both are hydrolyzed by acetyl cholinesterase
(B) Both inhibit nicotinic receptors
(C) Both may increase gastric motility
(D) Both may decrease sweating

Q. 65 An indirect acting cholinomimetic that crosses blood brain barrier (BBB) is:

(A) Muscarine (B) Neostigmine
(C) Physostigmine (D) Nicotine

Q. 66 Receptor actions of acetylcholine are mimicked by nicotine at which one of the following sites?

(A) Adrenal medullary chromaffin cells
(B) Urinary bladder smooth muscle
(C) Circular muscles of iris
(D) S.A. node

Q. 67 Muscarinic cholinoceptor agonists cause vasodilation through release of:

(A) Histamine (B) Acetylcholine
(C) Nitric oxide (D) Norepinephrine

62 (C) 63 (A) 64 (C) 65 (C) 66 (A) 67 (C)

Q. 68 Organ which received only parasympathetic innervations is:

(A) Ciliary muscles of the eye
(B) Ventricles
(C) Iris
(D) Gastrointestinal smooth muscles

Q. 69 Cholinomimetic drug preferred for the treatment of Alzheimer's disease is:

(A) Donepezil (B) Physostigmine
(C) Pyridostigmine (D) Demacarium

Q. 70 Oxybutynin works by:

(A) Inhibiting acetyl cholinesterase at muscarinic and nicotinic receptors
(B) Causing a neuromuscular blockade
(C) Antagonizing $alpha_1$ receptors
(D) Binding to muscarinic receptors on detrusor muscles

Q. 71 Which of the following drug is used to diagnose myasthenia gravis?

(A) Neostigmine (B) Bethanechol
(C) Edrophonium (D) Atropine

Q. 72 Neostigmine antagonizes non-depolarizing blockade by all of the following mechanism *except:*

(A) Decreasing the breakdown of ACh at the motor end plate
(B) Presenting K^+ efflux from the cell
(C) Increasing the release of ACh at the motor end plate
(D) Depolarization of the motor end plate

Q. 73 Pralidoxime (PAM-2) is not useful in the treatment of:

(A) Malathion (B) Parathion
(C) Paraoxon (D) Propoxur

Q. 74 Which neurotransmitter is released due to rise in blood pressure in the SA node?

(A) Acetylcholine
(B) Dopamine
(C) Norepinephrine (Noradrenaline)
(D) Epinephrine (Adrenaline)

68 (A) 69 (A) 70 (D) 71 (C) 72 (B) 73 (D) 74 (A)

Q. 75 The drug used to distinguish between myasthenic crisis (insufficient therapy) and cholinergic crisis (excessive therapy) is:

(A) Atropine (B) Edrophonium
(C) Physostigmine (D) Pyridostigmine

Q. 76 The true statement about parathion is:

(A) It is inactivated by conversion to paroxon
(B) It is less toxic than malathion
(C) It is poorly absorbed through skin and lungs
(D) Its toxicity may be reversed by pralidoxime, if treated early

Q. 77 The cause of death in organo phosphorus compound (OPC) poisoning is:

(A) Cardiac arrhythmia (B) Gastrointestinal bleeding
(C) Respiratory failure (D) Heart failure

Q. 78 Which one of the following is a direct acting cholinomimetic used for its mood elevating action and as an insecticide?

(A) Physostigmine (B) Nicotine
(C) Bethanechol (D) Neostigmine

Q. 79 The drug of choice for supraventricular tachycardia is:

(A) Neostigmine (B) Carbachol
(C) Adenosine (D) Edrophonium

Q. 80 The drug used to lower intra ocular pressure (IOP) after laser surgery is:

(A) Brimonidine (B) Apraclonidine
(C) Phenylephrine (D) Dipivefrin

Q. 81 The organophosphorus compounds produce irreversible inhibition of cholinesterase because:

(A) They bind to an allosteric site of the enzyme resulting in unfavorable confirmation of esteratic site to bind ACh
(B) Regeneration time of the phosphorylated enzyme is longer than the turnover time of the enzyme molecules
(C) Phosphorylation results in rapid degradation of enzyme molecule
(D) They are neither metabolized nor excreted from the body

75 (B) 76 (D) 77 (C) 78 (B) 79 (C) 80 (A) 81 (B)

Q. 82 Neostigmine would be expected to reverse which one of the following conditions?

(A) Paralysis of skeletal muscle induced by a competitive, non-depolarizing muscle relaxant
(B) Paralysis of skeletal muscle induced by a depolarizing muscle relaxant
(C) Cardiac slowing induced by stimulation of the vagus nerve
(D) Miosis induced by the bright light

Q. 83 Echothiophate is the preferred irreversible cholinesterase inhibitor for clinical use because:

(A) It acts very rapidly
(B) It has long duration of action
(C) It is the least toxic of all organophosphates
(D) It is highly lipid soluble and hence penetrate tissues better

Q. 84 Pralidoxime acts by:

(A) Reactivating cholinesterase enzyme
(B) Promoting synthesis of cholinesterase
(C) Promoting synthesis of acetylcholine
(D) Direct action on cholinergic receptors

Q. 85 The most common cause of death in belladonna poisoning in infants is:

(A) Dehydration (B) Hyperthermia
(C) Hypertension (D) Intraventricular heart block

Q. 86 Which of the following cause less or no cycloplegia?

(A) Atropine (B) Cyclopentolate
(C) Homatropine (D) Scopolamine

Q. 87 Anti muscarinic drugs can be used in all *except:*

(A) Hypertension (B) Motion sickness
(C) Parkinson's disease (D) Peptic ulcer

Q. 88 Which drug is preferred to be used as an adjuvant with levodopa in Parkinson's disease?

(A) Benztropine (B) Reserpine
(C) Timolol (D) Doxazocin

---

82 (A) 83 (B) 84 (A) 85 (B) 86 (B) 87 (A) 88 (A)

Q. 89 Which drug is preferred as an bronchodilator in patients with chronic obstructive pulmonary disease (COPD)?

(A) Albuterol (salbutamol) (B) Ipratropium bromide
(C) Pseudoephedrine (D) Theophylline

Q. 90 Agent which causes both cycloplegia and mydriasis on topical application in eye is:

(A) Atropine (B) Phenylephrine
(C) Prazosin (D) Carbachol

Q. 91 Atropine can be useful in combination with all *except:*

(A) Diphenoxylate in diarrhea
(B) Morphine in biliary colic
(C) Neostigmine in myasthenia gravis
(D) d-tubocurarine for skeletal muscle relaxants

Q. 92 Atropine does not antagonize the following features of anti-cholinesterase poisoning:

(A) Hypotension (B) Central excitation
(C) Muscle paralysis (D) Bronchoconstriction

Q. 93 Which of the following anticholinergic is preferred in pre-anaesthetic medication?

(A) Glycopyrrolate (B) Isopropamide
(C) Dicyclomine (D) Pirenzolate methylbromide

Q. 94 All anticholinergic agents produce central effects *except:*

(A) Atropine (B) Scopolamine
(C) Benztropine (D) Glycopyrrolate

Q. 95 Transient bradycardia caused by small doses of atropine is due to:

(A) Stimulation of vagal center
(B) Release of acetylcholine from nerve endings
(C) Blockade of M_1 receptors on post ganglionic parasympathetic neurons
(D) Inhibition of the enzyme cholinesterase

89 (B) 90 (A) 91 (D) 92 (C) 93 (A) 94 (D) 95 (C)

Q. 96 Atropine overdose may cause:

(A) Increased cardiac rate (B) Increased gastric secretion
(C) Papillary constriction (D) Urinary frequency

Q. 97 Skeletal muscle relaxant (SMR) with fastest onset of action is:

(A) Atracurium (B) Rocuronium
(C) Mivacurium (D) Pancuronium

Q. 98 All of the following skeletal muscle relaxants (SMRs) causes hypotension *except:*

(A) Tubocurarine (B) Atracurium
(C) Mivacurium (D) Rocuronium

Q. 99 Malignant hyperthermia following the use of inhalational anaesthetic agent and succinylcholine is due to defect in the:

(A) Nicotinic receptors
(B) Muscarinic receptors
(C) Due to release of transmitters from nerve ending
(D) Calcium channels

Q. 100 The drug which reduce muscle strength by interfering with the release of calcium from the sarcoplasmic reticulum is:

(A) Progabide (B) Dantrolene
(C) Baclofen (D) Glycine

Q. 101 All statements are true about succinylcholine *except:*

(A) It causes fasciculation
(B) It is hydrolyzed by both true and pseudo cholinesterase enzyme
(C) It is quaternary compound
(D) It has very brief duration of action

Q. 102 All is true about non-depolarizing skeletal muscle relaxants *except:*

(A) They are quaternary compounds
(B) They have small apparent volume of distribution
(C) Drugs excreted by kidney have shorter duration of action
(D) Drugs inactivated by plasma cholinesterase (pseudo ChE) have a shorter duration of action

---

96 (A) 97 (B) 98 (D) 99 (D) 100 (B) 101 (B) 102 (C)

Q. 103 Prolonged apnea may occur following administration of succinylcholine in a patient with hereditary deficiency of which of the enzyme?

(A) Glucose-6-phosphate dehydrogenase
(B) Plasma cholinesterase
(C) Cytochrome $P\text{-}450_{3A}$
(D) Acetyl cholinesterase

Q. 104 Dantrolene is the drug of choice to treat malignant hyperthermia caused by succinylcholine because it:

(A) Blocks Ca^{+2} release from sarcoplasmic reticulum
(B) Increases the rate of succinylcholine metabolism
(C) Inhibits succinylcholine binding to nicotinic receptors
(D) Acts centrally to reduce fever

Q. 105 Which of the following drug is used to reverse the effect of non-depolarizing skeletal muscle relaxants?

(A) Atropine (B) Neostigmine
(C) Physostigmine (D) Echothiophate

Q. 106 The short acting ganglionic blocking agent is:

(A) Atropine (B) Hexamethonium
(C) Trimetaphen (D) Nicotine

103 (B) 104 (A) 105 (B) 106 (C)

ANSWERS

Ans. 1 (D) Epinephrine, norepinephrine and dopamine are endogenous catecholamine while isoprenaline, dipivefrine, dobutamine, dopexamine, fenoldopam are synthetic one.

Ans. 2 (C) Metabolism is not the main mechanism for the termination of action for NE and E. The action terminated by (a) active reuptake into nerve terminal and then reuptake by storage vesicles (vesicular reuptake) (b) uptake into post synaptic non neuronal cell membrane and (c) metabolic degradation by mono amine oxidase (MAO) located intra neuronaly (intracellularly) and by catecholamine–o–methyl transferase (COMT) located intracellulary.

Ans. 3 (A) The major pathway of termination of action is reuptake into nerve terminals (also see Ans. 2).

Ans. 4 (B) Both alpha$_2$ and beta$_2$ receptors are located at post synaptic sites such as on many types of neurons in the brain. In contrast, alpha$_1$ and beta$_1$ receptors appear to be located mainly in the immediate vicinity of sympathetic adrenergic nerve terminals in peripheral target organs, strategically placed to be activated during stimulation of these nerves.

Ans. 5 (C) Beta$_2$ receptors are present predominantly on bronchi, coronary arteries, uterine smooth muscles and myocardium (though β_1 receptors are predominant) but beta$_1$ (solely) receptors are present at SA node and AV node. The innervations to skeletal muscle blood vessel is sympathetic in origin but cholinergic in character (but post synaptic receptors on smooth muscle is predominantly beta$_2$ in nature).

Ans. 6 (C) The excitatory response of alpha$_1$ receptor activation is mediated through IP$_3$ (Gq) and inhibitory is through increase in ionic permeability of K^+ ions. Alpha$_2$ receptor agonist act activating Gi receptors and decreases cAMP level. Phospholipase activity is involved with cholinergic drugs.

Ans. 7 (B) Beta agonist activates Gs-protein, resulting in stimulation of adenylyl cyclase, with increase in intracellular cAMP. Activation of Gq protein refers to the mechanism of action of muscarinic receptors.

Ans. 8 **(B)** Adrenergic drugs act through two types of receptors, *e.g.* alpha and beta receptors. Beta receptors are further divided into three subtypes, *e.g.* $beta_1$, $beta_2$ and $beta_3$. $Beta_1$ receptors are found mainly in heart and produce positive chronotropic and inotropic effects. $Beta_2$ receptors are mainly present in smooth muscles (bronchi, coronary arteries, uterus and gut) and cause muscle relaxation. $Beta_3$ receptors are present on adipocytes, activations of which promote lipolysis.

Ans. 9 **(D)** All muscarinic receptors belong to the family of G-protein coupled receptor. M_1, M_3 and M_5 act through inositol phosphate pathway and activate enzyme phospholipase-C IP_3 and DAG cascade. This triggers release of Ca^{2+} from storage vesicles. M_2 and M_4 receptor activation inhibits adenylate cyclase and thus reduce the intracellular cAMP. They do not have any action through potassium channels.

Ans. 10 **(B)** Both nicotinic receptors (Nm and Nn) subtype are the members of the 'ligand gated ion channel' family. These channels are normally closed but opens upon the binding of ACh or any cholinergic agonist. As the channel opens, Na^+ ions are permitted to flow down through their concentration gradient to cause depolarization.

Ans. 11 **(B)** The selective agonist at Nn receptor is DMPP (dimethyl-phenyl piperazinium) and epibatidine and antagonist are hexamethonium and trimethaphan. PTMA is the selective agonist at Nn receptor (phenyl trimethyl ammonium) and antagonists are bungarotoxin and dTC.

Ans. 12 **(A)** Muscarinic cholinergic receptors are both Gi (inhibitory-M_2 subtype) and Gq (M_1 subtype), coupled receptors while nicotinic receptors are ion channel receptors. Glucocorticoids and androgen both are cytosolic receptors.

Ans. 13 **(C)** Botulinum toxin blocks calcium-dependent exocytosis of acetylcholine from storage vesicles, producing paralysis. The condition is life threatening. Choline acetyltransferase is an enzyme catalyzing synthesis of acetylcholine.

Ans. 14 **(C)** Guanethidine blocks the release of norepinephrine from storage vesicles into the nerve terminals. Acetylcholine release can be blocked by botulinum toxin.

Ans. 15 (C) Sympathetic discharge causes constriction of the resistance vessels of the renal tissue and a fall in renal blood flow.

Ans. 16 (C) Epinephrine causes increase in free fatty acids by activating lipolysis of triglyceride in fat cells (through beta$_3$ receptors and thus decreases its level) and increase in blood glucose by glycogenolysis and increase in release of insulin (beta and alpha action).

Ans. 17 (C) Contraction of radial muscle of the eye is mediated through alpha receptors. All the other effects are mediated through beta receptors, so they are not blocked by phentolamine which is an alpha blocker.

Ans. 18 (D) Local anaesthetic with epinephrine as an adjuvant are contraindicated for surgeries of most facial structures, digits and the penis due to its vasoconstrictor effect, as these structure are supplied with end arteries.

Ans. 19 (A) Vascular smooth muscle tone is governed by the presence of alpha$_1$ and beta$_2$ receptors. Alpha$_1$ receptors (present predominantly in the skin, mucosal, splanchnic and renal blood vessles) stimulation increases arterial resistance and vasoconstriction. While beta$_2$ receptors promote smooth muscle relaxation.

Ans. 20 (B) Epinephrine (adrenaline) causes increase in the heart rate, force of contraction and conduction through beta$_1$ receptors while causes bronchodilation (not constriction) through beta$_2$ receptors present in bronchioles. Constriction of arterioles is mediated through alpha receptors (as mentioned in Ans. 19).

Ans. 21 (B) Amphetamine and other similar compounds act centrally to increase attention by acting on norepinephrine receptors.

Ans. 22 (B) Nasal decongestants, *e.g.* ephedrine, pseudo ephedrine, oxymetazoline, xylometazoline etc are non-catecholamine (synthetic) alpha$_1$ agonist. They have longer duration of action and used in rhinorrhoea. Fenfluramine is an anorectic agent.

Ans. 23 (D) Epinephrine is preferred drug in anaphylactic shock, cardiac arrest, and as vasoconstrictor for nasal oozing, with local anaesthetic agent. In acute attack of bronchial asthma (when given S.C.) it cause bronchodilation, though not used commonly now. For cardiogenic shock vasopressor, *e.g.* dopamine, dobutamine etc are preferred.

Ans. 24 (D) Mephentermine produces both cardiac stimulation and vasoconstriction by directly activating alpha and beta adrenergic receptors and by releasing NE. It increases cardiac output and systolic and diastolic BP. The direct positive chronotropic effect on heart is generally counter balanced by vagal stimulation due to rise in mean BP.

Ans. 25 (D) Ritodrine, a $beta_2$ agonist is used to suppress premature labor because of its ability to stop uterine contractions. Tamsulosin, a $alpha_1$ blocker is used for benign prostatic hypertrophy. Tolterodine, a muscarinic blocker is used for urinary incontinence.

Ans. 26 (D) Clonidine is a centrally acting $alpha_2$ agonist and reduces sympathetic activity, resulting in fall in BP and heart rate. It also activates the pre synaptic $alpha_2$ receptor present on sympathetic post ganglionic neurons and thus further suppress release of norepinephrine from peripheral nerve ending.

Ans. 27 (C) As mentioned above, by decreasing release of norepinephrine, it decreases sympathetic over activity and improve the symptoms in patients with opioid withdrawal.

Ans. 28 (A) Clonidine act at pre junctional $alpha_2$ adrenoceptors and is used to treat hypertension while methoxamine is non-selective alpha agonist. Metaproterenol is a selective $beta_2$ agonist and dobutamine is a relatively selective $beta_1$ agonist.

Ans. 29 (B) The activity of dobutamine is blocked by metoprolol, which is a selective $beta_1$ adrenergic receptor antagonist.

Ans. 30 (C) Dobutamine increases cAMP-mediated phosphorylation and the activity of calcium channels. It does not act on dopamine receptors; it act only on $beta_1$ receptors and produce mild tachycardia.

Ans. 31 (A) Stimulation of $beta_2$ receptors causes relaxation of smooth muscles. In liver $beta_2$ stimulation catalyses phosphorylase enzyme and thus promotes glycogenolysis and gluconeogenesis. The release of glucose is accompanied by an efflux of K^+, so there is hyperglycemia with brief hyperkalemia but later the K^+ released from liver is taken up by skeletal muscles and thus hyperkalemia is followed by hypokalemia.

Ans. 32 (B) Betaxolol is not a non selective, but is a cardio selective with no additional alpha blocking action. The drug is used in patient of glaucoma with diabetes, bronchial asthma or hypertension. It has cytoprotective action on retinal neurons, though less effective than timolol (as $beta_2$ are predominant on ciliary body) but better tolerated.

Ans. 33 (B) Sotalol is a water soluble beta blocker and is excreted in urine. It is a non selective beta blocker. It has an additional K^+ channel blocking and class III anti arrhythmic property independent of beta blocking activity.

Ans. 34 (D) Celiprolol and acebutolol are selective $beta_1$ antagonist with intrinsic sympathomimetic action. Celiprolol is partial $beta_2$ agonist. It also causes direct vasodilatation by releasing nitric oxide. So it is preferred in hypertensive patients having asthma. Acebutolol on other hand, is well absorbed but metabolized during first pass and converted into an active metabolite, *e.g.* diacetolol which has longer half life.

Ans. 35 (C) Sotalol is used in both ventricular tachyarrhythmias and atrial fibrillation or flutter. It prolongs APD of the heart. Incidence of torsade de pointes observed, usually with overdose. But occasionally, observed at low dosages, in patients with renal dysfunction because sotalol is eliminated by renal excretion in unchanged form. Propranolol, metoprolol, pindolol are extensively metabolized by hepatic enzymes. Other drugs which are excreted unchanged or minimally metabolized are atenolol and nidolol.

Ans. 36 (A) Carvedilol has unique pharmacological profile. It blocks $beta_1$, $beta_2$ and $alpha_1$ receptors. It causes vasodilatation. It also has anti oxidant and anti inflammatory effects. So have cardio protective effects.

Ans. 37 (B) Atenolol is water soluble selective $beta_1$ blocker, so does not cross BBB.

Ans. 38 (B) Propranolol and other beta blockers are rather contraindicated in variant angina. Because of beta blocking action, unopposed alpha receptor action is there which causes vasoconstriction and worsen the condition.

Ans. 39 (C) Timolol is a potent non selective beta receptor antagonist. It has no intrinsic sympathomimetic or membrane stabilizing activity, so it is used in CCF, HT, acute MI, migraine and glaucoma. But it should be avoided in bronchial asthma (also in CCF in susceptive patients).

Ans. 40 (C) Latanoprost is a prostaglandin analogue. It do not affect pupil size or accommodation. Brinzolamide and dorzolamide are topical carbonic anhydrase inhibitor. Acetazolamide is orally effective carbonic anhydrase inhibitor.

Ans. 41 (A) Propranolol (beta blocker) will not block the mydriasis by phenylephrine (as action is mediated through alpha receptors), vagal slowing induced by norepinephrine, nicotine induced hypertension, norepinephrine induced bradycardia. But it will block tachycardia by methacholine.

Ans. 42 (D) Timolol, a beta adrenergic blocker, reduces formation of aqueous humor and preferred drug in open angle glaucoma.

Ans. 43 (B) Pheochromocytoma is an adrenal tumor, secreting both epinephrine, norepinephrine in excess, so both beta blocker and alpha blocker in combination is used during removal of tumor.

Ans. 44 (D) Metabolic response of stimulation of beta receptors includes hyperglycemia due to glycogenolysis in liver ($beta_2$) and skeletal muscles ($alpha_1$ and $beta_2$), increase in free fatty acids due to lipolysis in adipose tissue (alpha and $beta_3$), inhibition of insulin release ($alpha_2$). So decrease insulin secretions is alpha receptor mediated not beta receptor mediated action.

Ans. 45 (D) Propranolol, a non selective beta blocker possess anti-hypertensive effect due to its effect on $beta_1$ receptor, and by decreasing plasma renin activity. It also decreases central sympathetic outflow.

Ans. 46 (C) Propranolol being a non selective blocker reduce unpleasant symptoms of sympathetic over activity, *e.g.* tachycardia irregular cardiac rhythm, tremors, sweating and raised BMR. It also inhibits the peripheral conversion of thyroxine to T3 (independent of beta receptor blockade action).

Ans. 47 (B) Indomethacin and others NSAIDs decreases or opposes the antihypertensive action of beta blockers.

Ans. 48 (C) Cardio selective beta blockers, *e.g.* metoprolol, atenolol, acebutolol, bisprolol, nebivolol possess all these features, but the selectivity is lost in higher doses. But partial agonist like pindolol activates beta$_1$ and beta$_2$ receptors submaximally. So withdrawal is less likely to exacerbate hypertension or angina in these agents, not with cardio selective drugs.

Ans. 49 (D) In MI, beta blockers are used as they decrease the mortality by preventing reinfarction, sudden ventricular fibrillation at the second attack of MI and limit infarction size by reducing O_2 consumption (myocardial salvage).

Ans. 50 (D) Beta-adrenergic antagonist, particularly propranolol, decreases plasma renin activity, tremors, heart rate and cardiac output. They should not be used in patients with diabetes, taking oral hypoglycemic drugs, as they decrease the hypoglycemic control. They inhibit glycogenolysis and delay recovery from hypoglycemia. They also mask the warning symptoms of hypoglycemia. Metoprolol, may be used in these patients.

Ans. 51 (D) Metoprolol is more selective at beta$_1$ adrenergic receptors, which are more abundant in heart than in lungs. So, it is less likely to produce bronchoconstriction.

Ans. 52 (C) Timolol is a non-selective beta blocker reduces intraocular pressure and is preferred because it has no local anaesthetic or intrinsic sympathomimetic activity and has longer duration of action.

Ans. 53 (C) Carvedilol does not have alpha agonistic action. It has combined beta blocker with alpha$_1$ beta$_1$ and beta$_2$ blocking action. It has more potent effect on beta rather than alpha receptors. The drug also has antioxidant property. All other statements are true.

Ans. 54 (C) Tamsulosin is selective alpha$_{1A}$ blockers while prazosin, indoramin and terazosin are non selective alpha$_1$ blockers. Being an alpha$_{1A}$ selective blocker, tamsulosin and silodosin (long acting analogue of tamsulosin) are used in benign prostatic hypertrophy.

Ans. 55 (A) Prazosin is a selective alpha$_1$ receptor antagonist. It causes marked postural hypotension at initial dose (first dose phenomenon). Yohimbine is a pre synaptic alpha$_2$ receptor antagonist.

Ans. 56 (A) Prazosin causes postural hypotension due to its first dose phenomenon.

Ans. 57 (B) Alpha$_1$ receptor antagonist, *e.g.* terazosin cause significant postural hypotension and should be prescribed carefully in elderly patients.

Ans. 58 (D) Blockade of alpha$_1$ receptors in the periphery causes vasodilatation and hypotension. Thus reflexly stimulate baro-receptors and cause sympathetic discharge. This in turn stimulates beta$_1$ receptors on the heart as alpha$_1$ receptors are blocked and produce tachycardia. Non-selective alpha blockade also block pre synaptic alpha$_2$ receptors which promote neuronal release of NE to produce more tachycardia and palpitation.

Ans. 59 (B) Urapidil has multiple effects and has alpha$_2$ agonist, beta$_1$ antagonist and 5 HT agonist action beside alpha$_1$ antagonist effect.

Ans. 60 (C) Yohimbine may be used to treat male sexual dysfunction and to treat diabetic neuropathy, though its mechanism and use is not established.

Ans. 61 (B) Ergotamine and ergotoxin are partial agonist and antagonist at alpha adrenergic serotonergic and dopaminergic receptors. It produces long lasting vasoconstriction which predominates on its alpha blocking actions.

Ans. 62 (C) Sildenafil acts by selectively inhibiting phosphodiesterase-5 (PDE-5) and enhancing nitric oxide (NO) action in corpus cavernosum. It does not cause priapism, but improve penile tumescene during sexual activity.

Ans. 63 (A) Labetalol is 5 times more potent in blocking beta than alpha receptors. Effect of labetalol resembles those of propranolol when used in low dose while at high dose they are like a combination of propranolol and prazosin.

Ans. 64 (C) Both increases gut motility.

Ans. 65 (C) Physostigmine is lipid soluble, naturally occurring anti ChE, thus enters in the CNS readily.

Ans. 66 (A) Nicotinic cholinergic receptors are present in adrenal medulla, while in all other, muscarinic cholinergic receptors are present.

Ans. 67 (C) The vascular endothelium releases nitric oxide by muscarinic cholinergic agonist. Nitric oxide activates guanylate cyclase and increases cGMP and sequestering calcium. This leads to relaxation of vascular smooth muscles.

Ans. 68 (A) Ciliary muscles of the eye have only parasympathetic innervations, while ventricles are having sympathomimetic innervations. Iris and smooth muscles of the GIT having both sympathetic and parasympathetic innervations.

Ans. 69 (A) Tacrine, a long acting reversible anti-cholinesterase, were used for palliative treatment of AD, but its use declines as it causes significant, though reversible hepatotoxicity. Donepezil, rivastigmine, galantamine are the newer reversible anti ChE having better penetration into CNS, less toxic and better tolerated, in AD but clinical results are modest and temporary.

Ans. 70 (D) Oxybutynin acts by binding to muscarinic receptors located on the detrusor muscle of the bladder, suppressing involuntary contraction of the muscle.

Ans. 71 (C) Edrophonium which will increase muscle strength in untreated patient, is preferred as it has a short duration of action.

Ans. 72 (B) Neostigmine is a quaternary ammonium drug having partial cholinergic agonist action in addition to inhibition of anti-cholinesterase enzyme. It stimulates nicotinic receptors and can depolarize the muscle end plate.

Ans. 73 (D) Pralidoxime is cholinesterase enzyme re-activator used in the treatment of organophosphorus compound (OPC) poisoning. It attaches with the anionic site of enzyme which is free in all OPC except in carbamates. Propoxur is a carbamate, attaches themselves with anionic as well as esteritic site of AChE. So anionic site is not free, thus pralidoxime is not helpful, rather may worsen the situation.

Ans. 74 (A) S.A. node is innervated by parasympathetic nerve endings, when BP increases, the vasomotor centre tries to return it to normal by slowing the heart rate and by releasing acetylcholine.

Ans. 75 (B) Edrophonium is short acting anti ChE. When it is given in the patients with cholinergic crisis it worsen the condition, but it is not dangerous as its action terminated early because of its short $t_{½}$, while it improve the symptoms of myasthenia crisis.

Ans. 76 (D) The organophosphorus compounds are rather activated by conversion to paroxon. Parathion is more toxic and highly lipid soluble, so absorbed well. Its toxicity is treated by pralidoxime, if given before 'aging'.

Ans. 77 (C) Respiratory failure due to neuromuscular paralysis is the important cause of death with OPC poisoning.

Ans. 78 (B) Nicotine is directly acting cholinomimetic alkaloid with mood elevation property.

Ans. 79 (C) Adenosine is used for SVT not cholinergic drugs.

Ans. 80 (A) Brimonidine is a selective $alpha_2$ adrenergic agonist. It is lipophilic and penetrates cornea easily. Apraclonidine, a selective $beta_2$ agonist also decreases formation of aqueous humor and may enhance uveoscleral outflow. Ocular and skin allergies are common with both these drugs but brimonidine is less likely to cause ocular allergy and is more commonly used. Other two drugs, *e.g.* phenylephrine and dipivefrin are more likely to cause toxicities and hyperemia.

Ans. 81 (B) OPC bind with the esteratic site of the cholinesterase enzyme which get phosphorylated. Hydrolysis of this becomes very slow or does not occur some time, so causes irreversible inhibition.

Ans. 82 (A) Neostigmine cause inhibition of cholinesterase enzyme and accumulates ACh. This leads to reversal of the action of the competitive non-depolarizing neuromuscular blocking agents.

Ans. 83 (B) Echothiophate is an organophosphorus compound. It is water soluble and as a solution (0.025-0.25%) is use in resistant cases of glaucoma, due to its potent and long acting (1-3 days) miotic effect. It is rarely used now-a-days.

Ans. 84 (A) Pralidoxime is a cholinesterase enzyme reactivator used in the treatment of organophosphorus compound poisoning.

Ans. 85 (B) The most dangerous effect in belladonna poisoning is hyperthermia in infants. Death due to increase in body temperatures (in excess of 42°C) have occurred after the use of atropine containing eye drops in children.

Ans. 86 (B) Cyclopentolate/tropicamide cause less or no cycloplegia and preferred mydriatic agents. Phenylephrine is preferred in elderly as mydriatic agent.

Ans. 87 (A) Anti muscarinic drugs are not used in hypertension.

Ans. 88 (A) Benztropine is used as an adjuvant for the treatment of parkinsonism which control the cholinergic symptoms and may reduce the dose of the levodopa.

Ans. 89 (B) Ipratropium as a nebulizer, is used extensively for COPD. Salbutamol (albuterol) can also be useful, but it may cause cardiac adverse effect.

Ans. 90 (A) Atropine causes mydriasis with cycloplegia while phenylephrine causes mydriasis without cycloplegia.

Ans. 91 (D) Atropine and its synthetic and semi-synthetic congeners are used in diarrhoea, in biliary colics (with morphine), in myasthenia gravis (to minimize muscarinic adverse effects) but not with dTC as muscle relaxant. Rather atropine is used for decurarization (after dTC and other skeletal muscle relaxants) to reverse the effect.

Ans. 92 (C) Signs and symptoms of OPC poisoning are due to both muscarinic and nicotinic receptor mediated. Diarrhoea, urination miosis, bronchoconstriction, lacrimation, salivation, sweating, bradycardia and hypotension are due to action on muscarinic receptors while fasciculation of skeletal muscle followed by muscle paralysis is due to nicotinic receptor stimulation. As atropine is anti muscarinic drug, it does not abolish action mediated through nicotinic receptors.

Ans. 93 (A) Glycopyrrolate, is preferred as a pre anaesthetic medication because it causes less tachycardia and reduces bronchial and salivary secretion more effectively. It does not cross BBB, so no CNS depressant effect is observed.

Ans. 94 (D) Atropine and scopolamine are tertiary ammonium compounds and lipid soluble anti-cholinergic. They cross BBB and have CNS effects. Benztropine, benzhexal, biperidin, cycrimine etc. are synthetic atropine compounds having weak peripheral anticholinergic effects, crosses BBB and act on the basal ganglion, so used in parkinsonism. Glycopyrrolate is a quaternary compound have more peripheral effects and does not crosses BBB, so no CNS effects are observed.

Ans. 95 (C) The most prominent effect of atropine on heart is to cause tachycardia. But blockade of muscarinic auto receptors (M_1) on vagal nerve ending, augment acetylcholine release and causes initial transient bradycardia on IM/SC injection.

Ans. 96 (A) Atropine poisoning causes tachycardia.

Ans. 97 (B) Rocuronium is having rapid onset of action (1-2 min) with intermediate duration of action (25-50 min). All the other have onset of action within 2-6 min and have duration of action of 35-100 min or more. Rapacuronium is also having shorter onset of action, but it is withdrawn due to its life threatening airway complications and bronchospasm.

Ans. 98 (D) Vecuronium and rocuronium show better cardio vascular stability due to lack of histamine release and ganglionic blockade action.

Ans. 99 (D) Malignant hyperthermia is a genetically inherited condition, as an autosomal dominant trait, caused by mutation and affect Ca^{2+} release channels of the sarcoplasmic reticulum. In these patients, it is triggered by SCh and has higher susceptibility when a combination of SCh and halothane is used.

Ans. 100(B) In case of malignant hyperthermia, dantrolene is used which directly acts on the contractile mechanism of voluntary muscles. It reduces depolarization induced Ca^{2+} release, from sarcoplasmic reticulum.

Ans. 101(B) Succinylcholine is a quaternary ammonium compound and depolarizing skeletal muscle relaxant. At NMJ it acts like an agonist of Ach, thus it causes transient fasciculation initially. Its action persists at NMJ for longer duration primarily as it is only hydrolyzed by pseudo cholinesterase and not by true cholinesterase.

Ans. 102(C) The SMR like d-Tubocurarine, pancuronium, doxacurium are excreted by kidney and have longer duration of action. Drugs which are excreted through bile, *e.g.* vencuronium, rocuronium have intermediate or shorter duration of action. Mivacurium is the only SMR metabolized by pseudo cholinesterase and have shorter duration of action.

Ans. 103(B) Succinylcholine is a short acting muscle relaxant. Plasma cholinesterase (pseudo cholinesterase) is responsible for the rapid inactivation of succinylcholine. Deficiency of this leads to persistent apnea, as its termination of action does not occur.

Ans. 104(A) In patient with malignant hyperthermia, a rare hereditary disorder, an impaired sarcoplasmic reticulum is unable to sequester calcium. The sudden release of calcium results in extensive muscle contraction and increase in body temperature. This can be reduced with dantrolene.

Ans. 105(B) Neostigmine is drug of choice for reversing the block produced by Nm blockers (long and intermediate acting), *e.g.* pancuronium vecuronium etc. It increases the availability of ACh by inhibiting the true AChE and due to its direct action at motor end plate. Reversal is not required for short acting agents, *e.g.* mivacurium. Sugammadex is a new drug introduced to reverse the blockade. It is not a cholinergic drug. It forms an inactive complex with these drugs rapidly, which is finally excreted in urine (FDA approval is pending).

Ans. 106(C) Trimethaphan is an ultra short acting ganglionic blocker, given I.V. They are used to control hypertension in patients with acute dissecting aortic aneurysm, hypertensive emergencies, to manage autonomic hyper-reflexia and acute pulmonary oedema. Though therapeutic uses of ganglionic blockers are declined but trimethaphan is still used in above mentioned conditions.

3

AUTACOIDS AND RESPIRATORY SYSTEM

HISTAMINE, ANTIHISTAMINES AND OTHER AUTACOIDS

Histamine

Histamine is a biogenic amine present in many animal and plant tissues. It is also present in venoms and stinging secretions. It is synthesized by decarboxylation of the amino acid, histidine. It is mainly present in storage granules of mast cells. It is also found in skin, lungs, liver, gastric mucosa, placenta, brain, CSF, bone marrow etc. It is one of the mediators involved in the inflammatory and hypersensitivity reactions.

Mechanism of Action and Effects

Histamine exerts its effects by binding to H_1, H_2, H_3 and H_4 receptors.

1. *H_1 Receptors:* Increases Ca^{2+}, IP_3 and DAG. Thus causes smooth muscle contraction, increase in capillary permeability. Its actions are blocked by anti histaminic drug.
2. *H_2 Receptors:* Increases cAMP and causes increase gastric acid secretion and its actions are blocked by cimetidine, ranitidine etc.
3. *H_3 Pre-synaptic (Auto Receptors):* Decreases cAMP and causes decrease histamine levels in brain, lungs, skin, and gastric mucosa. H_3 receptors present in CNS acts as auto receptors, they inhibits histamine release. H_3 receptors agonist prompt sleep while H_3 antagonist, *e.g.,* thioperamide causes wakefulness, improve cognitive function, enhance memory, learning.
4. *H_4 Receptors:* These are G_i coupled receptors, they decrease cAMP and Ca^{2+} influx. They are located on blood vessels.

Effects of Histamine

1. Dilatation of smaller blood vessels due to EDRF. IV infusion causes fall in B.P. and causes constriction of large arteries.
2. Increase capillary permeability and leads to exudation of plasma.

3. *Triple response:* (a) red spot due to capillary dilatation, (b) wheal due to exudates of fluid, (c) flare, *i.e.*, redness in the surrounding area and itching.
4. Bronchoconstriction.
5. Increase in gastric secretion (H_2 receptor mediated).
6. Inflammation promotes adhesion of leukocytes to vascular endothelium.

Uses

Histamine has no valid clinical use. It is used as a positive control injection for skin allergy testing.

Antihistamines (H_1-Antagonists/H_1 Blockers)

Classification

H_1 antagonist:

- *First generation:* Diphenhydramine, Dimenhydrinate, Promethazine, Cinnarizine (antivertigo), Cyclizine, Meclizine, Hydroxyzine, Pheniramine, Chlorpheniramine maleate, Cyproheptadine ,Triprolidine
- *Second generation:* Cetrizine, L-cetrizine, Azelastine, Mizolastine, Loratadine /Desloratidine, Fexofenadine, Terfenadine, Ebastine.

H_2 antagonist: Ranitidine, Famotidine etc.

H_3 antagonist: Thioperamide, Clopenpropit, Ciproxifen, Proxyfan.

H_4 antagonists: Impentamine, Iodophenpropit.

H_4 antagonist: H_4 receptors are hematopoietic origin and present in eosinophils mast cells, GI tract, basophils, T cells etc. Activation of H_4 receptors causes chemotaxis, secretion of cytokines. So H_4 antagonists are also useful in inhibition of allergic and inflammatory response.

Mechanism of Action of H_1 Blockers

H_1 antihistamines antagonize the effects of histamine by competitively blocking the H_1 receptors and yield an inactive conformation.

Pharmacological Actions

1. They causes CNS depression, sedation and drowsiness. Certain antihistamines have antiemetic and anti-parkinsonian effects.
2. They have anti-allergic action, hence most of the manifestations of type I reactions are suppressed.
3. *Anticholinergic actions:* They cause dryness of mouth, blurring of vision, constipation and urinary retention.

Pharmacokinetics

H_1 antihistamines are well absorbed after oral and parenteral administration. They are distributed widely throughout the body, metabolized extensively in the liver by microsomal P-450 enzyme and excreted in urine.

Adverse Effects/Drug Interaction

1. The common adverse effects are sedation, drowsiness, lack of concentration, headache, fatigue, weakness, lassitude, in-coordination, etc. Hence, H_1 anti-histamines should be avoided while driving or operating machinery.
2. Gastrointestinal side effects are nausea, vomiting, loss of appetite and epigastric discomfort.
3. Anticholinergic side effects such as dryness of mouth, blurring of vision, constipation and urinary retention. These effects are not seen with second generation anti-histamine.
4. Teratogenic effects have been noticed in animals with some of the agents.
5. Terfenadine is metabolized by cytochrome P-450 isoenzyme hence causes severe drug interaction with ketoconazole, erythromycin etc which inhibits cytochrome P-450 enzyme and may cause severe arrhythmias.

Uses

1. *Allergic diseases:* Pruritis, urticaria, dermatitis, rhinitis, common cold, conjunctivitis and angioneurotic edema respond to these drugs.
2. *Preanaesthetic medication (Promethazine).*
3. *Motion sickness:* Promethazine, diphenhydramine, dimenhydrinate, act probably on the vestibular apparatus or cortex. These drugs are also useful in morning sickness (doxylamine), drug induced and postoperative vomiting.
4. *Parkinsonism:* Promethazine, diphenhydramine or orphenadrine
5. *H_1 antihistamines* are used to control mild blood transfusion and saline infusion reactions (chills and rigors) and as adjunct in anaphylaxis.
6. *Vertigo:* Dimenhydrinate and meclizine.
7. *Antiemetic:* Promethazine.

8. *Sedative and hypnotic:* Promethazine and diphenhydramine are used to induce sleep, especially in children during minor surgical procedures.

Second Generation H_1 Antihistamines

They are highly selective for H_1 receptors and have the following advantages. They:

1. Have no anticholinergic effects.
2. Do not cross BBB, hence cause minimal/no drowsiness.
3. Do not impair psychomotor performance/donot potentiate the effect of alcohol or BZD.
4. Are relatively expensive.
5. Have additional anti-allergic mechanism by acting on leukotrienes or by anti-platelet activity.
6. Have narrow spectrum of action (poor antipruritic, antiemetic and anti-tussive).

Cetrizine is one of the commonly used second generation antihistamine. Incidence of cardiac arrhythmias is rare with this drug.

Uses

1. These agents are used in various allergic disorders, *e.g.* rhinitis, dermatitis, conjunctivitis, urticaria, eczema, drug and food allergies.
2. *Vertigo:* It is a sensation of rotation or movement of one's self or of one's surrounding in any plane.

   Anti-vertigo drugs are cinnarizine, promethazine, hyoscine, prochlorperazine, betahistine, thiazides, furosemide, corticosteroid etc.

Prostaglandins (PGs), Serotonin and Leukotrienes (Eicosanoids)

Prostaglandins: The main PGs in human being are PGE_2, PGF_{2alpha} and PGI_2(prostacyclin). Arachidonic acid is the precursor for the biosynthesis of all PGs. The enzyme cyclooxygenase (COX) is involved in the formation of PGs from arachidonic acid and lipo oxygenase for synthesis of leukotrienes.

Preparations, formulations and uses of PGs

Preparations	Formulations	Uses
Dinoprostone (PGE_2)	Vaginal tab Vaginal gel	Induction of labour Mid-term abortion
Dinoprost (PGF_{2alpha})	Intra amniotic injection	Mid-term abortion
Carboprost (15-methyl PGF_{2alpha})	IM, intra amniotic injection	Mid-term abortion, control of PPH
Gemeprost (PGE_2)	Vaginal pessary	Cervical priming in early pregnancy
Alprostadil (PGE_1)	Intravenous infusion Intracavernous injection	Maintenance of a patent ductus arteriosus in neonates with congenital heart disease Erectile dysfunction
Misoprostol (PGE_1)	Oral	Peptic ulcer Abortion
Epoprostenol (PGI_2)	Intravenous infusion	Pulmonary hypertension
Latanoprost (PGF_{2alpha})	Topical	Glaucoma

Adverse Effects: Nausea, vomiting, diarrhoea, fever and backache due to uterine contractions. Injections are painful due to sensitization of nerve endings.

5-Hydroxytryptamine (5-HT or Serotonin)

5-HT has diverse pharmacological and physiological roles in the body, which include (a) as a neurotransmitter in CNS, (b) as regulator of smooth muscle function in CVS and GIT, and (c) as regulator of platelet function.

5-HT Receptors

$5\text{-}HT_1$: Located mainly in CNS and function as pre-synaptic receptors (auto receptor), coupled with G-protein linked to adenylase cyclase.

$5\text{-}HT_{1A}$ and $5\text{-}HT_{1B}$: Involved in the regulation of mood and behavior.

$5\text{-}HT_{1D}$: Mediate cerebral vasoconstriction.

$5\text{-}HT_2$: Located in the periphery (smooth muscles and platelets). They are G-coupled receptors linked to IP_3 and DAG production.

$5\text{-}HT_{2A}$: Causes smooth muscle contraction and vasoconstriction.

$5\text{-}HT_3$: Occur in peripheral nervous system. They are directly linked to membrane ion-channels and have no involvement of any second messenger. It evokes pain.

5-HT_4 : Occurs in ENS as well as in CNS. It causes stimulation of peristalsis and gastric emptying.

Receptor	Agonist	Antagonist
5-HT_{1A}	Buspirone	Spipirone (5-HT_{1A})
5-HT_{1D}	Sumatriptan	Ergotamine (5-HT_{1A-1D})
	Almotriptan	
5-HT_2	LSD (non-selective)	Ketanserin (5-HT_{2A})
		Methysergide (5-HT_{2A-2C})
		Clozapine (5-HT_{2A-2C})
		Risperidone (5-HT_{2A-2C})
		Cyproheptadine (5-HT_{2A})
5-HT_3	2 methyl- 5-HT	Odansetron
		Granisetron
5-HT_4	Metoclopramide	
	Claspride	
	Mosapride	
	Tegaserod	
	Renzapride	

Leukotrienes: They play an important role in various physiological functions. They act through LT-receptors, *e.g.*, LTB_4, LTC_4, LTD_4 and LTE_4. They depresses myocardium. Bronchoconstriction and mediation of inflammation are other effects.

DRUG THERAPY OF BRONCHIAL ASTHMA AND COUGH

Drug Therapy of Bronchial Asthma

Asthma is a chronic inflammatory disease in which the patient suffers from reversible episodes of airways obstruction due to bronchial hyper-responsiveness.

The cardinal symptoms of asthma are breathlessness, wheezing, cough and chest tightness with worsening of these symptoms at night. In an acute attack, the respiratory rate is rapid and tachycardia is common.

Asthma may be described as:

a. **Extrinsic** when it is associated with exposure to specific allergen (pollen or house dust, mite).

b. **Intrinsic asthma** which have no identifiable external precipitating factor or immunological basis for asthmatic attack.

c. **Status asthmaticus** is a severe acute asthma, which is a life threatening condition involving exhaustion, cyanosis, bradycardia, hypotension, dehydration and metabolic acidosis.

d. **Cardiac asthma** is a bronchospasm precipitated by uncompensated congestive heart failure.

e. **Exercise induced.**

f. **Associated with COPD.**

Classification of Drugs Used to Treat Asthma

(A) Bronchodilators

i. *Selective beta$_2$ agonists (directly acting):* Salbutalmol (Albuterol), Terbutaline, Salmeterol, Formoterol, Bambuterol, Pirbuterol.

ii. *Nonselective sympathomimetics:* Epinephrine, Ephedrine, Isoprenaline, Orciprenaline (metaproterenol).

iii. *Anticholinergic:* Ipratropium, Tiotropium.

iv. *Methyl-Xanthine:* Theophylline, Aminophylline, Etophylline, Doxophylline.

(B) Corticosteroids

i. *Oral:* Prednisone, Methyl prednisolon.

ii. *Parenteral:* Methyl prednisolon, Hydrocortisone, Dexamethasone.

iii. *Inhalational:* Beclomethasone, Fluticasone, Triamcinolone, Budesonide, etc.

(C) Mast Cell Stabilizers: Sodium cromoglycate, Nedocromil, Ketotifen

(D) Leukotriene modulators:

i. *5-Lipoxygenase inhibitor:* Zileuton.

ii. *LTD$_4$ – receptor antagonists:* Zafirlukast, Monteleukast.

(E) Monoclonal anti IgE antibody – Omalizumab.

A. Bronchodilators

Selective Beta$_2$ Agonists

It is mainstay of modern bronchodilator therapy. They activate beta$_2$ adrenoceptors present on airway smooth muscle and:

a. Relax airway smooth muscle.
b. Inhibit the release of bronchoconstricting chemical mediators from the mast cells; and
c. Increase the mucociliary transport by increasing the ciliary activity.

Short acting selective $beta_2$ agonists are terbutaline, salbutamol; while salmeterol, bambuterol and formoterol are highly lipid soluble, long acting agents (half life 12 hours). When inhaled, these drugs produce effective bronchodilation with minimal cardiac stimulation (due to associated $beta_1$ stimulatory effect). Terbutaline is perhaps the only bronchodilator which can be used safely during pregnancy. The longer acting preparations are useful for treating nocturnal asthma or for long term prevention of asthma attacks.

The adverse effects by oral route are muscle tremors (due to direct stimulation of $beta_2$ receptors in skeletal muscle), tachycardia (due to stimulation of chronotropic $beta_2$ receptors and in high doses $beta_1$ receptors in the heart) and restlessness. Continued use of these agents usually results in desensitization / down regulation of $beta_2$ receptors that result in diminished responsiveness.

Non-Selective Sympathomimetics

Epinephrine is now rarely used, but was a drug of choice for the acute attack of asthma when $beta_2$ agonists were not available. Because it stimulates alpha, $beta_1$, as well as $beta_2$, receptors, its use is associated with troublesome adverse effects, *e.g.*, tachycardia, hypertension, worsening of angina and even arrhythmias. It is sometimes used (S.C.) to treat status asthmaticus because besides bronchodilation it also reduces pulmonary oedema.

Anticholinergic

These are less effective bronchodilators than $beta_2$ agonists. They cause bronchodilation by binding to M_3 receptors on airway smooth muscle and thereby preventing the action of acetylcholine released from parasympathetic nerves. They also decrease mucus secretion but have less drying effect on mucus and minimize the chances of forming mucus plugs (unlike atropine). They do not cross BBB and are devoid of CNS side effects. Tiotropium is a longer acting derivative of ipratropium. Combination of ipratropium with a $beta_2$ agonist works better in severe asthma and has longer duration of action than either drug alone.

Methylxanthines (Theophylline, aminophylline, doxophylline). They causes:

a. Inhibition of phosphodiesterase III (present in airway smooth muscle) and IV (present in eosinophil and mast cells), the two specific isoenzymes responsible for the metabolism of cAMP. The cAMP levels, therefore, get elevated leading to bronchodilation; and

b. Blockade of adenosine receptor present on airway muscles and those on mast cells.

Theophylline exhibits bronchodilator, anti-inflammatory and immunomodulatory effects with increased mucociliary clearance. Doxophylline is longer acting analogue of theophylline.

B. Corticosteroids

They provide long term stabilization of the symptoms due to their anti-inflammatory effects. Inhaled corticosteroids, along with $beta_2$ adrenoceptor agonists are the first choice drugs for chronic asthma. (1) they enhance $beta_2$ adrenergic receptor response by up regulating the $beta_2$ receptors in lung cells and leukocytes, (2) they inhibit the release of prostaglandins and leukotrienes and thus prevent smooth muscle contraction, vascular permeability and airway mucus secretion, and (3) they inhibit the formation and release of chemical mediators (from mast cells and eosinophils) so prevent recruitment, proliferation and activation of leukocytes.

Aerosol corticosteroids produce minimal systemic side effects which include dryness of mouth, voice changes and oral candidiasis.

Parenteral corticosteroids are used in severe acute asthma.

C. Mast Cell Stabilizers

These are non-bronchodilator, non-steroidal drugs used for prophylactic treatment of asthma available as metered-dose aerosol. Inhaled cromolyn sodium powder is used through a nebulizer.

Ketotifen is an oral antihistamine having cromolyn sodium like activity. It has a delayed onset of action and benefits are seen only after 6-12 weeks of treatment.

D. Leukotriene Modulators

Leukotriene (LT) are powerful mediators of inflammation, cause leukocyte recruitment, stimulate bronchoconstriction and increase capillary permeability leading to pulmonary edema.

The synthesis of leukotrienes can be blocked by inhibiting the 5-lipoxygenase enzyme by the drug zileuton, whereas the effects of leukotrienes on LT receptors can be blocked by drugs such as zafirlukast and montelukast. These are mainly used as the adjuvant with inhaled corticosteroids in poorly responding patients. Zileuton causes hepatotoxicity (hence withdrawn from several countries).

Zafirlukast administered 2 hours before meals, at 12 hourly intervals. Monteleukast is given once daily (usually, in the evening) and is quite safe.

They are used in children > 5 years of age.

E. Omalizumab

It prevents the binding of IgE to mast cell and thus prevents mast cell degradation but has no effect on IgE already bound to mast cells. It is administered parenterally and used in patients > 12 years of age.

Treatment of status asthmaticus:

1. Hydrocortisone IV.
2. Nebulized salbutamol + ipratropium bromide inhalation.
3. High flow humidified oxygen.
4. Salbutamol/terbutaline (IM/SC).
5. Intubation if needed.
6. Treatment of chest infection.
7. Correct dehydration and acidosis.

Drug Therapy of Cough

Cough is a physiologically useful protective reflex that clears the respiratory tract of the accumulated mucus and foreign substances. The non-productive cough is considered as serving no useful purpose, rather increases discomfort to the patient. For its treatment, anti-tussive agents are used. The productive cough is characterized by the presence of excessive sputum and may be associated with conditions such as chronic bronchitis and bronchiectasis. In this case, cough suppressants (anti-tussives) are not effective and are inappropriate but expectorants are used.

Expectorants increase the volume and decrease the viscosity of secretions to enhance the propulsion of these secretions upward and outward by ciliary movement and coughing.

Anti-Tussives

Centrally Acting Anti-Tussives

These include opioids like codeine and pholcodeine and non-opioids such as dextromethorphan, noscapine and benzonatate. They have central anti-tussive actions by virtue of suppressing cough center that mediates the cough reflex.

Pholcodeine is longer acting and better tolerated than codeine.

Dextromethorphan: It has least addiction liability, no analgesic action, least constipating effects and minimal drowsiness.

Noscapine: It is devoid of analgesic activity, drowsiness and addiction liability.

Benzonatate related to the local anaesthetic tetracaine. It not only suppresses the central cough center, but also inhibits the pulmonary stretch receptors.

Anti-tussives Having Peripheral Action

Prenoxdiazine relieves bronchospasm by inhibiting pulmonary stretch receptors.

Expectorants

They are:

a. **Mucokinetic Expectorants:** Stimulate the flow of respiratory tract secretions by stimulating the bronchial secretory cells (to increase the volume) and the ciliary movement to facilitate their removal and include essential volatile oils, ammonium chloride, sodium citrate, guaiacol and guaifenesin.
b. **Mucolytic Expectorants:** They alter the chemical characteristics of mucus to decrease its viscosity and to facilitate its removal by ciliary action or coughing and include acetylcysteine, carbocysteine, bromhexine and ambroxol.

Acetylcysteine is a mucolytic that decreases the viscosity of mucus by splitting the disulfide (S-S) bonds of mucoproteins.

Bromhexine depolymerises mucopolysaccharides of mucus and also breaks fibre network of tenacious sputum. Ambraxol is a metabolite of bromhexine.

Bronchodilators are also useful when cough is associated with bronchospasm. Decongestants, *e.g.* ephedrine, pseudoephedrine, phenylephrine are also added in cough mixtures.

MULTIPLE CHOICE QUESTIONS

Q. 1 The action of histamine that is not mediated through H_1 receptor is:

(A) Release of EDRF from vascular endothelium resulting in vasodilatation
(B) Direct action on vascular smooth muscle causing vasodilatation
(C) Bronchoconstriction
(D) Release of catecholamines

Q. 2 Histamine is involved as a mediator in the following pathological condition:

(A) Delayed hypersensitivity reaction
(B) Inflammation
(C) Carcinoid syndrome
(D) Variant angina

Q. 3 The drug that can directly release histamine from mast cells without involving antigen-antibody reaction is:

(A) Aspirin (B) Procaine
(C) Morphine (D) Sulfadiazine

Q. 4 Which anti-histamine have high anticholinergic activity:

(A) Diphenhydramine (B) Astemizole
(C) Cetrizine (D) Terfenadine

Q. 5 The conventional antihistamines possess the following activities *except:*

(A) Local anesthetic (B) Vasopressor
(C) Anti-arrhythmic (D) Anticholinergic

Q. 6 The second generation antihistamines have the following advantages *except:*

(A) Lack of anticholinergic side effects
(B) Lack of alcohol potentiating potential
(C) Recipient can drive motor vehicle
(D) Good anti-pruritic action

---

1 (B) 2 (B) 3 (C) 4 (A) 5 (B) 6 (D)

Q. 7 H_1 antihistaminic which is used topically in the nose for allergic rhinitis is:

(A) Loratidine (B) Cetrizine
(C) Terfenadine (D) Azelastine

Q. 8 The H_3 receptor agonist exhibit all of the following action *except:*

(A) Inhibition of H_1 receptor induced wakefulness
(B) Increase in H_1 mediated gastrin secretion
(C) Inhibition of H_1 mediated bronchoconstriction
(D) Negative chronotropic effect on atria

Q. 9 Histamine-3 (H_3) receptors are located pre-synaptically in the:

(A) Smooth muscles
(B) Gastric mucosa
(C) Brain and myentric plexus
(D) Cardiac muscle

Q. 10 All of the following effects are due to the activation of H_1 receptors *except:*

(A) Cardiovascular response
(B) Bronchoconstriction
(C) Pain and itching
(D) Contraction of smooth muscles of gut

Q. 11 The drug which is an agonist at H_2 receptors and antagonist at H_3 receptors is:

(A) Triploidine (B) Thioperamide
(C) Impromidine (D) Clobenpropil

Q. 12 Which subtype of histamine receptors function as pre-synpatic autoinhibitory receptor on histaminergic neurone?

(A) H_1 receptors (B) H_2 receptors
(C) H_3 receptors (D) H_4 receptors

Q. 13 Which tricyclic antidepressant is a potent antihistamine?

(A) Doxipen (B) Imipramine
(C) Amitriptyline (D) Nortriptyline

7 (D) 8 (B) 9 (C) 10 (A) 11 (C) 12 (C) 13 (A)

Q. 14 Which antihistamine cause potentially lethal ventricular arrhythmia with erythromycin?

(A) Cetrizine
(B) Terfenadine
(C) Loratidine
(D) Promethazine

Q. 15 The anti-histamine which is primarily excreted unchanged in urine is?

(A) Cetrizine (B) Terfenadine
(C) Diphenhydramine (D) Promethazine

Q. 16 Which antihistamine is a potential teratogenic?

(A) Fexofenadine (B) Diphenhydramine
(C) Cetrizine (D) Loratidine

Q. 17 Which of the following 5-HT receptors is not a G-protein coupled receptor?

(A) $5\text{-}HT_1$ (B) $5\text{-}HT_2$
(C) $5\text{-}HT_3$ (D) $5\text{-}HT_4$

Q. 18 Which of the following serotonergic receptor functions primarily as an auto receptor on neurons:

(A) $5\text{-}HT_{1A}$ (B) $5\text{-}HT_{2A}$
(C) $5\text{-}HT_3$ (D) $5\text{-}HT_4$

Q. 19 5-HT receptors appears to play a role in the following *except:*

(A) Regulation of normal B.P.
(B) Maintenance of circadian rhythm
(C) Haemostasis
(D) Causation of migraine

Q. 20 The 5-HT antagonist that has anti-hypertensive property is:

(A) Methysergide
(B) Cyproheptadine
(C) Ketanserin
(D) Ondansetron

14 (B) 15 (A) 16 (A) 17 (C) 18 (A) 19 (A) 20 (C)

Q. 21 Which of the following eicosanoid is generated through the lipo-oxygenase pathway?

(A) Prostaglandin E_2 (B) Thromboxane A_2
(C) Prostacyclin (D) Leukotriene C_4

Q. 22 The following prostanoid is a potent inducer of platelet aggregation:

(A) Prostacyclin (B) Prostaglandin E_2
(C) Prostaglandin D_2 (D) Thromoxane A_2

Q. 23 All of the following are indications for eicosanoids or their inhibitors *except:*

(A) Abortion
(B) Essential hypertension
(C) Patent ductus arteriosus
(D) Transposition of the great arteries

Q. 24 Misoprostol is a:

(A) Prostaglandin E_1 analogue
(B) Prostaglandin E_2 analogue
(C) Prostaglandin antagonist
(D) Antiprogestin

Q. 25 All of the following are correct statements *except:*

(A) PG and leukotrienes are derived from arachidonic acid
(B) COX-II is induced by cytokines at the site of inflammation
(C) COX-I is inducible enzyme
(D) Leukotrienes cause smooth muscle contraction

Q. 26 Which of the following statement is not correct regarding PGs?

(A) The human arteriolar smooth muscle is relaxed by PGE_2 and PGI_2 whereas TXA_2 and PGF_{2alpha} cause vasoconstriction
(B) PGE_1 has marked oxytocic action while PGF_{2alpha} has tocolytic action
(C) PGE_1 and PGI_2 inhibit platelet aggregation whereas TXA_2 facilitate aggregation
(D) PGE_2 is a bronchodilator whereas PGF_{2alpha} is a bronchoconstrictor

---

21 (D) 22 (D) 23 (B) 24 (A) 25 (C) 26 (B)

Q. 27 Prostaglandin E_2 is useful in:

(A) Dysmenorrhoea (B) Inflammation
(C) Peptic ulcer (D) Induction of abortion

Q. 28 Therapeutic uses of prostaglandin E_1 include all of the following *except:*

(A) Medical termination of pregnancy
(B) Impotence
(C) Primary pulmonary hypertension
(D) Maintenance of patent ductus arteriosus

Q. 29 All are true statement about TXA_2 is *except:*

(A) It is formed in platelets
(B) It is formed from PGG_2/H_2
(C) It is not prothrombotic
(D) Aspirin can inhibit its production

Q. 30 The drug of choice for controlling post partum haemorrhage is:

(A) Prostaglandin E_2 (B) Oxytocin
(C) Dihydroergotamine (D) Methylergonovine

Q. 31 Which of the following is most useful for reversing severe ergot induced vasospasm?

(A) Ergotamine (B) Methysergide
(C) Nitroprusside (D) Phenoxybenzamine

Q. 32 Which of the following steroid is preferred in status asthmaticus?

(A) Budesonide
(B) Beclomethasone dipropionate
(C) Fluticasone
(D) Hydrocortisone hemisuccinate

Q. 33 $Beta_2$ receptor mediated effects of terbutaline include all of the following *except:*

(A) Tremors (B) Mast cell stabilization
(C) Vasodilation (D) Free fatty acid release

---

27 (C) 28 (C) 29 (C) 30 (D) 31 (C) 32 (D) 33 (D)

Q. 34 All is true about ipratropium *except:*

(A) Produces slow but longer lasting bronchodilation
(B) Useful in chronic obstructive pulmonary disease
(C) Can be combined with beta adrenergic drugs
(D) High doses are required to cause bronchodilation

Q. 35 Which of the following statement is true regarding the mechanism of action of ipratropium?

(A) It acts centrally to decrease vagal ACh release
(B) It inhibits pulmonary ACh receptors
(C) It decreases mast cell release of histamine
(D) It blocks the action of histamine at H_1 receptor

Q. 36 All is true regarding theophylline dosage in bronchial asthma *except:*

(A) A loading dose is required to get therapeutic levels
(B) Smokers require higher maintenance dose
(C) Dose adjustment is not required in hepatic disease
(D) Children below 10 years of age require higher dose on weight basis than adults

Q. 37 Which of the following statement regarding the pharmacokinetics of theophylline is correct?

(A) It is primarily metabolized by the kidney
(B) Its metabolism depends on age
(C) It is poorly absorbed when given orally
(D) It has wide therapeutic index

Q. 38 Which of the following drug is not a bronchodilator?

(A) Theophylline
(B) Terbutaline
(C) Sodium cromoglycate
(D) Ipratropium bromide

Q. 39 Which of the following statement describe the action of theophylline?

(A) It stimulate cyclic AMP phosphodiesterase
(B) It is an adenosine receptor antagonist
(C) It does not cross the blood brain barrier
(D) It blocks the release of ACh in the bronchal tree

34 (D) 35 (B) 36 (C) 37 (B) 38 (C) 39 (B)

Q. 40 Major action of cromolyn sodium is:

(A) It blocks calcium channels in lymphocytes
(B) It blocks mediator release from mast cell
(C) It blocks phosphodiesterase in mast cell and basophil
(D) It causes smooth muscle relaxation in the bronchi

Q. 41 Which of the following is most likely to have adverse effects when used daily for prolonged period in children?

(A) Albuterol (salbutamol) by aerosol
(B) Cromolyn by inhaler
(C) Beclomethasone by aerosol
(D) Prednisolon by mouth

Q. 42 Which of the following anti-asthma drug is not indicated by oral route of administration in pregnancy?

(A) Albuterol (salbutamol) (B) Prednisolon
(C) Theophylline (D) Ipratropium bromide

Q. 43 Inflammation in the airways can be reduced by:

(A) Fluticasone (B) Budesonide
(C) Theophylline (D) Albuterol (salbutamol)

Q. 44 Which of the following is not a recognized action of albuterol (salbutamol)?

(A) Diuretic effect (B) Skeletal muscle tremors
(C) Tachycardia (D) Positive inotropic effect

Q. 45 In patients of bronchial asthma, inhaled corticosteroid achieve the following *except:*

(A) Reduce the need of bronchodilator medication
(B) Control an attack of refractory asthma
(C) Reduce bronchial hyperactivity
(D) Reverse diminished responsiveness to sympathomimetic bronchodilators

Q. 46 In bronchial asthma corticosteroids act by all of the following mechanisms *except:*

(A) Increasing cAMP in bronchial smooth muscle
(B) Decreasing capillary permeability
(C) Enhancing neuronal uptake of catecholamines
(D) Decreasing spasmogenic prostaglandin formation

---

40 (B) 41 (D) 42 (A) 43 (A) 44 (A) 45 (B) 46 (C)

Q. 47 Which of the following cannot be used in acute attack of bronchial asthma?

(A) Montelukast (B) Ipratropium
(C) Salmeterol (D) Beclomethasone

Q. 48 Which of the following is most likely causes alteration in liver enzyme (alanine aminotransferase)?

(A) Zileuton (B) Zafirlukast
(C) Albuterol (D) Sodium chromoglycate

Q. 49 Sodium cromoglycate has no role in the treatment of:

(A) Acute bronchial asthma
(B) Chronic urticaria
(C) Chronic allergic rhinitis
(D) Chronic allergic conjunctivitis

Q. 50 Release of histamine and leukotrienes from mast cell is prevented by:

(A) Zileuton (B) Zafirlukast
(C) Nedocromil sodium (D) Fexofenadine

Q. 51 Which of the following expectorants act both directly as well as reflexly on the airway mucosa?

(A) Potassium iodide
(B) Guaiphenesin
(C) Terpin hydrate
(D) Bromhexin

Q. 52 Mucokinetic is a drug which:

(A) Reduces mucus secretion
(B) Increases mucus secretion
(C) Makes respiratory secretions more watery
(D) Stimulates mucocillary activity of bronchial epithelium

Q. 53 Which of the following is not an anti-tussive?

(A) Chlophedianol
(B) Dextromethorphan
(C) Narcotine (noscapine)
(D) Dextropropoxyphene

---

47 (A) 48 (A) 49 (B) 50 (C) 51 (D) 52 (C) 53 (D)

Q. 54 Which drug is not used as an aerosol/inhalation in bronchial asthma?

(A) Zafirlukast (B) Salmeterol
(C) Budisonide (D) Ipratropium

Q. 55 Reflex bronchoconstriction is most likely to occur with the following form of inhaled antiasthma medication:

(A) Metered dose spray of drug in solution
(B) Dry powder rotacap
(C) Nebulizer
(D) Nebulizer with spacer

Q. 56 Which of the following drug is effective in dry cough?

(A) Dextromethorphan (B) Meperidine
(C) Levopropoxyphene (D) Dextropropoxyphene

54 (A) 55 (B) 56 (A)

ANSWERS

Ans. 1 **(B)** Both H_1 and H_2 receptors cause vasodilatation. H_1 receptors are present in the endothelium and cause vasodilatation by releasing NO. H_2 receptors present on the smooth muscles cause vasodilatation by direct action on muscles.

Ans. 2 **(B)** Histamine has been implicated as a mediator of vasodilatation and other changes that occur during inflammation. It promotes adhesion of leukocytes to vascular endothelium, sequestrating leukocytes at the inflammatory site. It also regulates micro circulation according to local needs.

Ans. 3 **(C)** A variety of stimuli, *e.g.,* tissue damage, antigen antibody reactions, polymers like dextran releases histamines. Some drugs, *e.g.,* morphine atropine, tubocurarine, vancomycin, polymyxin B directly release histamine without an immunological reaction.

Ans. 4 **(A)** First generation anti-histamine, *e.g.,* diphenhydramine, promethazine, pheneramine etc. have high anti-cholinergic activity as compare to second generation anti-histamines, *e.g.,* cetrizine, terfenadine etc.

Ans. 5 **(B)** Anti-histamine possess anticholinergic, allergic, anti-parkinsons, anti-motion sickness, local anaesthetic activity, sedative, anti-arrhythmic, antivertigo activity. They are not, vasopressor agent, but causes fall in blood pressure.

Ans. 6 **(D)** Second generation anti-histamines have all advantages mentioned over conventional anti-histaminics but they have poor anti pruritic action as compare to first generation anti-histamines.

Ans. 7 **(D)** Azelastin has good topical activity and also shown to down regulate intracellular adhesion molecule-1 (ICAM-1) expression on nasal mucosa.

Ans. 8 **(B)** H_3 receptors act as presynaptic receptors and decrease the release of histamine and other neurotransmitters. They antagonize H_1 mediated wakefulness and broncho-constriction decrease gastrin release (not increase) and produce negative chronotropic effect.

Ans. 9 **(C)** H_1 receptors are expressed mainly in CNS especially in basal ganglion, hippocampus and cortex.

Ans. 10 (A) Bronchoconstriction and contraction of the gut smooth muscles are mediated by H_1 receptors. Other less prominent effects are oedema and stimulation of nerve ending produces pain and itching. Response like vascular dilation is mediated by both H_1 and H_2 receptor stimulation.

Ans. 11 (C) H_3 antagonist, *e.g.*, impromidine and burimamide had mixed effects as agonist on H_2 receptor and antagonist to H_3 receptors. But now specific H_3 antagonist are available (in Phase II/III trials), *e.g.*, Thioperamide, Clobenpropit, Ciproxifen and Proxyfen.

Ans. 12 (C) H_3 receptor subtype functions as presynaptic autoreceptors (auto-inhibitory) on histaminergic neurons and modulate the release of other neurotransmitters.

Ans. 13 (A) Doxipen is one of the most potent anti-histamines and is about 800 times more potent than diphehydramine, so effective in chronic urticaria.

Ans. 14 (B) Terfenadine and astemizole are metabolized by cytochrome to active metabolite and induces fatal arrhythmia. Chances of toxicity increases with erythromycin which inhibit cytochrome enzyme (Cyp-3A) and hence both are withdrawn.

Ans. 15 (A) Cetrizine, loratidine and fexofenadine are well absorbed and are excreted mainly in the unmetabolized form. Cetrizine and loratidine are excreted primarily into the urine while fexofenadine excreted in the feces.

Ans. 16 (A) Azelastine, hydroxyzine and fexofenadine showed teratogenic effects in animal studies while others, *e.g.*, chlorpheniramine maleate, deiphenhydramine, cetrizine and loratidine did not show any teratogenic effect.

Ans. 17 (C) 5-HT_1, decrease cAMP production, 5-HT_2 generate IP_3/DAG while 5-HT_4 increases cAMP as second messenger. But 5-HT_3 is a ligand gated cation (Na^+, K^+) channel which on activation elicits fast depolarization.

Ans. 18 (A) 5-HT_{1A} receptors function as auto receptors in brain and inhibit firing of 5-HT neurons or release of 5-HT from nerve endings.

Ans. 19 (A) 5-HT, being a precursor of melatonin, regulate or maintain circadian rhythm. It is also cause migraine, raynaud's phenomenon, variant angina, carcinoid tumor etc. It may show triphasic response (early fall, brief rise, followed by prolonged fall) in BP but is not involved in the physiological regulation of BP. It is also responsible for pre-eclamptic rise in BP.

Ans. 20 (C) Ketanserin has anti-hypertensive property. Increased responsiveness to 5-HT and its reduced uptake and clearance by platelet is observed in hypertensive patient.

Ans. 21 (D) The cycloxygenase (COX) pathway generates eicosanoids with a ring structure (PG, TXs and prostacyclin) while lipo-oxygenase (LOX) produces open chain compounds, *e.g.*, leukotrienes (LTS).

Ans. 22 (D) TXA_2 is a potent inducer of platelet aggregation, while PGI_2 (prostacyclin) is a potent inhibitor of platelet aggregation PGD_2 has anti-aggregatory action but less potent than PGI_2. PGE_2 has inconsistent effects.

Ans. 23 (B) All are the indications of PG (eicosanoids) or their inhibitors but not essential hypertension. PG is useful in the treatment of pulmonary arterial hypertension.

Ans. 24 (A) Misoprostol, rioprostil are PGE_1 analogue, enprostil is PGE_2 analogue used in peptic ulcer. NSAIDs are inhibitors or antagonist of PG.

Ans. 25 (C) COX II normally present in insignificant amount but is inducible by cytokines and other stimuli during the inflammatory response. COX I is a constitutive enzyme in most cells and its activity is not changed once the cell is fully grown and not inducible.

Ans. 26 (B) PGE_2 mainly causes softening of cervix and is utilized for cervical ripening while PGF_2 alpha is an oxytocic agent and can be used for the induction of abortion.

Ans. 27 (C) PGE_2 markedly reduces acid secretion in the stomach. PGE_2 and PGI_2 also increase mucus production and mucosal blood flow. Increase synthesis of PGE_2 and PGF_2 alpha during menstruation causes dysmenorrhoea. PGE alpha and PGE_2 used for induction of labor and not for abortion. PG cannot be used as anti-inflammatory drug as PGE_2 and PGI_2 sensitize pain receptors to mediate pain.

Ans. 28 (C) PGE_1 is (Alprostadil) is used to maintain PDA, in impotence and for medical termination of pregnancy. Misoprostol (PGE_1) is used with mifepristone to induce abortion. PGI_2

(epoprostenol) lowers peripheral, pulmonary and coronary resistance and used in PAH.

Ans. 29 (C) TXA_2 is produced inside the platelets with the help of TXA_2 synthetase. It is formed from cyclic endoperoxides (PGG_2/H_2) with the help of an enzyme cyclooxygenase. Aspirin inhibits its production by inhibiting COX enzyme. It causes aggregation of platelets therefore is prothrombotic.

Ans. 30 (D) All the natural ergot alkaloid markedly increases the motor activity of the uterus and causes increased in contraction (both frequency and force) involving both upper and lower segment and thus useful for PPH. Ergonovine and its semisynthetic derivative is more active and less toxic among all ergot alkaloids.

Ans. 31 (C) Sodium nitroprusside is used in case of acute or chronic poisoning of ergot. Precordial pain, transient tachycardia or bradycardia, as a result of coronary vasospam occurs in poisoning. Treatment include anti-coagulant, LMWH, dextran, and potent vasodilator, *e.g.*, sodium nitroprusside intravenously.

Ans. 32 (D) Hydrocortissone is preferred agent in status asthmaticus. It acts rapidly and can be given intravenously. Dexamethasone, Betamethasone etc can be used but they have marked selective glucocorticoid action, long acting and causes marked suppression of pituitary-adrenal axis. Budesonide and Fluticasone have high topical systemic potency ratio (better than beclomethasone) so used as inhation glucocorticoid.

Ans. 33 (D) $Beta_2$ receptors mediated actions includes relaxation of respiratory, uterine and vascular smooth muscle, increases glucogenolysis due to effect on liver and causes tremor due to action of skeletal muscles. Lipolysis or increase FFA release action is mediated through $beta_3$ receptors mainly.

Ans. 34 (D) Ipratropium is more selective anticholinergic which can be used in bronchial asthma and are valuable for patients who are intolerant of inhaled beta agonist, though they are less effective than beta agonist. Long acting tiotropium is approved as a treatment of COPD. It causes bronchodilation at a lower dose than that needed to cause an increase in heart rate.

Ans. 35 (B) Ipratropium is an ACh receptor anatagonist. It is poorly absorbed and does not cross BBB so have no CNS effect. It does not block release of histamine from mast cells through H_1 receptor.

Ans. 36 (C) Theophylline is well absorbed and distributed in all tissue and 50% is protein bound, having $t_{1/2}$ 7-12 hours, so loading dose is required to get therapeutic effect. Clearance is increased through the induction of hepatic enzyme in smokers, so they require higher maintenance doses. Children clear theophylline faster than adults so require higher doses on weight basis. Dose adjustment is required in hepatic disease as theophylline is extensively metabolized in liver by demethylation and oxidation. Only 10% is excreted unchanged. Its kinetic also changes from first order to zero order as its metabolic enzymes are saturable so chances of toxicity is more.

Ans. 37 (B) Metabolism of theophylline depends on age. It has narrow safety of margin and may cause toxicity related with GIT, CNS and CV system (also see Ans. 36).

Ans. 38 (C) Sodium cromoglycate is mast cell stabilizer. It is non-bronchodilating, non-steroidal drug used for prophylactic treatment of asthma and is available as metered dose aerosol.

Ans. 39 (B) Theophylline acts through various mechanisms but the adenosine receptor antagonist activity and the inhibition of the phosphodiesterase are the best understood.

Ans. 40 (B) Sodium cromoglycate (cromolyn sodium) is a synthetic derivative which inhibits degranulation of mast cells as well as other inflammatory cells by trigger stimuli. So the release of histamine, LTS, PAF, IL etc is restricted.

Ans. 41 (D) Steroids, when used for prolonged period orally are likely to have adverse effects while incidences are less when used as aerosols form in the treatment of bronchial asthma.

Ans. 42 (A) There are no adequate and well controlled data regarding the use of albuterol in humans but animal data shows, that it is teratogenic in mice.

Ans. 43 (A) Systemic steroid therapy, *e.g.*, with fluticasone improve airflow, reduce asthma exacerbation and may influence airway remodeling, and retarding disease progression in a better way than $beta_2$ agonist or any other drug. Budesonide is a topically used steroid not absorbed when given orally.

Ans. 44 (A) $Beta_2$ agonists cause smooth muscle relaxation. Though salbutamol is selective $beta_2$ agonist, but in moderate to higher doses, it may stimulate $beta_1$ cardiac receptors. But diuretic effect is not a $beta_2$ receptor mediated action. Theophylline (methyl xanthine) possesses diuretic effect.

Ans. 45 (B) Inhaled steroids suppress bronchial inflammation, increase peak expiratory flow rate, reduce the need of $beta_2$ agonist and prevent episodes of acute asthma but they have no role in acute attack or in status asthmaticus.

Ans. 46 (C) Corticosteroids are not bronchodilators but they reduce bronchial hyperactivity, musocal oedema and suppress inflammatory response and have more sustained symptomatic relief.

Ans. 47 (A) It is the most commonly used drugs in the allergic asthma especially in children. It is leukotriene antagonist and blocks the occurrence of bronchoconstriction. They are ineffective once bronchoconstriction occurs.

Ans. 48 (A) Zileuton, among leukotrienes antagonist (montelukast and zafirlukast) is hepatotoxic, thus not used commonly. Sodium chromoglycate is not absorbed orally and given as an aerosol through inhaler. Only a small fraction of inhaled drug is absorbed systemically. It is rapidly excreted unchanged. Albuterol (salbutamol) also do not alter hepatic enzyme.

Ans. 49 (B) Sodium cromoglycate inhibits the release of histamine etc from mast cell. Exact mechanism is not known but it may involve a delayed Cl-channel in the membrane of these cells. However, Ag:Ab reaction is not interfered. It does not antagonize the constrictor action of histamine so ineffective during attack. It can be used in allergic rhinitis, conjunctivitis but not in urticaris which may involve antigen-antibody reaction.

Ans. 50 (C) Sodium cromoglycate and nedocromil inhibit the release of histamine from mast cells.

Ans. 51 (D) Bromhexin expectorant (mucolytic agent and mucokinetic) capable of inducing thin copious bronchial secretion. It depolymerises mucopolysaccharides directly as well as by liberating lysosomal enzymes. So network of fibres in tenacious sputum is broken.

Ans. 52 (C) Mucokinetics are drugs which increases bronchial secretion or reduce its viscosity and facilitating its removal by coughing.

Ans. 53 (D) Codeine, pholcodeine (but not dextropropoxphene) belong to opioids have anti-tussive effect. Non opioids, *e.g.*, noscapine, dextromethorphan, chlophedianol are also have centrally anti-tussive action.

Ans. 54 (A) Zafirleukast or leukotrine antagonists are used orally in allergic bronchial asthma.

Ans. 55 (B) Dry powders inhalers (rotacap) are used by puncturing the capsule and the aerosols are inhaled by inspiratory air flow. It require high velocity inspiration so not useful in children, elderly and very sick patients. It also causes cough and bronchoconstriction.

Ans. 56 (A) Dextromethorphan is synthetic, has selective anti-tussive action devoid of constipating and addicting action (as with codeine) and effective in dry cough.

4

DRUGS USED IN THE TREATMENT OF GASTROINTESTINAL DISORDERS

DRUG TREATMENT OF PEPTIC ULCER

Peptic ulcer is caused due to imbalance between the aggressive factors and the defense mechanism. Aggressive factors are H. pylori infection, acid secretion, pepsin and various drugs, *e.g.*, alcohol NSAIDs, histamine stress, coffee etc. Defensive factors are gastric mucous secretion, bicarbonates, tight sphincters between stomach and duodenum, prostaglandins, vasculature and normal cell renewal process.

Objectives of therapy are:

a. Relief of pain.
b. Promotion of ulcer healing.
c. Prevention of recurrence and complications.

Classification of Drugs Used in Peptic Ulcer

1. **Drugs that inhibit gastric acid secretion (Anti-secretary agents)**
   a. *Proton pump inhibitors (PPIs):* Omeprazole, Lansoprazole, Pantoprazole, Rabeprazole, Esomeprazole.
   b. *H_2 receptor antagonists:* Cimetidine, Ranitidine, Famotidine, Roxatidine, Nizatidine, Ebrotidine.
   c. *Anti-muscarinic agents (Anticholinergic agents):* Pirenzepine, Telenzepine,Propantheline, Oxyphenonium.
   d. *Prostaglandin analogues:* Misoprostol, Enprostil, Rioprostil, Arbaprostil.
2. **Drugs that enhance mucosal defense**
   a. *Prostaglandin analogues:* Misoprostol and its analogue (cyto protective).
   b. *Ulcer protective:* Sucralfate, Colloidal bismuth subcitrate (CBS).
   c. *Ulcer healing:* Carbenoxolone sodium.
3. **Drugs that neutralize gastric acid (Antacids)**
   a. *Systemic antacids:* Sodium bicarbonate, Sodium citrate.

b. *Non-systemic antacids:* Magnesium hydroxide, Magnesium trisilicate, Aluminum hydroxide gel, Calcium carbonate.

4. **Anti H. pylori drugs:** Amoxycillin, Clarithromycin, Metronidazole, Tindazole, Tetracycline.
5. **Prokinetics:** Cisapride, Metoclopramide, Domperidone (less useful).

Proton Pump Inhibitors (PPIs)

Proton pump H^+ K^+-ATPase is a membrane bound enzyme that plays an important role in the final step of gastric acid secretion. PPIs are the most powerful inhibitors of gastric acid secretion (both fasting and meal stimulated). They are prodrugs and are activated to sulfenamide and sulfenic acid at acidic pH. The activated form binds covalently with SH groups of the proton pump (selectively) and irreversibly inactivates it. So acid secretion resumes only when new H^+-K^+ ATPase molecule is synthesized. PPIs are administered orally about 30 minutes before food. They are highly bound to plasma proteins; extensively metabolized in the liver and metabolites are excreted in urine. **Rabeprazole** and **pantoprazole** are also available in IV formulation.

Adverse Effects

PPIs are generally well tolerated. The side effects are headache, diarrhea and abdominal pain. Skin rashes and arthralgia can rarely occur. Reduction in Vitamin B_{12} absorption from food, increased risk of infection due to bacterial colonization, gastric carcinoid tumor formation (in animals) may occur.

Drug Interactions

PPIs may interfere with the absorption of ketoconazole, digoxin and iron by decreasing the gastric acid secretion. Omeprazole may inhibit the metabolism of certain drugs, *e.g.*, warfarin, diazepam, phenytoin, etc. by inhibiting cytochrome P-450 enzymes and enhance the toxicity of these drugs.

Therapeutic Uses

1. Peptic ulcer:
   a. H. Pylori associated ulcer.
   b. NSAIDs associated ulcer.
   c. Prevention of re-bleeding from peptic ulcer.

2. Gastroesophageal reflux disease (GERD).
3. Zollinger-Ellison syndrome.
4. Non-ulcer dyspepsia.
5. Stress ulcers (Curling's ulcer).
6. Aspiration pneumonia.

H_2 Receptor Antagonists (H_2 Blockers)

Mechanism of Action

H_2 receptor antagonists competitively block the H_2 receptors on parietal cell and inhibit gastric acid production. They suppress the secretion of acid in all phases (basal, cephalic and gastric). They mainly suppress nocturnal acid secretion. They also reduce acid secretion stimulated by ACh, gastrin, food, stress etc. They are rapidly and completely absorbed after oral administration. Bioavailability varies from 50-60% -90%. They are minimally metabolized, major portion excreted unchanged in urine and bile.

Ranitidine: It is more potent, has longer duration of action, does not inhibit hepatic microsomal enzymes, hence drug interaction are rare. It has no anti-androgenic effect. It does not cross the BBB and hence CNS side effects are rare.

Nizatidine: It has higher bioavailability (almost 100%).

Drug interaction: Antacids reduces the absorption of all H_2 antagonists.

Therapeutic Uses

1. Peptic ulcer.
2. Zollinger-Ellison syndrome.
3. Gastroesophageal reflux disease (GERD)–Omperazole is preferred.
4. Stress ulcers/Non-ulcer dyspepsia.
5. H_2 blockers are used preoperatively.
6. Pruritis-along with H_1 antagonists.

Anticholinergic Agents

Pirenzepine, a selective M_1 receptor blocker, inhibits acid and pepsin secretion without producing side effects on the pupil, heart, bladder and bowel. It poorly penetrates BBB, therefore, CNS side effects are rare. Pirenzepine is less effective than H_2 blockers. It also have narrow therapeutic index, so not used as a first line drug.

Drugs that Enhance Mucosal Defense

Prostaglandin Analogues

Misoprostol is a synthetic PG analogue (PGE_1). It is effective orally for the prevention and treatment of NSAID induced gastric and duodenal ulcers. It inhibits gastric acid secretion by decreasing cAMP levels in the parietal cells. It increases mucus and bicarbonate secretion, increases mucosal blood flow, thus produces cyto protective effect. They strengthen gastric mucosal barrier with a reduction in H^+ ion back diffusion. They also increase renewal process. Natural PG has short t½ so their analogues (enprostil and rioprostil) are used. PGs are contraindicated in pregnancy.

Ulcer Protective

Sucralfate

It is a complex of aluminium hydroxide and sulphated sucrose. First, in acidic environment of the stomach, sucralfate undergoes extensive polymerization to form a sticky gel that adheres to the ulcer base and protects it. Secondly, it precipitates proteins at the ulcer base and forms a barrier against acid and pepsin. It stimulates the release of PGs and epidermal growth factor locally and thus produces cytoprotective effect. It also increases mucus and bicarbonate secretion and enhances mucosal defense and repair. It reduces the absorption of drugs such as digoxin, tetracycline, ketoconazole, fluoroquinolones, etc. Since it requires pH <4 for activation, concurrent administration of antacids, H_2blockers or PPIs should be avoided.

Sucralfate is effective for the prevention of bleeding from stress ulcers and to reduce the risk of aspiration pneumonia.

Colloidal–Bismuth Sub-citrate (CBS)

They have negligible neutralizing capacity. They act by:

1. React with protein in the base of the ulcer and protect it from peptic digestion.
2. Stimulate the secretion of mucus and bicarbonate through increase in PGE_2.
3. Have anti H. pylori effect that is directly kill the organism and detaches H. pylori from surface of mucosa, thus prevent relapse.

Antacids

Antacids are weak bases that neutralize gastric acid and thus raise the gastric pH. They do not affect acid production rather, reflexes more gastrin and cause rebound increase in gastric acid secretion.

Systemic Antacids

Sodium Bicarbonate ($NaHCO_3$)

It is very effective and rapidly neutralizes gastric acid, but the duration of action is short. The disadvantages of $NaHCO_3$ are:

i. It is highly water soluble and rapidly absorbed from the gut.
ii. It releases CO_2 that can cause abdominal distension and belching.
iii. It may cause metabolic alkalosis; and
iv. It produces rebound acidity.

It should be avoided in patients with hypertension and congestive cardiac failure (CCF).

Non-Systemic Antacids

They are water insoluble and largely unabsorbed. The cation (Al^{3+}, Mg^{2+}, Ca^{2+}) form chloride salt in stomach during neutralization. When they reaches to alkaline pH of the intestine, they dissociated and combined with bicarbonate and regenerate original salt. So HCO_3^- is not available for absorption, hence, there is no systemic alkalosis.

Combination of antacids produces various beneficial effects.They are:

1. Aluminium salts cause constipation and magnesium salts cause diarrhea, so combination of these two can counteract the adverse effects of each other.
2. Magnesium hydroxide has rapid onset of action, but aluminium hydroxide acts slowly, the combined product produces rapid and sustained effect.
3. Dose of individual antacid is reduced, hence systemic toxicity is minimized.

Oxethazine

It resemble with lignocaine, causes mucosal anaesthesia, so useful in reflux esophagitis when combined with antacids.

Anti-H. Pylori Agents

H. pylori, a gram negative, rod shaped bacteria, associated with gastritis, duodenal ulcer, gastric ulcer and gastric carcinoma (hostile environment of stomach). It attaches to epithelium, have high urease activity. Ammonia produced by urease activity may directly damage the cells.

Many regimens are available for the eradication of H. pylori. Combination therapy (triple/quadruple) is always recommended as single drug therapy is ineffective and chances of development of resistance are more. The objectives of combination therapy are:

- To prevent or delay the development of resistant organism.
- To prevent relapse.
- To promote rapid ulcer healing; and
- To eradicate H. pylori infection.

A. Triple therapy regimen for 14 days includes:

Omeprazole (lansoprazole)	20 mg B.D. (30 mg B.D.)
+ Clarithromycin	500 mg B.D.
or Amoxicillin	1000 mg B.D.
+ Metronidazole	500 mg B.D.
Or Tinidazole	1000 mg/day
Or tetracycline	500 mg QID

This regimen causes 90% eradication of H. pylori.

B. Quadruple therapy (for 14 days)

(a)	PPI (Omeprazole)	20 mg BD
	+Metronidazole	500 mg TDS
	+Bismuth sub salicylate	525 mg QID
	+Tetracycline	500 mg QID
(b)	H_2 antagonist (Ranitidine)	150 mg BD
	+ Bismuth sub salicylate	525 mg QID
	+Metronidazole	250 mg TDS
	+Tetracycline	500 mg QID

ANTI-EMETIC DRUGS

The drugs which are used to prevent or control vomiting are called antiemetic drugs.

Classification

1. **Anticholinergic:** Scopolamine (hyoscine), Dicyclomine.
2. **Antihistamines (H_1 blockers):** Dimenhydrinate, Diphenhydramine, Cyclizine, Meclizine, Hydroxyzine and Promethazine, Doxylamine.
3. **5-HT_3receptor antagonists:** Ondansetron, Granisetron, Dolasetron and Palonosetron.
4. **Prokinetic drugs:** Metoclopramide, Domperidone, Cisapride, Mosapride and Tegaserod.
5. **Neuroleptics:** Chlorpromazine, Fluphenazine, Prochlorperazine and Haloperidol.
6. **Adjuvant antiemetic:**
   a. *Glucocorticoids:* Betamethasone, Dexamethasone and Methylprednisolone.
   b. *Benzodiazepines:* Lorazepam and Alprazolam.
   c. *Cannabinoids:* Dronabinol.
   d. *Vitamin B_6* (Pyridoxine).

Anticholinergic

Scopolamine is the drug of choice to prevent motion sickness. It blocks the afferent impulses to the vomiting centre by its anticholinergic action. Scopolamine is not effective for other types of vomiting. It has brief duration of action and has other anti-cholinergic side effects.

Antihistamines (H_1 Blockers)

H_1 blockers are mainly useful for the prevention of motion sickness. They are also effective in morning sickness, postoperative and other types of vomiting. Their antiemetic effect is due to sedative and central anticholinergic properties. Cyclizine has the shortest duration of action (8 hours), and meclizine has the longest duration of action (24 hours).

5-HT_3 Receptor Antagonists

Their antiemetic effect is mainly due to the blockade of 5-HT_3 receptors on vagal afferents in the gut. In addition, they also block 5-HT_3 receptors in the CTZ and solitary tract nucleus (STN). 5-HT_3 antagonists are well-absorbed after oral administration, ondansetron and other undergoes extensive first pass metabolism. The metabolites are excreted in the urine and faeces. These agents are also available for intravenous administration.

Granisetron is more potent than ondansetron. Palonosetron is more efficacious and longer acting than all three drugs and have long plasma half life, *i.e.*, 40 hours.

Uses

1. For prevention as well as the treatment of anti-cancer drug induced nausea and vomiting (cellular damage due to cytotoxic drugs causes release of various mediators including 5-HT from intestine, which causes vomiting), in post-operative and post-radiation vomiting and to control vomiting in children with cyclic vomiting syndrome.
2. $5\text{-}HT_3$ antagonists are also effective in post-operative vomiting, due to overdose of drugs, uremia and some neurological disorders.

Side Effects

They may cause headache, dizziness and constipation, prolongation of QT interval (especially with dolasetron).

Prokinetic Drugs

Metoclopramide

Metoclopramide is a D_2receptor antagonist, $5\text{-}HT_4$ agonist and $5\text{-}HT_3$ antagonist. It has two important actions:

Central Actions

Metoclopramide blocks D_2 receptors in CTZ. At high concentrations, it also blocks $5\text{-}HT_3$ receptors.

Prokinetic Effect on Upper GIT

Metoclopramide causes release of ACh from myenteric neurons and has prokinetic effect on upper GIT and enhances the rate of gastric and duodenal emptying. These effects may be due to cholinergic, serotonergic ($5\text{-}HT_4$ agonist action), antidopaminergic effects, and it also has direct action on the smooth muscles of upper GIT. Thus, it:

1. Increases the tone of the lower esophageal sphincter (LES).
2. Increase the tone and amplitude of antral contractions.
3. Relax the pyloric sphincter and duodenal bulb.
4. Increase the peristalsis of small intestine and promotes forward propulsion of the content of the upper GIT.

Pharmacokinetics

It rapidly absorbed after oral administration. It has a short half life of 4 hours; poorly bound to plasma proteins; crosses BBB and placenta. Most of the drug is excreted unchanged in urine. In renal diseases, the dose of metoclopramide should be reduced to half of the usual dose.

Adverse Effects

Drowsiness, dizziness and diarrhea are common. Extra pyramidal symptoms, occur due to blockade of D_2 receptors in basal ganglia, disappear after withdrawal of the drug. Long-term use may lead to gynaecomastia, galactorrhoea and menstrual irregularities by blocking the inhibitory effect of dopamine on prolactin release.

Uses

1. *As an antiemetic:* Vomiting due to gastrointestinal disorders, drug induced, post-operative, migraine, radiation sickness and cancer chemotherapy.
2. It is less effective against motion sickness and vomiting due to labyrinthine disorders.
3. It may be used in gastroesophageal reflux disease (GERD) but is less effective than PPI and H_2 blockers.
4. To alleviate symptoms associated with gastric stasis in patients with diabetes, post-operative or idiopathic gastroparesis.
5. Metoclopramide has been used in the treatment of intractable hiccups.

Domperidone

Its antiemetic and prokinetic effects are due to blockade of dopamine (D_2) receptors in upper GIT (also act on CTZ not protected by BBB). It is less potent and less efficacious than metoclopramide. It does not cross the BBB and hence extra pyramidal side effects are rare, but it increases the prolactin level. Domperidone is usually administered orally, have extensive first pass effect; preferred antiemetic in children. Side effects are dry mouth, diarrhoea, headache, skin rashes, galactorrhoea and menstrual irregularities. Cardiac arrhythmias have developed on rapid I.V. injection (so no IV preparations are available).

Uses

Domperidone is used in L-dopa induced vomiting. Other indications are similar to metoclopramide.

Cisapride

Because of its serious cardiac toxicity specially when used with drugs inhibiting CYP3A4, *e.g.*, macrolides, it is withdrawn.

Mosapride

A congener of cisapride with action similar effect on LES tone (as with metoclopramide, domperidone) due to 5-HT_4 agonist and 5-HT_3 antagonist action.

Tegaserod

It is selective 5-HT_4 partial agonist with no action on 5-HT_3 receptors. It also increases colonic Cl^- (and water) secretion so used in IBS (constipation predominant).

Neuroleptics

They are potent anti-emetics. They act by blocking D_2 receptors in the CTZ. In addition, they have anticholinergic and antihistaminic actions.

Prochlorperazine is commonly used as an antiemetic.

Uses

1. Drug induced vomiting.
2. Vomiting due to gastroenteritis.
3. Morning sickness.

Drugs Used in Different Types of Emesis

- During pregnancy–doxinate (anti-histamines are preferred).
- Vomiting due to radiation sickness/chemotherapy–Ondansetron is preferred.
- Motion sickness–scopolamine, promethazine is preferred.

Adjuvant Anti-Emetics

a. **Cannabinoids (Dronabinol):** It is the principal psychoactive component of marijuana and is used to prevent cancer chemotherapy induced vomiting in patients refractory to other antiemetic. It produces serious side effects such as sedation, hallucinations, disorientation, increased appetite and drug dependence, hence kept as a reserve drug.
b. **Benzodiazepines:** Lorazepam and alprazolam are used to control psychogenic and anticipatory vomiting due to their sedative, amnesic and anti-anxiety effects.

c. **Corticosteroids:** Dexamethasone augments the anti-emetic effect of other primary drugs.

d. **Pyridoxine (Vitamin B_6).**

DRUGS USED IN DIARRHEA AND INFLAMMATORY BOWEL DISEASE

Management of Diarrhea

1. **Non-specific therapy**
   a. Oral and parenteral rehydration solutions.
   b. Anti-motility and anti-secretary agents.
      i. *Opioid:* Codeine, Diphenoxylate, Loperamide.
      ii. *Alpha adrenergic receptor agonists:* Clonidine.
      iii. *Octreotide.*
2. **Specific therapy:** Antimicrobial agents.

Anti Motility and Anti Secretary Agents

Loperamide

It is an opiate analogue and has more potent anti diarrheal effect than morphine. By interacting with μ opioid receptors in the gut, loperamide reduces GI motility and increases the anal sphincter tone. It also has anti secretary activity against cholera and some forms of Escherichia coli toxin. It poorly penetrates the BBB and has no abuse potential.

Anti-motility drugs produce only symptomatic relief in diarrhea and should be avoided in acute infectious diarrheas.

Pharmacotherapy of Inflammatory Bowel Disease (IBD)

IBD includes Crohn's disease and ulcerative colitis, which are characterized by diarrhea, bleeding, abdominal discomfort, anaemia and weight loss.

Drug Used in IBS

1. **5-Aminosalicylic acid (5-ASA) agents:** Sulphasalazine, Mesalazine, Olsalazine.
2. **Antibiotics:** Metronidazole, Ciprofloxacin.
3. **Glucocorticoids:** Prednisolone, Methylprednisolone, Hydrocortisone.
4. **Immunomodulators:** Azathioprine, 6 Mercaptopurine, Methotrexate, Infliximab.

Sulphasalazine

It is a prodrug and is composed of sulphapyridine and 5-aminosalicylic acid (5-ASA). On oral administration sulphasalazine reaches the colon, where it is broken down by colonic bacteria to 5-ASA and sulphapyridine. The released 5-ASA acts locally by inhibiting the production of inflammatory mediators such as interleukin (IL-1), tumor necrosis factor (TNF alpha), leukotrienes (LTs), etc. Sulphapyridine gets absorbed and causes many side effects like nausea, vomiting and headache.

Mesalazine and Olsalazine

Mesalazine is a 5-ASA. Olsalazine is composed of two molecules of 5-ASA with a linkage and given as special formulations (delayed release capsules or pH dependent tablets). Mesalazine can be administered as suppository or enema. Mesalazine and olsalazine have a lower incidence of side effects than sulphasalazine.

DRUGS USED IN CONSTIPATION (LAXATIVES)

Laxatives (Purgatives, Cathartics)

Laxatives–they have mild action with soft but formed stool.

Purgatives–strong action with evacuation of watery stool.

Classification

1. **Bulk purgatives:** Dietary fibers; Bran, Methylcellulose, Ispaghula (isabgol).
2. **Stool softeners:** Docusates (DOSS), Liquid paraffin.
3. **Stimulant or irritant purgatives:** Phenolphthalein, Bisacodyl, Castor oil.
4. **Anthraquinone derivatives:** Senna, Cascara.
5. **Osmotic/Saline purgatives:** Magnesium sulphate, Magnesium hydroxide, Sodium phosphate, Sodium sulphate, Sodium potassium tartarate, Lactulose.
6. **Prokinetic agents:** 5-HT_4 agonist, Tegaserod.

Bulk Forming Laxatives

They are indigestible, hydrophilic substances which absorb water, swell up and increase the bulk of the stools. They cause mechanical distension, so stimulate peristalsis and promote defecation. Drawback of bulk formatting laxatives are, they are unpalatable and large quantity is required.

Stool Softners

They lower the surface tension of stool, thereby cause the accumulation of fluid and fatty substance and thus soften the stools. They emulsify the colonic content and increases penetration of water into feces.

Liquid Paraffin

It penetrates and softens the stools in 2-3 days. It also has lubricant effect and thus helps in smooth defecation. It is a preferred laxative in patients with cardiac disease and pregnancy.

Adverse Effects of Liquid Paraffin

1. Lipid pneumonia.
2. Malabsorption of vitamin A, D, E and K (fat soluble vitamins).
3. Leakage of fecal matter through anal sphincter may lead to soiling of clothes.

Stimulant (Irritant) Purgatives

These agents have direct action on enteric neurons and GI mucosa. They increase prostaglandin and cyclic adenosine monophosphate (cAMP) levels, but inhibit Na^+- K^+ -ATPase activity in the intestinal mucosa. This causes an increased secretion of water and electrolytes by the mucosa and thus stimulates peristalsis. The site of action is on large intestine.

Osmotic (Saline) Purgatives

Osmotic/saline purgatives are the most powerful and rapid acting agents. When given orally, they are not absorbed from the gut. They remain in the lumen and exert osmotic effect. They draw water into the lumen, distend the bowel, which then stimulates peristalsis. To mask the bitter taste, they are often administered with fruit juice.

Prokinetic Agent

Tegaserod, a partial 5-HT_4 agonist, exhibits prokinetic activity by stimulating peristalsis. It is effective in the treatment of constipation predominant irritable bowel syndrome.

Contraindications of laxatives:

1. Patient with undiagnosed abdominal pain.
2. Organic constipation due to stricture or obstruction in bowel.

Uses of Purgatives with Preparation of Choice

1. Acute functional constipation–Bulk laxatives.
2. To avoid straining during defecation in patients with cardiovascular disease, eye surgery, hernia–Bulk laxatives.
3. In patients with hepatic coma to reduce the blood ammonia level—lactulose.
4. Preoperatively in bowel surgery, colonoscopy and abdominal X-ray Osmotic purgatives or bisacodyl.
5. Following certain anthelmintics (*e.g.* for Taenia solium) Osmotic purgatives to expel the worm segments.
6. In drug poisoning to wash out the poisonous material from the gut Osmotic purgatives.

MULTIPLE CHOICE QUESTIONS

Q. 1 The H_2 receptor antagonist which has maximum oral bioavailability is:

(A) Nizatidine (B) Famotidine
(C) Ranitidine (D) Zolentidine

Q. 2 Antacids decrease the bioavailability of all of the following drugs *except:*

(A) Iron (B) Tetracycline
(C) Isoniazid (D) Quinolone

Q. 3 All of the following are congeners of prostaglandin useful in the therapy of peptic ulcer *except:*

(A) Rioprostil (B) Misoprostil
(C) Enprostil (D) Alprostadil

Q. 4 All of the following are rapidly acting antacids *except:*

(A) Calcium carbonate (B) Magnesium hydroxide
(C) Aluminium hydroxide (D) Sodium bicarbonate

Q. 5 Which of the following is long acting H_2 blocker?

(A) Cimetidine (B) Nizatidine
(C) Ranitidine (D) Famotidine

Q. 6 All are the correct statements regarding H_2 blockers *except:*

(A) Increase healing rate of peptic ulcer
(B) Prevent relapse
(C) Decrease all phases of acid secretion
(D) Produce healing in early carcinoma

Q. 7 All drug can be used in case of gastroesophageal reflux disease (GERD) during pregnancy *except:*

(A) Antacids (B) Sucralfate
(C) Ranitidine (D) Omeprazole

Q. 8 Aluminium hydroxide can be used in:

(A) Renal stones (B) Chronic renal failure
(C) Hyperphosphatemia (D) Osteomalacia

---

1 (A) 2 (C) 3 (D) 4 (C) 5 (D) 6 (D) 7 (D) 8 (C)

Q. 9 Concurrent use of antacids decreases the effectiveness of all *except:*

(A) Colloidal bismuth (B) Sucralfate
(C) Carbenoxolone (D) Pirenzepine

Q. 10 Ranitidine is given by intravenous infusion in the following condition:

(A) For rapid relief of gastric ulcer pain
(B) NSAIDs induced ulcer
(C) Prophylaxis of gastric mucosa erosion in patients with extensive burns
(D) Reflux oesophagitis

Q. 11 Which of the following drug inhibits round the clock gastric output?

(A) Ranitidine
(B) Cimetidine
(C) Omeprazole
(D) Pirenzepine

Q. 12 Misoprostol is a:

(A) Prostaglandin E_1 analogue
(B) Prostaglandin E_2 analogue
(C) Prostaglandin antagonist
(D) Anti progestin

Q. 13 All drugs can be used in the treatment of H. pylori infection *except:*

(A) Omeprazole (B) Metronidazole
(C) Amoxicillin (D) Mosapride

Q. 14 True statement regarding the use of combination of ranitidine and sucralfate is:

(A) Ranitidine decrease the action of sucralfate
(B) Combination of these two produces serious side effect like agranulocytosis
(C) Ranitidine decreases the gastric pH, so sucralfate is not able to act
(D) Sucralfate inhibits absorption of ranitidine

9 (D) 10 (C) 11 (C) 12 (A) 13 (D) 14 (D)

Q. 15 Gynaecomastia may be caused by:

(A) Cimetidine (B) Ranitidine
(C) Famotidine (D) Nizetidine

Q. 16 True statement about omeprazole is:

(A) It may cause leiomyosarcoma
(B) It is a nitro source
(C) May induce carcinoid tumors in rats
(D) It is more frequently used by the IV route than orally

Q. 17 The correct statement about magaldrate is:

(A) It is a mixture of magnesium sulphate and aluminium hydroxide
(B) It has a rapid as well as sustained acid neutralizing action
(C) Its acid neutralizing capacity is 2-3 mEq/gm
(D) It causes systemic alkalosis

Q. 18 In peptic ulcer antacids are now primarily used for:

(A) Prompt pain relief
(B) Ulcer healing
(C) Preventing ulcer relapse
(D) Control of bleeding from the ulcer

Q. 19 Which of the following is not true of anti H. pylori therapy?

(A) Two weeks regimen is less efficacious than one week regimen
(B) Resistance to any single antimicrobial drug develops rapidly
(C) Concurrent suppression of gastric acid enhances efficacy of the regimen
(D) Colloidal bismuth directly inhibits H. pylori but has poor patient acceptability

Q. 20 The primary mechanism by which prostaglandins promote ulcer healing is:

(A) Inhibition of gastric acid secretion
(B) Augmentation of bicarbonate buffered mucus layer covering gastro duodenal mucosa
(C) Increased bicarbonate secretion in gastric juice
(D) Increased turnover of gastric mucosal cells

15 (A) 16 (C) 17 (B) 18 (A) 19 (A) 20 (B)

Q. 21 The following anti ulcer drug does not act by reducing the secretion of or neutralizing gastric acid:

(A) Magaldrate
(B) Sucralfate
(C) Misoprostol
(D) Omeprazole

Q. 22 Proton pump inhibitors are most effective when they are given:

(A) After meals
(B) Shortly before breakfast
(C) Along with H_2 antagonist
(D) During prolonged fasting period

Q. 23 The antacid preferred for heartburn for long term in patients with hypertension is:

(A) Sodium bicarbonate
(B) Calcium carbonate
(C) Magnesium hydroxide
(D) Combination of magnesium hydroxide and aluminium hydroxide

Q. 24 Pharmacological effects of H_2-receptor antagonists include all of the following *except:*

(A) Inhibition of gastric acid secretion by histamine
(B) Inhibition of acid secretion elicited by gastrin and muscarinic agonist
(C) Inhibition of basal, nocturnal and stimulated acid secretion
(D) Reduction of both volume of gastric acid secretion and its H^+ ion concentration

Q. 25 Oral prostaglandin analogue useful in peptic ulcer is:

(A) Prosten E_2 (B) 15 methyl PGE_1
(C) 15 methyl PGF_2 alpha (D) PGE_2

Q. 26 Which one of the following agent suppress emetic (CTZ) centre and useful during pregnancy?

(A) Prochlorperazine (B) Metoclopramide
(C) Cyclizine (D) Trifluoperazine

21 (B) 22 (B) 23 (D) 24 (D) 25 (D) 26 (C)

Q. 27 The most dependable emetic used to expel ingested poison is:

(A) Intramuscular emetine
(B) Oral syrup ipecacuanha
(C) Intramuscular apomorphine
(D) Oral bromocriptine

Q. 28 The most effective drug preferred for short brisk journies is:

(A) Promethazine (B) Cinnerizine
(C) Domperidone (D) Hyoscine

Q. 29 Phenothiazines (chlorpromazine and its congeners) suppress vomiting of following etiology *except:*

(A) Motion sickness (B) Radiation sickness
(C) Post anaesthetic (D) Uremic

Q. 30 The drug which act as prokinetic, blocks both D_2 as well as 5-HT_3 receptors and increase in acetylcholine release is:

(A) Cisapride (B) Prochlorperazine
(C) Metoclopramide (D) Domperidone

Q. 31 Which antiemetic selectively blocks levodopa induced vomiting without blocking its anti-parkinsonian action?

(A) Metoclopramide (B) Cisapride
(C) Domperidone (D) Ondansetron

Q. 32 True statement regarding prokinetic is that they:

(A) Act as adjuvant to proton pump inhibitors
(B) Blocks dopamine D_2 receptors
(C) Promotes healing of esophagitis
(D) Activate muscarinic M_3 receptors

Q. 33 Ondansetron is effective as an antiemetic in all of the following *except:*

(A) Cisplatin induced vomiting
(B) Radiotherapy induced vomiting
(C) Postoperative vomiting
(D) Motion sickness

27 (C) 28 (D) 29 (A) 30 (C) 31 (C) 32 (A) 33 (D)

Q. 34 Which drug is used to control cancer chemotherapy induced vomiting not controlled by metoclopramide alone?

(A) Amphetamine
(B) Dexamethasone
(C) Hyoscine
(D) Cyclizine

Q. 35 The antibiotic which acts as a prokinetic agent by stimulating motilin receptor is:

(A) Tetracycline
(B) Streptomycin
(C) Erythromycin
(D) Ciprofloxacin

Q. 36 All of the following drugs can be used in motion sickness *except:*

(A) Hyoscine
(B) Dicyclomine
(C) Domperidone
(D) Promethazine

Q. 37 Which laxative to be avoided in renal failure?

(A) Liquid paraffin
(B) Magnesium sulphate
(C) Methyl cellulose
(D) Bisacodyl

Q. 38 Overuse of irritant purgative will cause:

(A) Spastic colon
(B) Electrolyte depletion
(C) Melanosis coli
(D) Vitamin D deficiency

Q. 39 All is true about liquid paraffin *except:*

(A) Lubricates feces
(B) Increases absorption of Vitamin A
(C) May cause aspiration pneumonia
(D) Can be given during pregnancy

Q. 40 Irrespective of the type, all laxative exerts the following action:

(A) Increase the content of solids in the feces
(B) Increase the water content of feces
(C) Reduce absorption of nutrients
(D) Increase intestinal motility

Q. 41 Which purgative may cause cardiac toxicity when used for long period (regularly)?

(A) Bisacodyl
(B) Liquid paraffin
(C) Methyl cellulose
(D) Phenolphthlein

---

34 (B) 35 (C) 36 (C) 37 (B) 38 (A) 39 (B) 40 (B) 41 (D)

Q. 42 Stimulant purgatives are contraindicated in which of the following condition?

(A) Bed ridden patients (B) Before abdominal radiography
(C) Spastic constipation (D) Atonic constipation

Q. 43 Saline osmotic purgatives are used for:

(A) Treatment of constipation
(B) Prevention of constipation in patients of piles
(C) Avoidance of straining at stools in patients of hernia
(D) Tapeworm infestation: following niclosamide administration

Q. 44 The laxative which is helpful in managing chronic hepatic encephalopathy is:

(A) Glycerin (B) Lactulose
(C) Sorbitol (D) Mannitol

Q. 45 The success of oral rehydration therapy of diarrhea depends upon the following process in the intestinal mucosa:

(A) Sodium pump mediated Na^+ absorption
(B) Glucose coupled Na^+ absorption
(C) Bicarbonate coupled Na^+ absorption
(D) Passive Na^+ diffusion secondary to nutrient absorption

Q. 46 Oral rehydration therapy has following beneficial *effects:*

(A) Stops further diarrhea
(B) Restores hydration and electrolyte balance
(C) Hastens clearance of the entero pathogen
(D) Obviates the need for specific antimicrobial therapy

Q. 47 Which of the following statement is not true about loperamide?

(A) It is absorbed and exerts centrally mediated anti diarrheal action
(B) It acts on the opioid receptors in the gut
(C) It increases tone and segmenting activity of the intestine
(D) It inhibits intestinal secretion by binding to calmodulin in the mucosal cells

---

42 (C) 43 (D) 44 (B) 45 (B) 46 (B) 47 (A)

Q. 48 Atropine is added to diphenoxylate in anti diarrheal preparation mainly to:

(A) Potentiate is anti diarrheal action
(B) Block its cholinergic side effects
(C) Discourage abuse of this opioid preparation
(D) Reduce systemic absorption of diphenoxylate

Q. 49 Drug of choice in ulcerative colitis is:

(A) 5-aminosalicylic acid (B) Sucralfate
(C) Metronidazole (D) Misoprostol

Q. 50 The therapeutic effect of sulfasalazine in ulcerative colitis is exerted by:

(A) Inhibitory action of unabsorbed drug on the abnormal colonic flora
(B) Breakdown of the drug in colon to release 5-aminosalicylic acid which suppresses inflammation locally
(C) Release of sulfapyridine having antibacterial property
(D) Systemic immuno modulatory action of the drug

Q. 51 Which of the following drug would be best to use to treat irritable bowel syndrome (IBS)?

(A) Infliximab (B) Diphenoxylate
(C) Tegaserod (D) Orlistat

Q. 52 The following drugs are used in obesity *except:*

(A) Orlistat
(B) Silbutaramine
(C) Olestra
(D) Neuropeptide Y (NPY) antagonist

48 (C) 49 (A) 50 (B) 51 (C) 52 (D)

ANSWERS

Ans. 1 (A) Nizatidine and roxatidine, both have maximum oral bioavailability (>90%) as compare to ranitidine and famotidine (around 50%) but roxatidine is more potent than nizatidine.

Ans. 2 (C) By forming inert complexes, Al^{3+}, Ca^{2+} and Mg^{2+} group of antacids decrease the absorption and bioavailability of tetracycline, fluroquinolones, itraconazole, digoxin and iron salts. They also decrease the absorption of acidic drugs like barbiturates phenytoin and NSAIDs, so should not be given within 2 hours of administration of these drugs. But antacid do not affect the absorption of isoniazid.

Ans. 3 (D) Misoprostol is a methyl analogue of PGE_1 while enprostil and rioprostil are PGE_2 analogue useful in peptic ulcer. Alprostadil is used in congenital heart disease (CHD).

Ans. 4 (C) Sodium bicarbonate, calcium carbonate, magnesium salts are rapidly acting antacids while aluminium hydroxide is having slow and sustained effect.

Ans. 5 (D) Famotidine exhibits longer duration of action despite an elimination t ½ of 2.5 – 3.5 hours. Some inverse antagonistic action also has been demonstrated with famotidine.

Ans. 6 (D) H_2 blocker suppresses all phases of acid secretion (basal, psychic, neurogenic and gastric) in dose dependent manner but basal nocturnal secretion is suppressed more completely. It also decreases the secretary response due to ACh, histamine, gastrin, insulin, alcohol food etc. The acid volume, pepsin content, and intrinsic factor secretion is also reducing without causing Vitamin B_{12} deficiency even after prolonged use. But it is not effective in carcinoma.

Ans. 7 (D) Mild cases of GERD during pregnancy should be treated with antacids and sucralfate. But if symptoms persist ranitidine (having the establish data) to be used among H_2 antagonists. Proton pump inhibitors should be avoided (Omeprazole have FDA category C), but in complicated cases lansoprazole is preferred (based on animal data).

Ans. 8 (C) Aluminium hydroxide is useful in hyperphophatemia as it binds with phosphates in the intestine and prevents its absorption and hypophosphatemia occurs on regular use.

It causes osteomalacia. It is excreted by kidney and may cause encephalopathy, osteoporosis in renal failure so not used in chronic renal failure. It is also not a very potent drug to be used in Z.E. syndrome.

Ans. 9 **(D)** Antacids reduces the effectiveness of sucralfat, colloidal bismuth carbonate and carbenoxolone, as for their action acidic pH is required while pirenzepine action is receptor (M_1) mediated and its effect is not affected by change in pH.

Ans. 10 **(C)** Intravenous ranitidine is indicated as an infusion for prophylaxis of stress ulcer (with extensive burn which may cause bleeding) or in ZE syndrome.

Ans. 11 **(C)** Omeprazole cause dose dependent suppression of gastric acid secretion without anti cholinergic or H_2 blockade action. It is powerful inhibitor of gastric acid and totally abolish HCl secretion, both resting as well as that stimulated by food etc.

Ans. 12 **(A)** Misoprostol is a PGE_1 analogue. Prostaglandins play an important role in gastric defense mechanism. They inhibit acid secretion (PGE_2) by inhibiting production of gastrin, cAMP, increase mucosal blood flow and have cyto protective role. PGE_2 have very short half life, misoprostol is stable analogue of PGE_1 and helps in healing of ulcer (NSAIDs and smoking induced).

Ans. 13 **(D)** Treatment of H. pylori includes triple drug combination therapy which include omeprazole, clarithromycin amoxicillin or metronidazole, but not mosapride (for details see text).

Ans. 14 **(D)** Sucralfate inhibits absorption of ranitidine. Sucralfate act by polymerization in acidic medium and form sticky like gel over ulcer crater which act as physical barrier. Dietary and mucosal proteins also get absorbed over this coat forming another layer of protection. It may stimulate mucosal PGE_2 synthesis and bicarbonate secretion. It also helps in mucosal repair and ulcer healing. It reduces the upper GIT bleeding in critically ill patients (as other acid inhibitory therapy may cause or increase the risk of nosocomial pneumonia).

Ans. 15 (A) Cimetidine but not other H_2 antagonist has anti androgenic effect, increases plasma prolactin and inhibits degradation of estradiol. So may cause gynaecomastia, loss of libido and impotence.

Ans. 16 (C) Omeprazole, a proton pump inhibitor, causes marked and long lasting acid suppression. This raise the gastrin secretion which stimulates hyperplasia and gastric carcinoid tumors may develop in areas of hyperplasia (proved in female rats).

Ans. 17 (B) Magaldrate is a hydrated complex of aluminium magnesium hydroxide sulfate. When it reacts with HCl, it rapidly releases aluminium hydroxide and magnesium hydroxide which have prompt and sustained neutralizing effect.

Ans. 18 (A) Antacids are used OTC for treatment of intermittent heart burn and dyspepsia.

Ans. 19 (A) Two weeks triple drug therapy with omperazole is more efficacious than one weak therapy. This triple regimen prevents/delays the development of resistance with antimicrobial. Omeprazole potentiate the action of this therapy by increasing gastric pH (see text also).

Ans. 20 (B) Prostaglandin analogue prompt ulcer healing by making bicarbonate/mucus layer on ulcer.

Ans. 21 (B) Sucralfate act by making physical barrier and covering ulcer crater.

Ans. 22 (B) Proton pump inhibitors, *e.g.*, omeprazole, are prodrug and converted into active metabolite in presence of acidic pH and are more effective in acidic pH.

Ans. 23 (D) Both sodium carbonate and calcium carbonate are not for long term use. Also sodium bicarbonate is contraindicated in hypertension. The combination of magnesium and aluminium salt is the best choice as it provide balance between the diarrhea associated with magnesium hydroxide and constipation with aluminum hydroxide.

Ans. 24 (D) H_2 receptor antagonists are effective in reducing gastric secretion not only by histamine stimulation but by gastrin, food, alcohol etc. It reduces volume of gastric acid but not H^+ ion concentration.

Ans. 25 (D) PGE_2 markedly reduces the acid secretion in the stomach, increases mucous production and mucous blood flow and are anti ulcerogenic but are short acting.

Ans. 26 (C) Morning sickness (in pregnancy) is due to the effect of increased estrogen levels on CTZ and causes hyperemesis. Anti histamines, *e.g.*, doxylamine, cyclizine, meclizine can be used (doxylamine is safest). All other are not the preferred drugs.

Ans. 27 (C) Intramuscular apomorphine is used to expel ingested poison. Ipecacuanha also a potent emetic but less dependable then parenteral apomorphine but it is safer than apomorphine.

Ans. 28 (D) Hyoscine is useful in motion sickness due to stimulation of vestibular nuclei (centrally acting anticholinergics are effective).

Ans. 29 (A) Phenothiazines are not effective in vomiting due to motion sickness, where hyoscine is more effective.

Ans. 30 (C) Metoclopramide is a D_2 and 5-HT_3 receptor antagonist, and 5-HT_4 agonist. Being a D_2 receptor antagonist, it increases ACh release while 5-HT_4 agonist causes prokinetic effect. Thus it increases LES tone, facilitate gastric peristalsis and increase gastric motility.

Ans. 31 (C) Domperidone is a peripheral D_2 receptor blocker so can be used to prevent emetic side effect of levodopa and bromocriptine.

Ans. 32 (A) Prokinetic agents stimulate GIT motility, increase LES pressure, increase gastric emptying, and stimulate small intestinal movement (hence effective in paralytic ileus, enhance colonic transit (useful in constipation), so act as adjuvant to PPI in GERD for acid suppression.

Ans. 33 (D) Ondansetron or 5-HT_3 antagonists, is not effective in motion sickness. It does not block dopamine receptor or apomorphine or motion sickness induced vomiting.

Ans. 34 (B) Adjuvant anti emetics, *e.g.*, corticosteroids, benzodiazepines cannabinoids can be used in chemotherapy induced emesis not respond to metoclopramide or ondansetron.

Ans. 35 (C) Macrolide antibiotics like erythromycin, azithromycin and clarithromycin directly stimulate motilin receptors on GIT smooth muscles and promote upper gastrointestinal motility, increase LES tone and stimulate small intestine contractility, but have no effect on colonic motility.

Ans. 36 (C) Domperidone is a D_2 blocker and does not possess anti cholinergic effects. For a drug to be useful in motion sickness, it must have central anti cholinergic action.

Ans. 37 (B) Osmotic purgatives (saline purgatives), *e.g.*, magnesium sulfate, magnesium hydroxide are hyperosmolar agents and may lead to intravascular fluid depletion and electrolyte imbalance. They (magnesium salts) should not be used in hypertension, CCF and in patients with renal insufficiency due to risk of hypermagnesaemia.

Ans. 38 (A) Irritant purgatives, *e.g.*, bisacodyl sodium sulfate can cause colonic atonys steatorrhoea and hypokalemia on prolonged or overdosing.

Ans. 39 (B) Liquid paraffin is a fecal lubricant and make stool soft by retarding water absorption though used occasionally, it is useful where straining at defecation is avoided, *e.g.*, during pregnancy. But it decreases the absorption of fat soluble vitamins (A, D, E and K) as they are carried away with stools. It also leads to aspiration lipid pneumonia. It may interfere with healing in the ano rectal region.

Ans. 40 (B) All laxative/purgative increases water content of feces by osmotic action, decreasing absorption or by increasing propulsive activity allowing less time for absorption of salt and water and causes laxative effect.

Ans. 41 (D) Phenolphethalein causes cardiac toxicity and is carcinogenic.

Ans. 42 (C) Stimulant purgative should not be used in spastic constipation.

Ans. 43 (D) Saline purgatives or senna may be used to flush out the dead worm and the anthelmintic drug.

Ans. 44 (B) In hepato encephalopathy there is a severe hepatocellular damage and several toxic metabolites from the colon (NH_3) get accumulated in the blood leading to CNS toxicity. Lectulose is degraded to lactic acid and converts NH_3 to ionized NH_4^+ salt which is then excreted.

Ans. 45 (B) The molar ratio of glucose (higher than Na^+) will be utilized which helps in absorbing Na^+ in the intestinal secretion in addition to present in ORS.

Ans. 46 (B) ORS restores hydration and electrolyte balance.

Ans. 47 (A) Loperamide is an opiate analogue with major peripheral μ (mu) opioid and weak anticholinergic property. Because of its poor water solubility, little is absorbed from the intestine and entry in brain is negligible. So CNS effects are rare. All such drugs are useful in traveler's diarrhea.

Ans. 48 (C) Opioid agonists, *e.g.*, loperamide, diphenoxylate, difenoxin and racecadortil act by stimulating mu (μ) receptors. They have negligible analgesic activity, does not cross BBB, so devoid of abuse liability. But higher doses of diphenoxylate may depresses CNS and exhibit dependence liability, so small doses of atropine is added, which provide antispasmodic effect, as well as prevents possible abuse effect of diphenoxylate due to undesirable effects.

Ans. 49 (A) Amino salicylates, *e.g.*, sulfasalazine, olsalazine balsalazine and mesalamine (a new drug) they have only topical anti-inflammatory action when giving orally. They inhibit PG synthesis as well as production of cytokines which is responsible for inflammation. Anti diarrhoeal should be avoided in the patients of ulcerative colitis as they can lead to perforation of colon.

Ans. 50 (B) 5 amino salicylic acid suppress inflammation locally.

Ans. 51 (C) Tegaserod has 5-HT_4 receptor agonist and promotes gastric emptying facilitate small and large bowel transit. Antiemetic/prokinetic drugs have been shown to provide some relief of IBS (constipation predominant) while infliximab is a biological agent used in the treatment of inflammatory bowel disease.

Ans. 52 (D) Neuropeptide Y is appetite stimulant, decreases energy expenditure. It is a co-transmitter in sympathetic neuron and suppresses sympathetic activity. NPY receptors are G-protein coupled receptors. While all other suppress appetite and used in the obesity.

5

CARDIOVASCULAR SYSTEM

DIURETICS AND ANTI-DIURETICS

Diuretics

Kidney is the excretory organ of our body which serves the important functions of excretion of waste products (urea, uric acid), regulation of fluid volume and electrolyte content of the extracellular fluid. **Diuretics** are the agent which increases urine and solute excretion. These drugs can modify renal function directly or indirectly by modifying renal circulation and filtration. Diuretics may be classified as follows:

1. **High efficacy diuretics:** These agents act on ascending limb of Henles' loop (High ceiling or loop diuretic): Furosemide, Bumetanide, Piretanide, Ethacrynic acid, Torsemide, Azosemide, Tripamide.
2. **Moderate efficacy diuretics:** These agents act on distal convoluted tubule.

   Thiazides: Chlorothiazide, Hydrochlorothiazide, Polythiazide, Bendroflumethiazide, Cyclopenthiazide, Chlorthalidone, Clopamide, Indapamide, Metolazone, Xipamide.
3. **Low efficacy diuretics:** These agents act at cortical collecting tubule.They may be:
   - *Potassium sparing diuretics:* Triamterene, Amiloride, Spironolactone, Indacrinone, Canrenone.
   - *Carbonic anhydrase inhibitors:* These agents act on proximal tubule: Acetazolamide, Methazolamide, Dorzolamide, Dichlorophenamide.
   - *Osmotic diuretic:* Mannitol, Urea, Glycerol.
4. **Newer agents:** Vasopressin antagonist–Tolvaptan, conivaptan, Lixivaptan.

High Ceiling or Loop Diuretics

Furosemide is the most commonly used loop diuretic. Loop diuretics have rapid onset and short duration of action. They are called high ceiling because their dose response curve is steep and by increasing the dose, the maximal Na^+ excretion reaches upto 30-40% in comparison to 10-12% caused by thiazides.

Mechanism of Action

Furosemide acts by inhibiting NaCl reabsorption in the thick ascending limb of the Henle's loop. It bind to the Na^+ -K^{+}-2Cl symporter and interfere its function and results in inhibition of transport of electrolytes (reabsorption). Thus, increases the excretion of Na^+ and Cl^- in the urine.

Other Actions: Loop diuretics also enhance the excretion of K^+, Ca^{++} and Mg^{+++} (by inhibiting reabsorption).They increase the excretion of HCO_3 and phosphate. They are powerful stimulator of renin release. They also alter renal haemodynamic and increases total renal blood flow. Furosemide causes hyperglycemia. They increase reabsorption of uric acid in the proximal tubule.

Intravenous administration of furosemide causes venodilation and reduces left ventricular filling pressure. This effect may be mediated by P.G. It thus relieves pulmonary congestion in congestive heart failure and in pulmonary edema even before the onset of diuresis.

Furosemide is rapidly absorbed orally (bioavailability is 60%), have low lipid solubility, highly bound to plasma proteins, metabolized in the liver by conjugation and excreted in urinc mainly unchanged. Plasma half life is 1-2 hours (prolonged in patients with renal and hepatic disease).

Bumetanide is 40 times more potent than furosemide. Bioavailability is 80% and is better tolerated. **Ethacrynic** acid is irritant and causes adverse effects and hence is not commonly used.

Torsemide: It is longer acting and therefore can be given once a day, preferred in patients with heart failure.

Adverse Effects

1. Electrolyte imbalance: Hyponatraemia, hyperuricaemia, hypocalcaemia (hypercalciuria), hypomagnesaemia, hypokalemia and metabolic alkalosis. Hypokalemia may precipitate cardiac arrhythmias.

2. Dehydration hypovolaemia and hypotension (by overjudicious use).
3. Ototoxicity.
4. Hyperglycemia and hyperlipidaemia.
5. GIT disturbances.
6. Allergic reactions: Skin rash, photosensitivity.

Uses

1. Edema: Acute pulmonary edema/Cerebral edema.
2. Acute left ventricular failure following MI.
3. Forced diuresis in case of poisoning.
4. Hypertension.
5. Hypercalcaemia and renal calcium stones.
6. Along with blood transfusion in severe anaemia to prevent overload.

Drug Interactions

1. They potentiate the actions of all hypertensives.
2. They enhance digitalis toxicity.
3. Probenecid decreases diuretic effect by reducing concentration in tubular fluid.
4. Indomethacin and other NSAIDs cause loss of response probably by interfering with the formation of vasodilatory prostaglandins.

Thiazides

Mechanism of Action

The primary site of action of thiazide diuretics is the cortical diluting segment or the early distal convoluted tubule. They are of moderate efficacy because 90% of the filtered sodium is already reabsorbed before reaching to the distal tubule. These groups of drugs block Na^+/Cl^- co-transport system in the early distal tubule (proximal to the sodium and potassium exchange region). They also inhibit carbonic anhydrase activity and increase bicarbonate loss (weak action). Thiazides also enhance excretion of Mg^+ and K^+. But they inhibit urinary excretion of Ca^{++} and uric acid resulting in hypercalcaemia and hyperuricaemia. Excessive loss of sodium, chloride and potassium causes hypokalemic hypochloremic alkalosis.

Other effects: Hyperglycemia, hyperlipidemia.

Thiazides are well absorbed orally, and are rapidly acting, their action starts within one hour. They are distributed throughout the extracellular space and are concentrated in kidney. Protein binding is variable. Most of the drug excreted unchanged in urine.

Adverse Effects

Most of the adverse effects of thiazides are similar to those of loop diuretics, *e.g.,* electrolyte imbalance (hypokalemia, hyperuricaemia and hyponotraemia alkalosis etc.) but they cause hypercalcaemia, hypomagnesaemia and hyperglycemia.

Uses

1. Essential hypertension.
2. Congestive heart failure and edema.
3. Nephrogenic diabetes insipidus.
4. Idiopathic hypercalciuria and renal stones formation.

Indapamide is particularly suitable in hypertension because it is claimed to lower blood pressure in subdiuretic doses.

Potassium Sparing Diuretics

These agents inhibit sodium absorption in the distal tubule and collecting duct and indirectly suppress the secretion of potassium.

Spironolactone is an aldosterone antagonist. As major amount of Na^+ is already reabsorbed in the proximal parts, spironolactone has low efficacy. Spironolactone inhibits Na^+/K^+ exchange by antagonizing the action of aldosterone by competing for intracellular mineralocorticoid receptor in distal tubule. This results into an inhibition of the sodium retaining action of aldosterone. Spironolactone also reduces H^+, K^+ loss and uric acid excretion. It enhances the excretion of calcium by a direct action on the renal tubules. It is excreted in urine and in bile, thus undergoes enterohepatic circulation.

Adverse effects include gynaecomastia, drowsiness, hyperkalemia, metabolic acidosis and skin rashes.

Amiloride and **Triamterene** are directly acting agents which enhance Na^+ excretion and reduce K^+ loss by acting on ion channels in the distal tubule and collecting duct.

Uses of Potassium Sparing Diuretics

1. With thiazide and loop diuretics to counteract K^+ loss (Amiloride and triamterene are used).
2. Edema (spironolactone).
3. Hypertension with heart failure.
4. Primary or secondary aldosteronism.
5. Hepatic cirrhosis/cystic fibrosis.

Carbonic Anhydrase Inhibitors

Carbonic anhydrase inhibitors block sodium bicarbonate reabsorption in the proximal tubule and cause excretion of HCO_3. They are weak diuretics.

Acetazolamide is a sulfonamide derivative which inhibits carbonic anhydrase enzyme and enhances excretion of sodium, potassium, bicarbonate and water. The loss of bicarbonate in urine makes urine alkaline. This leads to metabolic acidosis and decreases the activity of acetazolamide, so, it is self limiting diuretic.

Adverse Effects

1. Metabolic acidosis due to HCO_3^- loss.
2. Renal stones Ca^{++} is lost with HCO_3^- resulting in hypercalciuria. This excess Ca^{++} may precipitate, resulting in the formation of renal stones.
3. Hypokalemia, drowsiness and allergic reactions can occur.

Uses

1. Glaucoma: It decreases IOT.
2. Alkalinization of urine.
3. Metabolic alkalosis.
4. Mountain sickness.
5. Epilepsy.

Contraindications: Hepatic disease, COPD (acidosis is severe).

Osmotic Diuretics

These agents are solutes which are pharmacologically inert, non-metabolized and freely filtered at the glomerulus. They are not reabsorbed.

Mannitol is pharmacologically inert substance. When given IV, mannitol gets filtered by the glomerulus but not reabsorbed. It expands extracellular fluid volume, increase GFR, decrease renin release and increase renal blood flow. It causes water to be retained in the proximal tubule and descending limb of Henle's loop by osmotic effect resulting in water diuresis.

Uses

1. Threatened acute renal failure: To maintain urine volume and prevent oliguria in conditions like massive haemolysis and shock (not helpful when renal failure already occurred).
2. To reduce intracranial and intraocular pressure following head injury and glaucoma respectively.

Glycerol is effective orally. It reduces intraocular and intracranial pressure.

Drug Interactions with Diuretics

1. Furosemide highly protein bound and may compete with drugs like warfarin and clofibrate for protein binding sites.
2. Other ototoxic drugs like aminoglycosides; should not be used with loop diuretics.
3. Hypokalemia induced by diuretics enhance digitalis toxicity.
4. Diuretics enhance lithium toxicity by reducing renal excretion of lithium.
5. Oral potassium supplements should be avoided with potassium sparing diuretics.

Anti-Diuretics

Anti-diuretics are drugs that reduce urine volume. These include:

1. Anti-diuretic hormone (ADH) or Vasopressin.
2. Thiazide diuretics.
3. Miscellaneous: Chlorpropamide, Carbamazepine.

Anti-diuretic hormone (ADH) is secreted by the posterior pituitary along with oxytocin. ADH is released in response to two stimuli, *i.e.*, dehydration and rise in plasma osmolarity. ADH acts on by three receptors V_{1a}, V_{1b} and V_2 receptors.

V_{1a}, receptors are present in vascular and other smooth muscles, kidneys and anterior pituitary. They act mainly through the phospholipase C-IP_3/DAG pathway and release Ca^{2+}. V_{1b} receptors are responsible for the release of ACTH.

V_2 receptors are present in collecting duct in the kidneys. They regulate their water permeability through cAMP production.

ADH enhances water reabsorption by acting on the collecting duct. ADH activates the V_2 receptors present on the cell membrane of the collecting duct and increases the water permeability of these cells. ADH also causes vasoconstriction and raises BP mediated by V_1 receptors. It also acts on other smooth muscles to increase peristalsis in the gut and contracts the uterus. It may play a part in pathogenesis of depression. Stimulation of V_2 receptors increases circulating levels of factor VIII.

Vasopressin is given parenterally as injection SC/IM/IV.

Uses

1. Diabetes insipidus.
2. Bleeding esophageal varices (Terlipressin).
3. Before abdominal radiography.
4. Haemophilia and von Willebrand's disease.
5. Post-operative ileus and abdominal distension.
6. Bed wetting in children and nocturia in adults.
7. Cyclophosphamide included haemorrhagic cystitis.

Desmopressin is selective for V_2 receptors and is longer acting. It is given as nasal spray. **Terlipressin** is synthetic prodrug of vasopressin and longer acting while **felypressin** is short acting is used with local anesthetics to prolong the duration of action.

Absolute contraindications: Acute renal failure and psychogenic polydipsia.

DRUGS USED IN ANGINA PECTORIS AND MYOCARDIAL INFARCTION

Angina pectoris is characterized by sudden, severe, sub sternal discomfort or pain which may radiate to the left shoulder and along the flexor surface of the left arm which is relieved by rest.

When the oxygen supply to the myocardium is insufficient for its needs, myocardial ischemia develops. This may be due to atheromatous changes in coronary lumen, vasospasm of coronary artery and severe chronic hypertension. The anginal pain occurs due to imbalance between the oxygen requirement and supply to the ischemic area of myocardium. Pain is due to accumulation of metabolites in the cardiac muscle.

Three forms of angina are:

1. **Classical angina** (stable angina, angina of effort, exertional angina): Pain is induced by exercise or emotion and relieved by rest or by nitrates.

2. **Variant or Prinzmetal's angina** occurs at rest or during sleep and is caused by spasm of the coronary artery. This may be superimposed with atheromatous stenosis.
3. **Unstable angina** It occurs with minimum exertion or at rest and need hospitalization. It is mostly due to rupture of an atheromatous plaque with progressive occlusion of the coronary artery.

In angina, drugs are used to improve the balance between oxygen supply and demand either by increasing oxygen supply to the myocardium (coronary dilation) or by reducing the oxygen demand (reducing preload/afterload/heart rate or all of these) or combination of both.

Classification of Anti Angina Drugs

1. *Organic nitrates:* Nitroglycerine, Isosorbide dinitrate, Isosorbide mononitrate, Penta erythritol tetranitrate, Erythrityl tetranitrate.
2. *Calcium channel blockers:* Verapamil, Diltiazem, Amlodipine, Nifedipine.
3. *Beta blockers:* Propranolol, Atenolol, Metoprolol, Nadolol, Celiprolol.
4. *Potassium channel openers:* Nicorandil.
5. *Miscellaneous:* Dipyridamole, Aspirin, Trimetazidine, Ticlopidine, Lidoflazine, Oxyfedrin, Pentoxiphylline, Ranolazine, Clopidogrel.

Organic Nitrates

Mechanism of action: They are converted to nitric oxide which activates vascular guanylyl cyclase. This in turn increases the synthesis of cGMP. This cGMP catalyse the phosphorylation of protein kinases and causing relaxation of the vascular smooth muscles through inhibition of Ca^{2+} entry. Formation of PGE_2 or PGI_2 and membrane hyperpolarization also contribute to its action.

Nitrates are predominantly venodilators. Venodilation reduces venous return to the heart, decrease cardiac work thereby reducing preload. Arteriolar dilation reduces vascular resistance thus decreasing afterload (cardiac work). As both preload and afterload are reduced, workload of the heart is decreased thereby reducing oxygen requirement of the heart. They also cause dilatation of large coronary (epicardial) arteries, collateral vessels and redistribution of the coronary blood flow with improved perfusion to ischemic areas. They increase exercise tolerance.

In variant angina, nitrates relieve vasospasm due to coronary vasodilatation. Nitrates also cause dilation of blood vessels in the skin resulting in flushing; dilatation of the meningeal vessels results in headache but have no direct effect on heart. Bronchial smooth muscles are also relaxed.

Nitrates are well absorbed orally but they undergo extensive first pass metabolism. They are inactivated in liver by glutathione organic nitrate reductase.

Nitrates are available for oral, sublingual, parenteral use and as ointment and transdermal patches for topical use. Topical preparations are used for the prevention of nocturnal episodes of angina.

Adverse Effects

Throbbing headache is common; flushing, sweating, palpitation, weakness, postural hypotension and rashes can occur. By adopting proper dosing schedule, tolerance can be avoided.

Uses

1. Angina.
2. Cardiac failure.
3. Myocardial infarction (IV nitroglycerine is used).
4. Cyanide poisoning.
5. Oesophageal spasm.

CALCIUM CHANNEL BLOCKERS (CCBs)

CCBs relax the arterioles leading to a decrease in the peripheral vascular resistance and a reduction in the afterload. Reflex tachycardia can occur particularly with dihydropyridines. But CCBs also depress the myocardial contractility thereby reducing the heart rate and force of contraction. This results in reduced cardiac workload and oxygen consumption. CCBs also dilate the coronaries thereby increasing the coronary blood flow. CCBs are used for the prophylaxis of exertional angina.

Beta Blockers

Beta blockers reduce the frequency and severity of attacks of exertional angina by reducing heart rate and myocardial contractility. Thus, are useful in the prevention of angina. They are used for the long term prophylaxis of classical angina and may be combined with nitrates. Beta blockers should always be tapered after prolonged use. They are not useful in variant angina.

Potassium Channel Openers

Nicorandil is an arterial and venous dilator. Opening of the ATP sensitive K^+ channels results, in efflux of K^+, leading to hyperpolarization and therefore relaxation of the vascular smooth muscles. In addition, it also acts through NO like nitrates.

Adverse effects are headache, flushing, palpitation, dizziness and hypotension.

Pinacidil is similar to nicorandil. It is useful in angina and hypertension.

Miscellaneous

Dipyridamole is a coronary vasodilator but it diverts the blood from ischemic zone (steal phenomenon) and is therefore not beneficial. It inhibits platelet aggregation for which it is used in post MI and post stroke patients for prevention of coronary and cerebral thrombosis.

Aspirin: Low dose aspirin is recommended to prevent myocardial infarction.

Trimetazidine is a calcium channel blocker claimed to have a protective effect on the ischemic myocardium.

Ranolazine is a new drug which spare free fatty acid oxidation and shifts ATP production to more O_2 efficient carbohydrate oxidation.

Beneficial Combinations of Drugs in Angina

1. **Nitrates + beta blockers:** Very effective in exertional angina. Reflex tachycardia due to nitrates is countered by beta blockers. Ventricular dilatation due to beta blockers is opposed by nitrates.
2. **Nifedipine + beta blockers:** The anti-anginal effects are additive. Reflex tachycardia due to nifedipine is countered by beta-blockers.
3. **Nitrates + CCBs:** Nitrates decrease preload, CCBs reduce after-load and the combination reduces cardiac workload effective in vasospastic angina.
4. **CCBs + beta blockers + Nitrates:** If the angina is not controlled by 2 drug combinations, 3 drugs can be used.

Unstable Angina

Patients with unstable angina are at a high risk of developing MI or sudden death and need hospitalization and rigorous treatment for its prevention.

Drugs used in unstable angina are:

1. Aspirin.
2. Heparin.
3. Nitrates: Intravenous nitroglycerine.
4. Beta adrenergic blockers and calcium channel blockers.

Drugs Used in Myocardial Infarction

Coronary heart disease is the most important cause of premature deaths.

Myocardial infarction results from prolonged myocardial ischemia and precipitated by sudden occlusive coronary thrombus at the site of pre-existing plaque.

Immediate Treatment

1. *Analgesia:* (a) Morphine or pethidine. Diazepam may also be given to reduce anxiety and produce sedation.(b) Sublingual nitroglycerine.
2. *Oxygen.*
3. *Thrombolytics:* Streptokinase /Anistreplase/Alteplase/Reteplase/ Urokinase.
4. *Aspirin:* After hospitalization.
5. *Nitrates and vasodilators.*
6. *Other drugs:* (i) Beta adrenergic blockers (ii) Anti-emetics (iii) Anti-arrhythmic, Dopamine to treat hypotension.
7. *Anti-coagulants:* Heparin/ LMWH.

Long Term Treatment

Long term administration of low dose aspirin, a beta adrenergic blocker and an ACE inhibitor, oral anti-coagulants are useful in reducing long term mortality in myocardial infarction.

Calcium Channel Blockers

The depolarization of the cardiac and vascular smooth muscle cells depend on the entry of extracellular calcium into the cell through the calcium channels. Intracellular calcium is also increased by receptor-mediated action, *i.e.*, agonist induced calcium release. This calcium triggers the release of intracellular calcium from the sarcoplasmic reticulum. All these calcium ions bring about contraction of the cardiac and vascular smooth muscle cells. In the vascular smooth muscle, two regulating mechanisms are there to control Ca^{2+} influx, *i.e.,* inward movement of Ca^{+2} through voltage sensitive channels and excitation contraction coupling through phosphorylation of myosin light chain.

Calcium Channels

A. Voltage dependent channels are influenced by high K^+ levels or depolarizing external stimuli. They are again divided into 'L' (long lasting or slow channels), 'N' (neuronal) and T (transient or fast) subtypes based on their voltage sensitivity and conductance. T and L channels are present in cardiac and vascular smooth muscles while N channels are seen only in nerves.
B. Receptor operated channels increases calcium influx in response to various hormones.
C. Stretch operated channels are present in blood vessels and increase calcium influx on being stretched.

Calcium channel antagonists inhibit the entry of calcium by blocking the L type of calcium channels.

Calcification of CCBs

1. *Dihydropyridine (DHP) compounds:* Nifedipine, Nimodipine, Nisoldipine, Nitrendipine, Nicardipine, Amlodipine, Felodipine, Isradipine Lercandipine.
2. *Benzothiazepine compounds:* Diltiazem.
3. *Phenyl alkylamines:* Verapamil, Gallopamil, Tiapamil.
4. *Miscellaneous:* Bepridil.

These drugs decreases calcium current and calcium entry into cardiac and vascular smooth muscle cells resulting in the following effects:

1. **Vascular smooth muscle:** Relaxation of the arteriolar smooth muscles results in reduced peripheral vascular resistance and blood pressure (nifedipine is more effective).
2. **Heart:** CCBs depress myocardial contractility, reduce heart rate and in higher doses they slow AV conduction (Negative inotropic effect, more with verapamil).
3. **Coronary circulation:** CCBs dilate the coronary vessels, increasing the coronary blood flow. Hence they are useful in variant angina.
4. **CCBs** relax the uterus and may be useful in premature labour.

Nicardipine has selective action on coronary vessels having less inotropic effect on the heart. **Amlodipine** produces less reflex tachycardia, has slow onset and longer duration of action. **Nimodipine** is highly lipid soluble, crosses the BBB and relaxes the cerebral blood vessels, so can be used in subarachnoid haemorrhage to reduce vasospasm. **Lacidipine** exert more marked vascular protection. **Isradipine** can be used in patients with AV block.

Pharmacokinetics: CCBs are well absorbed but undergo extensive first pass metabolism. So, oral bioavailability is reduced. They are all highly plasma protein bound (70-90%) and are metabolized in the liver. In patients with hepatic cirrhosis, both bioavailability and half life are increased.

Therapeutic Uses of CCBs

1. **Angina pectoris:** In prinzmetal/variant angina–Verapamil and amlodipine are used.
2. **Hypertension.**
3. **Arrhythmias.**
4. **Peripheral vascular disease** (intermittent claudication).
5. **Other uses:**
   a. Hypertrophic cardiomyopathy.
   b. Migraine.
   c. Subarachnoid hemorrhage.
   d. Preterm labour.
   e. Diabetic nephropathy.
   f. Cardiac transplantation.

Drug Interactions: Verapamil and diltiazem should be avoided in patients receiving beta adrenergic blockers because of the myocardial depressant effects get added up.

Verapamil can precipitate digoxin toxicity by reducing its excretion. It also inhibits CYP3A isoenzyme and therefore potentially increases blood levels of atrovastatin and other drugs metabolized by CYP3A enzyme.

Contraindications: CCBs are contraindicated in unstable angina (unless combined with beta-blockers) digitalis toxicity, patients of systolic heart failure, sinus bradycardia, WPW syndrome, sick sinus syndrome and early phase of acute MI.

ANTI-HYPERTENSIVE DRUGS

Hypertension is an elevation of systolic and/or diastolic blood pressure (SBP/DBP) above 140SBP/90DBP. Based on the degree of severity, hypertension can be graded as:

- *Normal:* SBP <120 and DBP <80 mm of Hg.
- *Prehypertensive:* SBP 120-139 or DBP 80–89 mm of Hg.
- *Hypertension stage I:* SBP 140-159 or DBP 90–99 mm of Hg.
- *Hypertension stage II:* SBP >160 or DBP >100 mm of Hg.
- *Hypertensive emergency:* DBP more than 115.

Prolonged hypertension damages the blood vessels of the heart, brain and the kidneys which may result in several complications like stroke, coronary artery disease or renal failure.

Classification of Drugs Used in Hypertension

1. **Diuretics:**
   a. *Thiazides:* Hydrochlorothiazide, Chlorthalidone, Indapamide.
   b. *Loop diuretics:* Frusemide (Furosemide), Bumetamide, Torsemide.
   c. *Potassium sparing diuretics:* Spironolactone, Amiloride, Triamterene.
2. **Angiotensin converting enzyme inhibitors:** Captopril, Enalapril, Lisinopril, Ramipril, Perindopril, Fosinopril, Trandolapril, Quinapril, Benazepril.
3. **Angiotensin II receptor antagonists:** Losartan, Candesartan, Valsartan, Eprosartan, Irbesartan, Telmisartan.
4. **Sympatholytic agents:**
   a. *Centrally acting drugs:* Clonidine, Methyldopa, Guanabenz, Guanfacine.
   b. *Adrenergic neuron blockers:* Guanithidine, Reserpine.
   c. *Ganglion blockers:* Trimethaphan.
   d. *Adrenergic receptor blockers:*
      i. *Alpha blockers:* Prazosin, Terazosin, Doxazosin, Phenoxybenzamine, Phentolamine.
      ii. *Beta blockers:* Propranolol, Atenolol, Esmolol, Metoprolol.
      iii. *Alpha and beta blockers:* Labetalol, Carvedilol.
5. **Calcium channel blockers:** Verapamil, Nifedipine, Nicardipine, Nimodipine, Amlodipine, Felodipine, Diltiazem.
6. **Vasodilators:**
   a. *Arteriolar dilators:* Hydralazine, Minoxidil, Diazoxide, Fenoldopam.
   b. *Arteriolar and venous dilators:* Sodium nitroprusside.

7. **Renin antagonist:** Aliskiren.
8. **Potassium channel opener:** Nicorandi, Pinacidil.

Clinical Classification

a. *First line drugs (most commonly used) used in the treatment of mild to moderate hypertension:* ACE inhibitors, beta blockers, calcium channel blockers and diuretics (ABCD).

b. *Second line drugs used in moderate hypertension:* Centrally acting drugs (Clonidine), alpha blocker or adrenergic neuron blocker (Reserpine).

c. *Third line drugs used in severe hypertension:* Drugs acting on vessel wall (Hydralazine, Minoxidil).

d. *Drugs used in hypertensive emergency, e.g.,* Sodium nitroprusside, Diazoxide, Labetalol, Trimethaphan.

Diuretics

Diuretics enhance the excretion of sodium and water resulting in:

1. Decrease plasma volume and decrease cardiac output thus decrease BP.
2. Decrease body sodium, cause relaxation of vascular smooth muscles (due to Na^+ depletion in the vascular smooth muscle), and decrease TPR thus decrease BP.

Thiazide diuretics are the first line anti-hypertensive drug.

Indapamide is useful in hypertension because it lowers BP in sub-diuretic doses.

Loop diuretics, *e.g.*, furosemide are powerful diuretics, their antihypertensive efficacy is low. They are used only in hypertension with chronic renal failure, congestive heart failure, and in patients with azotemia or refractory edema.

Advantages

They are cheap, moderately potent, have good oral absorption and have no effect on capacitance vessels, so postural hypotension is rare.

Disadvantages

Electrolyte imbalance, allergic reaction may observe. They may be combined with a K^+ sparing diuretic to avoid hypokalemia.

Angiotensin Converting Enzyme Inhibitors (ACEI)

Angiotensin II is a powerful vasoconstrictor and stimulates aldosterone which raises the BP by increasing the plasma volume. ACE inhibitors prevent the formation of angiotensin II and aldosterone. There is vasodilatation and decrease in TPR resulting in a fall in BP. ACEI also degrades bradykinin, which is a potent vasodilator. This also contributes to the fall in BP. They increase plasma renin activity, decrease in salt and water retention and increase serum potassium. They decrease arteriolar tone and systemic arterial resistance and thus causes fall in B.P. The blood flow to the kidneys, brain and heart increases due to selective vasodilatation and thus maintains adequate blood supply to these vital organs.

Pharmacokinetics: ACE inhibitors are generally well absorbed. Food reduces its bioavailability, partly metabolized and excreted through the kidney so dose should be reduced in renal dysfunction.

Adverse Effects

Persistent dry cough due to increase bradykinin levels, hypotension, hyperkalemia, dysgeusia, skin rashes and angioneurotic edema, bone marrow depression are common adverse effects. They can cause headache nausea, abdominal pain, proteinuria and acute renal failure and rarely neutropenia. Neutropenia is more common in patients with collagen disease. They are teratogenic.

Advantages of ACEI

Effective and safe anti-hypertensive, no electrolyte imbalance, no postural hypotension, safe in diabetes, asthma, can be used in CCF.

Uses

1. Hypertension: ACE inhibitors are presently the first line anti-hypertensive drug.
2. CCF/Myocardial infarction (LVF).
3. Coronary artery disease.
4. Chronic renal failure and scleroderma renal crisis.
5. Diabetic nephropathy/retinopathy.

Precautions and Contraindications

- ACE inhibitors are contraindicated in pregnancy, in patients with renal artery stenosis as they can cause renal failure in them.
- ACE inhibitors should not be combined with K^+ sparing diuretics.
- At the first sign of angioedema, ACE inhibitors should be stopped.
- ACE inhibitors may enhance plasma levels of digoxin and lithium.

Angiotensin II Receptor Blockers (ARBs)

Losartan is first orally effective AT_1 receptor antagonist. There are, two subtypes of angiotensin II receptors, *e.g.*, AT_1 and AT_2. AT_1 receptors are present in vascular and myocardial tissue, brain, kidney and glomerular cells. Losartan has high affinity for AT_1, receptors when compared to AT_2 receptors. By blocking AT_1 receptors, losartan blocks the effect of angiotensin II and thus relaxes vascular smooth muscles, promotes salt and water excretion and reduces plasma volume.

The main advantage of ARBs over ACE inhibitors is that there is no increase in bradykinin levels and not associated with adverse effects like dry cough and angioedema.

ARBs are contraindicated in pregnancy because of their teratogenic potential. They may precipitate renal failure.

They are used in:

1. Hypertension.
2. Cardiac failure.
3. Myocardial infarction.
4. Diabetic neuropathy (may be combined with ACEI).

Sympatholytics Drugs

Drugs Acting Centrally

Clonidine is a selective $alpha_2$ agonist. Stimulation of $alpha_2$, receptors in the CNS (in the vasomotor centre and hypothalamus), decreases central sympathetic outflow. Thus, causes fall in BP and reduction in heart rate (bradycardia). Clonidine cause initial presser effect during rapid IV administration.

Adverse effects include drowsiness, dryness of mouth, nose and eyes; parotid gland swelling and pain, fluid retention, constipation and impotence. Sudden withdrawal of clonidine will lead to rebound hypertension. Bradycardia may occur in patients with SA node and AV nodal disease. It is available as oral, transdermal as well as parenteral preparations.

Uses

1. Mild to moderate hypertension.
2. Opioid/alcohol withdrawal.
3. Diabetic neuropathy.
4. With general anaesthetics.
5. Used as substitute for morphine for intrathecal injections.
6. Attenuate hot flushes and other vasomotor symptoms of menopausal syndrome.

Alpha methyl dopa is a prodrug. It is metabolised in the CNS to alpha methyl norepinephrine which stimulate $alpha_2$ receptors and resulting in the reduction in sympathetic outflow and fall in BP. Cardiac output and renal blood flow are well maintained.

Uses

Alpha methyl dopa is used in mild to moderate hypertension along with a diuretic. It is safe to be used in hypertension during pregnancy.

Ganglionic Blockers

These drugs block both sympathetic and parasympathetic ganglia resulting in decreased sympathetic tone and a fall in BP. But they produce several side effects and are not used now. Trimethaphan is the only ganglionic blocker used intravenously to produce controlled hypotension during certain surgeries. It is also used in hypertensive emergencies (malignant hypertension).

Adrenergic Neuron Blockers

Guanethidine: It is a potent drug. It depletes norepinephrine from the sympathetic nerve ending (tissue store). This leads to fall in C.O.P., but no change in TPR.

Reserpine: In the adrenergic neurons, it binds to the vesicles that store monoamines like norepinephrine, dopamine and 5-HT and destroys these vesicles. It thus depletes the stores of these monoamines and reduces BP. It has the advantages of being inexpensive, effective, long acting (once daily dose) and generally well tolerated when given with a diuretic. It is not preferred due to its adverse effects.

Adverse Effects

The common adverse effects are sedation, depression, EPS, breast carcinoma, aggravation of peptic ulcer, nasal stiffness.

Adrenergic Receptor Blockers

Beta blockers are mild anti-hypertensive; they reduce the BP due to reduction in HR and fall in the cardiac output. They also lower plasma renin activity and have an additional central anti-hypertensive action. They are suitable for combination with other anti-hypertensive particularly with drugs that cause tachycardia. They are thus the first line anti-hypertensive drugs in mild to moderate hypertension. Atenolol or other cardio selective drugs are the preferred beta blocker because of the advantages like once a day dosing, absence of CNS side effects and $beta_1$ selectivity.

Alpha blockers, phenoxybenzamine and phentolamine are used in the treatment of hypertension due to pheochromocytoma. Prazosin, terazosin and doxazosin dilate both arterioles and venules, thus peripheral vascular resistance is decreased leading to a fall in BP with mild tachycardia.

Advantages of Alpha Blocker

Renal flow and GFR is maintained, improve carbohydrate metabolism, effect on lipid profile (decrease LDL) helps in LVH by decreasing both preload and afterload. So, they are useful anti-hypertensive in patient with gout, diabetes and hyperlipidaemia.

Alpha and beta blockers are used IV in the treatment of hypertension in pheochromocytoma and in hypertensive emergencies.

Calcium Channel Blockers

They dilate the arterioles resulting in reduced peripheral vascular resistance. They are not preferred in patients who also have left ventricular hypertrophy and previous myocardial infarction. CCBs are particularly effective in elderly patients.

CCBs may be used as monotherapy in mild HT or in moderate to severe HT along with other anti-hypertensives. Details already discussed earlier.

Vasodilators

Vasodilators relax the vascular smooth muscles thus reducing BP due to decreased peripheral vascular resistance. Salt and water retention and reflex tachycardia are common with vasodilators.

Hydralazine is a directly acting arteriolar dilator with little effect on capacitance vessels. The fall in BP is associated with tachycardia, renin release and fluid retention. Coronary, cerebral and renal blood flow is increased. So, it is useful in hypertension with renal dysfunction. It has more effect on DBP than SBP. Activation of K^+ channels (thus hyperpolarization) and generation of nitric oxide is main mechanism

Adverse effects are headache, dizziness, flushing, palpitation, nausea, hypotension and salt and water retention. It may precipitate angina in some patients because of increased demand of O_2 due to reflex tachycardia and decreased myocardial blood supply due to peripheral vasodilatation. Serum sickness and lupus erythematosus may occur and is more common in slow acetylators.

Minoxidil a directly acting arteriolar dilator used in severe hypertension. It acts by opening K^+ channels in the smooth muscles. It also reduce calcium uptake. It is reserved for uncontrolled severe hypertension or hypertension associated with chronic renal failure. Minoxidil can cause fluid retention, tachycardia and angina. It stimulates the growth of hair on prolonged use.

Diazoxide is an arteriolar dilator causes Na^+ and water retention when used for longer period.

Fenoldopam: It is a dopamine agonist (D_1) causes peripheral vasodilatation and natriuresis.

Sodium nitroprusside is a rapidly acting vasodilator and it relaxes both arterioles and venules. Both peripheral resistance and cardiac output are reduced resulting in lower myocardial oxygen consumption. Nitroprusside acts through the release of nitric oxide which activates guanylyl cyclase, resulting in the formation of cGMP which relaxes the vascular smooth muscles. This enzyme is different from those that produce NO with nitrates. On IV administration, its action is rapid (acts within 30 seconds) and short acting (duration is 3 minutes). This makes it suitable for use in hypertensive emergencies with close monitoring.

Adverse reactions are palpitation, sweating, weakness, nausea, vomiting and hypotension.

Uses

1. Nitroprusside is the drug of choice in hypertensive emergencies.
2. It is used in situations where short-term reduction of myocardial workload is required as in myocardial infarction.
3. Acute MR.
4. HT with acute MI or LVF.

Vasodilators are contraindicated in:

a. Patients with aortic aneurysm.
b. Elderly patients.
c. As monotherapy.
d. Patients with coronary artery disease.
e. Pregnancy.

CARDIAC GLYCOSIDES AND TREATMENT OF CARDIAC FAILURE (CHF)

The myocardium has two types of cells, *i.e.,* contracting cells and the conducting cells. The contracting cells participate in the pumping action of the heart. Parts of the conducting tissue have the characteristic property of automaticity. **Automaticity** is the ability of the cell to generate electrical impulses spontaneously. **Excitability** is the ability of the cell to undergo depolarization in response to a stimulus. **Contractility** is the ability of the myocardium to adequately contract and pump the blood out of the heart.

Congestive cardiac failure (CCF) is one of the common causes of morbidity and mortality. In congestive cardiac failure, the heart is unable to provide adequate blood supply to meet the body's oxygen demand. This causes pulmonary edema, dyspnoea, liver enlargement and peripheral edema. As a compensatory mechanism, there is stimulation of the sympathetic system, renin angiotensin system and release of atrial natriuretic peptides which help in maintaining the cardiac output. These peptides increase renal excretion of salt and water and dilate vascular smooth muscles.

In low output failure the metabolic demands of the body are limited but the heart is unable to meet them. This could result from ischemic heart disease, hypertension, valvular and congenital heart diseases. High output failure results from anaemia, thyrotoxicosis, beriberi and certain congenital heart diseases. In this condition the metabolic need of the body are excessive, and even increased cardiac output is insufficient to meet them.

Drugs Used in Heart Failure

A. Drugs with Positive Inotropic Effects:

a. *Cardiac glycosides:* Digoxin, Digitoxin and Oubain.
b. *Phosphodiesterase III inhibitors:* Inamrinone, Milrinone, Levosimendan, Amrinone, Piroximone.
c. *Beta adrenergic agonists:* Dopamine, Doubtamine, Dopexamine.
d. *Natriuretic peptide:* Nesiritide.

B. Drugs Without Positive Inotropic Effects:

a. *Diuretics:* Furosemide, Torasemide, Spironolactone.
b. *ACEI:* Enalapril, Lisinopril.
c. *ATBs:* Losartan.

d. *Beta-adrenergic receptor antagonist:* Metoprolol, Carvedilol.
e. *Vasodilators:* Hydralazine, Isosorbide dinitrate, Sodium nitroprusside.

Cardiac Glycosides

Pharmacological Actions

1. Cardiac Actions

- *Positive inotropic effect:* They increase the force of contraction of the heart, the stroke volume increases and thereby the cardiac output. The systole is shortened and the diastole is prolonged which allows more rest and ventricular filling to the heart.
- The heart rate is reduced due to increased vagal tone, decreased sympathetic overactivity due to improved circulation and by a direct action on SA and AV nodes.
- *Blood pressure:* No significant effect is seen.
- Coronary circulation improves due to increased cardiac output and prolonged diastole.

2. Extra Cardiac Actions

It opposes compensatory sympathetic activity in heart failure.

- It causes diuresis, which relieves edema.
- High dose stimulate CTZ resulting in nausea and vomiting.

Mechanism of action: Cardiac glycosides inhibit the enzyme Na^+-K^+ ATPase also called the 'sodium pump' present on the cardiac myocytes. Inhibition of this pump results in an increase in the intracellular Na^+ and Ca^{++}. Thus more calcium is available for contraction, resulting in increased force and velocity of contraction. Thus an increased amount of calcium is released during each action potential resulting in an increased force and velocity of contraction. Extracellular K^+ promotes dephosphorylation of ATPase and decrease the affinity of ATPase for cardiac glycosides. The binding of glycosides to Na^+ - K^+ ATPase is slow even after intravenous injection and therefore, inotropic action takes hours to develop.

Pharmacokinetics: Digoxin is well absorbed. Presence of food in the stomach delays absorption. Plasma $t_{1/2}$ of digitoxin is 5–9 days. Oubain is the most potent and digitoxin is the least potent. Digoxin is excreted unchanged in urine, while digitoxin is actively metabolized by hepatic microsomal enzyme.

Digitalization: Response to digitalis develops over 5–7 days with the maintenance dose as given in mild to moderate cases of CCF.

Adverse Effects: Cardiac glycosides have a low safety margin and adverse effects are common. These includes:

Extra Cardiac: Anorexia, nausea, vomiting and diarrhea are the first symptoms to appear. Weakness, confusion, hallucinations, blurred vision and gynaecomastia can occur.

Cardiac Toxicity: Arrhythmias of any type including extra systoles, bradycardia, pulses bigeminy and AV block can occur.

Treatment of Toxicity

- Stop digitalis.
- Oral or parenteral K^+ supplements (for tachyarrhythmias).
- IV lignocaine (for ventricular arrhythmias).
- Bradycardia is treated with atropine.
- Supraventricular arrhythmias with propranolol.
- In severe toxicity anti-digoxin immunotherapy (anti-digoxin antibodies) is now available.

Uses

1. Congestive cardiac failure.
2. Cardiac arrhythmias– Atrial fibrillation (AF), Atrial flutter (AFl), Paroxysmal supraventricular tachycardia (PSVT).

Precautions and Contraindications to Digitalis Therapy

- Hypokalemia.
- MI, thyrotoxicosis, patients with AV-block and elderly.
- Acid base imbalance.
- WPW syndrome.

Other Positive Inotropic Drugs

Phosphodiesterase Inhibitors

Amrinone and milrinone: These drugs inhibit the enzyme phosphodiesterase resulting in increase cAMP levels. They increase the force of contraction and also cause vasodilatation. They may be used for short periods in severe heart failure. Milrinone has shorter $t_{1/2}$ and fewer side effects.

Other drugs used in CCF are discussed earlier.

Treatment of CCF

A. *To relieve symptoms of congestion and improve cardiac performance:*

   a. Inotropic drugs, *e.g.*, digitalis, dobutamine/dopamine, amrinone/milrinone.

   b. Diuretics.

   c. Vasodilators, *e.g.*, ACEI, ARBs, nitrates, hydralazine, nitroprusside.

   d. Beta blockers.

B. *To arrest progression of disease:*

   a. ACEI/ARBs.

   b. Beta blockers.

   c. Spironolactone.

ANTI-ARRHYTHMIC DRUGS

Arrhythmia is an abnormality of the rate, rhythm or site of origin of the cardiac impulse or an abnormality in the impulse conduction. Cardiac arrhythmias may be due to abnormal generation or conduction of impulses.

Mechanism of Genesis of Arrhythmias

A. *Due to disturbed impulse formation or automaticity:* SA node has the highest automaticity in normal cardiac cells, but abnormal automaticity of other areas (other than SA node) of junctional tissue may cause arrhythmia.

B. *Due to abnormal conduction:* This is commonly referred as re-entry disturbances. It may be:

   a. *Partial or complete block of AV conduction* (ectopic beats).

   b. *Re-entry phenomenon:* Normally the conduction of impulse from AV node to ventricle through purkinji fibers is unidirectional in both branches. But due to myocardial ischemia or injury (depressed area), it is directed to adjacent excitable tissue and reach after some time taking circuitous route through normal tissue. This leads to ventricular tachycardia.

Graphical Representation of Myocardial Action Potential is shown in Fig. 5.1.

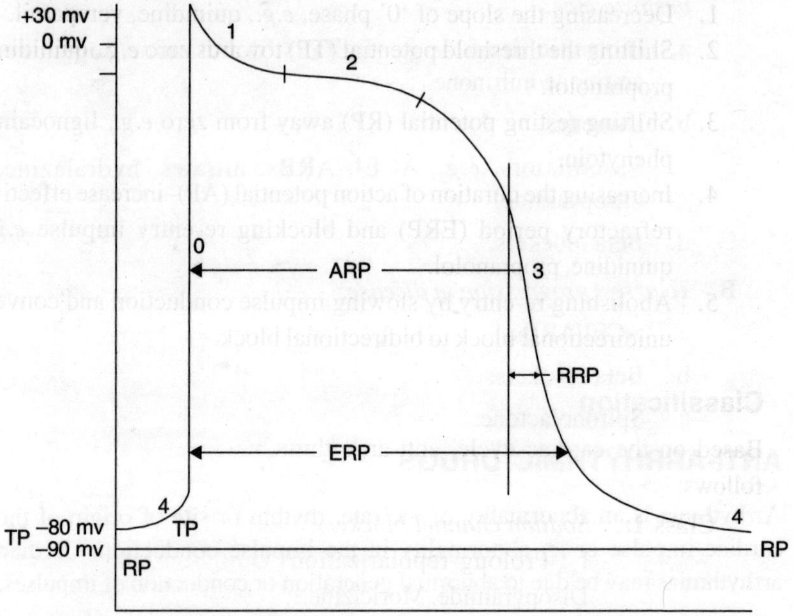

ERP - Effective refractory period
ARP - Absolute refractory period
RRP - Rapid repolarization

RP - Resting potential
TP - Threshold potential

Fig. 5.1: Myocardial action potential

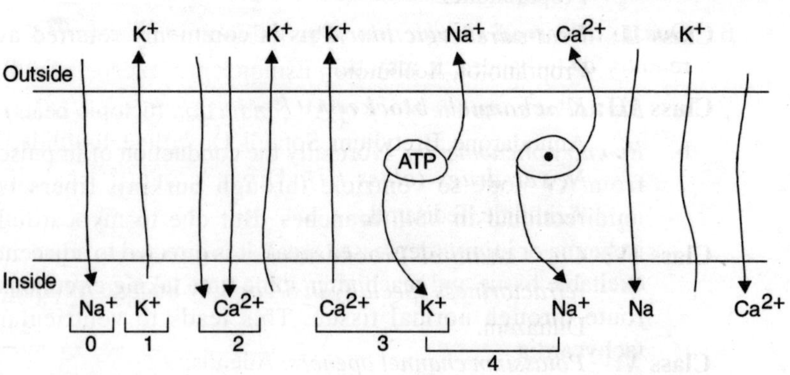

Fig. 5.2: Ionic movement during difference phases of action potential

Mechanism of Action of Anti-arrhythmic Drugs

Anti-arrhythmic drugs may act by:

1. Decreasing the slope of '0' phase, *e.g.*, quinidine, verapamil.
2. Shifting the threshold potential (TP) towards zero *e.g.*, quinidine, propranolol.
3. Shifting resting potential (RP) away from zero *e.g.*, lignocaine, phenytoin.
4. Increasing the duration of action potential (AP)–increase effective refractory period (ERP) and blocking re-entry impulse *e.g.*, quinidine, propranolol.
5. Abolishing re-entry by slowing impulse conduction and convert unidirectional block to bidirectional block.

Classification

Based on the cardiac cycle, anti-arrhythmic drug can be classified as follows:

Class I: *Sodium channel blockers:*

I_A: Prolong repolarization: Quinidine, Procainamide, Disopyramide, Moricizine.

I_B: Shorten repolarization: Lignocaine, Mexiletine, Phenytoin.

I_C: Little effect on repolarization and markedly decrease the rate of phase '0' depolarization: Encainide, Flecainide, Propafenone.

Class II: *Beta-adrenergic blockers (reduce sympathetic tone):* Propranolol, Acebutolol, Esmolol, etc (except sotalol).

Class III: *K^+ channel blockers (Prolong repolarization):* Amiodarone, Bretylium, Sotalol, Dofetilide, Ibutilide.

Newer drugs (class III): Dronedarone, Vernakalent, Azimilide, Tedisamil.

Class IV: *Ca^{++} channel blockers (Prolong conduction and refractoriness specially in SA and AV nodes):* Verapamil, Diltiazem.

Class V: *Potassium channel openers:* Adenosine.

Sodium Channel Blockers

Mechanism of Action: All drugs in Class I block the sodium channels and prevent the inward movement of Na^+ ions. Sodium channel blockers preferentially bind Na^+ channels in the open and inactivated state and thus interfere with depolarization.

Class I_A drugs block Na^+ channels and depress phase '0' depolarization.

Quinidine: By blocking Na^+ channels, it depresses all cardiac properties, *e.g.*, automaticity, excitability, conduction velocity and prolongs repolarization. It thus has membrane stabilizing activity. It also blocks potassium channels.

Quinidine also has vagolytic and adrenergic-blocking properties. It is also a skeletal muscle relaxant.

Pharmacokinetics: Quinidine is rapidly absorbed, having variable bioavailability, plasma half life is 7-9 hours, 90% bound to plasma proteins, metabolized in the liver by hydroxylation and excreted in the urine (20% unchanged.

Adverse Effects

Cardiac: Quinidine itself can cause arrhythmias (ventricular tachycardia) and heart block, hypotension, prolongation of QT interval and torsade de pointes.

Non-cardiac: Diarrhea, nausea, vomiting and hypersensitivity reactions including thrombocytopenia and rarely bone marrow depression, hepatitis and idiosyncratic reactions.

Drug Interactions

- Quinidine is a microsomal enzyme inhibitor. It raises the plasma levels of propafenone and reduces the conversion of codiene to morphine thereby decreasing its analgesic efficacy.
- Microsomal enzyme inducers like phenytoin and phenobarbitone enhance metabolism of quinidine resulting in therapeutic failure.
- Quinidine reduces the clearance of digoxin thereby precipitating digoxin toxicity.

Due to large number of adverse effect and availability of better drugs quinidine is not used commonly.

Procainamide has short half life, no interaction with digitalis, weak vagolytic properties and is not an alpha blocker. It is better tolerated, higher doses can cause hypotension, heart block and torsade de pointes.

Disopyramide has significant anticholinergic properties.

Class I_A drugs are useful in almost all types of arrhythmias (atrial fibrillation and atrial flutter).

Class I_B drug: They shorten the action potential duration and selectively act on diseased or ischemic tissue.

Lignocaine suppresses the electrical activity of the arrhythmogenic tissues. Lignocaine is used in the treatment of ventricular arrhythmias associated with AMI and with cardiac surgery. Lignocaine is not useful in atrial arrhythmias.

Phenytoin useful in digitalis induced cardiac arrhythmias and ventricular arrhythmias in children.

Mexiletine can be used orally. It is used as an alternative to lignocaine in ventricular arrhythmias.

Class I_C Drugs: They are most potent and powerful sodium channel blockers. They may be used in severe ventricular arrhythmias and to maintain sinus rhythm in atrial fibrillation refractory to other drugs.

Class II Drugs: Beta blockers like propranolol exert anti-arrhythmic effect due to blockade of cardiac beta receptors.

Cardio selective beta blockers like atenolol and metoprolol are used in the treatment and prevention of supraventricular arrhythmias especially those associated with exercise, emotion or hyperthyroidism and digitalis induced ventricular arrythmias.

Class III Drugs: These drugs prolong the action potential duration and refractory period by blocking the potassium channels.

Amiodarone: It acts by multiple mechanisms. It prolongs APD by blocking Ca^{2+} channels, blocks sodium channels, blocks beta adrenergic receptors (having properties of all four classes of anti-arrhythmic drugs).

Adverse Effects: Heart block, cardiac failure, hypotension, bluish discoloration of the skin, hypothyroidism, gastrointestinal disturbances, hepatotoxicity, pulmonary fibrosis, myopathy, peripheral neuropathy are common adverse effects.

Amiodarone is used in:

(1) Life-threatening ventricular arrhythmias specially post myocardial infarction and associated with CCF.

(2) In preventing recurrences of paroxysmal AF or Aflutter.

Bretylium used in resistant ventricular arrhythmias. Newer class III drugs also act on K^+ channels and have less adverse effects.

Dofetilide is a newly introduced and selective K^+, channel blocker. It has no other actions as it is a pure K^+ channel blocker and prolongs APD. It is used orally in atrial fibrillation to convert and to maintain sinus rhythm. The only adverse effect known is torsade de pointes in 1% patients.

Ibutilide used as intravenous infusion to quickly convert atrial flutter/fibrillation to sinus rhythm.

Class IV Drugs: Calcium channel blockers inhibit the inward movement of calcium (verapamil and diltiazem) and have prominent cardiac effects through AV node and increase the refractory period of nodal tissue.

Adenosine is a potassium channel opener having large number of the effects including adenosine-sensitive inward rectifier potassium opener with inhibition of the sinus and AV node. It enhance potassium conductance and inhibition of cAMP induced calcium flux and suppression of calcium dependent action potential. It is used in PSVT.

DRUG THERAPY OF DYSLIPIDAEMIA

Hypolipidaemic Drugs

Lipids and proteins form complexes called lipoproteins and circulate in the blood vessels. There are four types of lipoproteins: Low density lipoproteins (LDL), High density lipoproteins (HDL), Very low density lipoproteins (VLDL), Chylomicrons (CM).

LDL is the primary carrier of cholesterol while VLDL carries triglycerides. Hyper lipoproteinaemias (HPL) are conditions in which the concentration of cholesterol or triglyceride (TG) carrying lipoproteins in the plasma is elevated above normal. Increase in lipoproteins can hasten the development of atherosclerosis and is a risk factor for myocardial infarction and ischemic cardiac diseases. Increase in VLDL, LDL (rarely CM) are atherogenic while HDL may be protective as it facilitate removal of CH from tissue.

Hypolipidaemics Drugs

1. **HMG CoA reductase inhibitors:** Lovastatin, Simvastatin, Pravastatin, Atorvastatin, Rosuvastatin, Fluvastatin.
2. **Fibric acids derivatives:** Gemfibrozil, Clofibrate, Fenofibrate, Bezafibrate, Ciprofibrate.
3. **Bile acid binding resins:** Cholestyramine, Colestipol, Plant sterols, Colesevelam.
4. **Antioxidant:** Probucol, Omega-3 fatty acid.

5. **Miscellaneous:** Nicotinic acid, Neomycin, Gugulipid, Ezetimibe
6. **Newer drugs:** Torcetrapib, Anacetrapib.

HMG CoA Reductase Inhibitors (Statins)

3-Hydroxy 3-methylglutaryl CoA (HMGCoA) reductase is the rate controlling enzyme in the biosynthesis of cholesterol. Statins inhibits this enzyme and biosynthesis of cholesterol (CH). This leads to the depletion of intracellular pools of cholesterol which in turn increase the expression of LDL-receptors. This enhances the removal of circulating LDL and LDL precursors. They also reduce hepatic VLDL synthesis and reduced TG levels.

Lovastatin and its congeners are competitive inhibitors of the enzyme HMGCoA and inhibit the conversion of HMG-CoA to mevalonic acid. They lower plasma LDL cholesterol and triglycerides. The concentration of HDL cholesterol (the protective lipoprotein) increases by 10%. Atorvastatin is most potent, long acting with additional anti-oxidant property.

Pharmacokinetics: Statins are well absorbed when given orally but may undergo extensive first pass metabolism in the liver by the Cyt P450 (except atorvastatin). Food enhances their absorption. Simvastatin is a prodrug converted to its active metabolite in the liver.

Adverse Effects

These include GI disturbances, headache, insomnia, vertigo rashes, and rarely angioedema. They increase the level of hepatic enzymes. Statins rarely causes muscle tenderness and myopathy with inflammation of the skeletal muscles leads to muscle pain and weakness.

Uses

Statins are used in patients with MI, angina, stroke and transient ischemic attacks to lower cholesterol levels in primary hyperlipidaemias.

Contraindications are active liver disease, pregnancy, with drugs like cyclosporine, macrolide and azol antifungal.

Fibric Acids (Fibrates)

Fibric acids enhance activity of the enzyme lipoprotein lipase which degrades VLDL resulting in lowering of triglycerides. They also increase HDL levels. Fibrates also inhibit coagulation and promote thrombolysis, which also account for their beneficial effects. Many effects of these agents are affected by binding to peroxisome proliferators activator receptor (PPARs). All are well absorbed orally and highly protein bound drugs.

Adverse Effects

GI upset, skin rashes, headache, myositis, muscle cramps and blurred vision. Fibrates can cause rhabdomyolysis particularly in patients with renal failure and when used with statins.

Bezafibrate is, similar to gemfibrozil and has greater LDL lowering effects.

Contraindications are hepatic dysfunction, renal dysfunction and gallbladder disease.

Bile Acid Binding Resins

Bile acid binding resins are not absorbed but they bind bile acids in the intestine and increase their excretion by preventing their reabsorption. Bile acids are required for intestinal absorption of cholesterol and up regulation of LDL receptor activity. Thus plasma cholesterol and LDL levels fall. Bile acid binding resins are unpleasant to take; they may cause GI upset, constipation and piles. They also bind with fat soluble vitamins and many drugs like warfarin, chlorothiazide, digoxin in the intestines thereby reducing their absorption. They can be used along with lovastatin or nicotinic acid.

Probucol lowers LDL and HDL cholesterol and has antioxidant properties. It is generally not preferred.

Nicotinic acid inhibits triglyceride synthesis in the liver and VLDL production by inhibiting the mobilization of fatty acid from adipose tissue, thus resulting in a decrease in LDL and increase in HDL cholesterol. Adverse effects include flushing, dyspepsia, dryness and pigmentation of the skin.

Niacin is used in hypertriglyceridaemia with low HDL levels.

Omega 3 fatty acid: Fish oil contain PUFA (poly unsaturated fatty acids) and used as prophylaxis in high risk patients of coronary artery disease with hyperlipidaemia.

Gugulipid obtained from 'gum guggul' lowers plasma cholesterol and triglycerides. It is well tolerated but can cause diarrhea.

Ezetimibe act by inhibiting intestinal absorption of cholesterol.

Newer agents: Cholesterol ester transfer proteins (CETP) inhibitor, *e.g.*, torcitrapib, anacetrapib results in increase in HDL-CH and decrease in LDL-CH levels.Combination of two lipid lowering agent is very useful.

PLASMA EXPANDERS

Plasma expanders are high molecular weight substances which when infused IV exert osmotic pressure and remain in the body for a long time to increase the volume of circulating fluid.

The plasma expanders used are dextrans, gelatin polymer, hydroxyethyl starches, polyvinyl pyrrolidone and human albumin.

Dextrans (Dextran 70 mol. wt. 70,000 and dextran 40 mol. wt. 40,000) are polysaccharides obtained from sugar beat. Their osmotic pressure is similar to that of plasma proteins. **Dextran 70** effectively expands the plasma volume and remains so for 24 hours. It interferes with coagulation, blood grouping and cross matching. One gram of dextran in circulation maintains 20 ml of plasma volume. **Dextran 40** is faster but shorter acting. It can improve microcirculation in shock by preventing rouleax formation of RBCs and have an anti-sludging effect. It can block renal tubules resulting in renal failure, though rare. Allergic reactions are common as dextrans are antigenic.

Dextrans have a long shelf life (10 years). Dextran should not be used:

a. If the urinary output is less than 1500 ml/day.
b. For more than 5 days.
c. When blood urea is 60 mg % or higher.
d. Patients allergic to dextran, with cardiac failure and with severe anaemia.

Dextrans are used in burns, endotoxic shock and extensive tissue damage.

Gelatin products have a molecular weight of 30,000 and have duration of action of 12 hours. They do not interfere with coagulation, blood grouping and cross-matching. They can rarely cause urticaria, allergic reactions and bronchospasm.

Hydroxyethyl starch (Hetastarch) maintains blood volume for a long period. Allergic reactions are rare and it does not interfere with coagulation.

Polyvinyl pyrrolidone (PVP): It is not preferred due to various disadvantages, *e.g.*, it provokes histamine release and interferes with blood grouping. Human albumin is obtained from pooled human blood. It is given as 5% or 20% solution. It is non-antigenic, does not interfere with coagulation, blood grouping or cross-matching.

Human albumin is used in edema, burns, hypovolaemic shock, hypoproteinaemia, acute liver failure and in dialysis.

Uses of Plasma Expanders

These are used as plasma substitutes in hypovolaemic shock burns and in extensive fluid loss, as an emergency measure to restore plasma volume in whole blood loss but they do not have oxygen carrying capacity.

DRUGS ACTING ON BLOOD AND BLOOD FORMING ORGANS

In the blood two sets of factors, *i.e.*, pro-coagulant and anti-coagulants are present. Coagulation of blood in vessels does not occur due to presence of anti-coagulant. Three basic mechanisms which prevent the blood loss from smaller vessels are: (1) vascular spasm caused by damage to smooth muscle; (2) platelet plug formation; and (3) blood coagulation.

COAGULANTS AND ANTI-COAGULANTS

Coagulants (Haemostatic Agents)

Local Haemostatics (Styptics)

These drugs are used locally to control bleeding from capillaries and minute vessels, *e.g.*, tooth sockets, open wound etc. Most of them provide a network of fibrin which promotes coagulation. These are:

Astringents, Adrenaline, Thrombin, Fibrin glue, Gelatin, Calcium alginate, Oxidized cellulose and Russel's viper venom.

Systemic Agents

Vitamin K

It is a fat-soluble vitamin, which promotes coagulation. It is required for the synthesis of clotting factors. Vitamin K exists in different forms: **vitamin K_1** is obtained from the plant and animal sources; **vitamin K_2** is produced by intestinal bacteria and is stored in hepatic tissue; whereas **vitamin K_3** is a synthetic form. All the three forms of vitamin K (K_1, K_2 and K_3) are naphthoquinone derivatives. Vitamin K is found in green leafy vegetables butter, meat, milk, liver and pears. Daily intake for an adult is 50-100 mcg/day. Vitamin K_1 and K_2 require the presence of bile for their absorption while water-soluble forms can be absorbed in the absence of bile. There is no proper storage of vitamin K in the body. It is metabolized in liver and the conjugated glucuronide are excreted in bile and urine.

Actions

Vitamin K acts as a cofactor in the hepatic synthesis of certain clotting factors (factor II, VII, IX and X). It is also required for the gamma carboxylation of glutamic acid residues of osteocalcin, which is important for bone development. Deficiency of vitamin K is manifested as increased bleeding tendency and hypoprothrombinaemia.

Uses

1. For prevention and treatment of bleeding associated with vitamin K deficiency.
2. In obstructive jaundice with hemorrhagic symptoms–vitamin K_1 is preferred parenterally, vitamin K_3 can be given orally.
3. Vitamin K_1 (1 mg phytonadione, I.M.) is given routinely to all neonates to prevent bleeding, as the intestinal flora which is necessary for the synthesis of vitamin K is not developed.
4. To control bleeding due to oral anti-coagulant therapy, phytonadione (vitamin K_1) is used.
5. Vitamin K_1 is used in salicylate poisoning with hemorrhagic complications.

Adverse Reactions

Oral vitamin K is safe. Reactions to I.V. injection include flushing, sweating, dyspnoea, cyanosis, collapse and anaphylactic reaction. Menadione may cause haemolysis, hyperbilirubinaemia and kernicterus in newborn, hence is not used.

Other systemic procoagulants are: Fibrinogen, Anti-hemophilic factor, Ethamsylate and Desmopressin, Amino caproic acid, Aprotinin, Rutin etc.

Anti-Coagulants

Anti-coagulants are drugs that prevent or reduce the coagulability of blood.

Classification

1. **Drugs used in vitro:**
   A. Heparin.
   B. Sodium citrate: Used in blood banks to store the blood.

C. Sodium oxalate and sodium edetate are used as an anti-coagulant in laboratory.

2. **Drugs used in vivo:**

A. Parenteral anti-coagulants:

i. *Heparin and low molecular weight heparins (LMWHs): e.g.,* Enoxaparin, Dalteparin, Tinzaparin and Ardeparin.

ii. *Heparinoids:* Heparan sulphate, Lepirudin and Danaparoid, Hirudin, Bivalirudin, Argatroban.

B. Oral anti-coagulants:

i. *Coumarin derivatives:* Warfarin, Dicumarol, Acenocoumarol.

ii. *Indandione derivatives:* Phenindione.

Heparin

Heparin is a mixture of sulfated mucopolysaccharides with a molecular weight ranging from 10,000–40,000. Antithrombin III inhibits activated clotting factors X_a, II_a, IX_a XI_a, XII_a and XIII_a by forming stable complexes with them. Under physiological condition, these interactions are slow. But heparin accelerates the activity of plasma anti-thrombin III 1000 times. At low concentration, heparin selectively inhibits the conversion of prothrombin to thrombin. Heparin thus prevents further thrombus formation, but it does not have thrombolytic action. Both thrombin (IIa) and factor Xa are sensitive to the inhibitory effect of heparin-AT III complex. Heparin in high doses has anti-platelet action and, thereby, prolongs the bleeding time. Heparin reduces the blood lipid level by releasing lipoprotein lipase from vessel wall and tissues.

Pharmacokinetics

Heparin is not absorbed after oral administration because of its high negative charge and large molecular size. Therefore, it must be given parenterally (intravenously or subcutaneously). Heparin is highly protein bound. It does not cross the BBB or placental barrier and is safe during pregnancy. It is rapidly inactivated in the liver by heparinase and the metabolites are excreted in urine.

During heparin therapy, the activated partial thromboplastin time (aPTT) monitoring is necessary, and it should be maintained at 1.5–2.5 times of the normal value.

Adverse Effects

1. *Bleeding:* Heparin has a narrow therapeutic dose range and bleeding is the main side effect. Protamine sulphate is a specific

heparin antagonist used for bleeding due to heparin overdose especially in cardiac / vascular surgery (need to terminate heparin action rapidly).

2. Heparin induced thrombocytopenia.
3. Hypersensitivity reactions.
4. Osteoporosis.

Low Molecular Weight Heparins (LMWHs)

These are fractionated heparin with low molecular weight. LMWHs produce anti-coagulant effect mainly by inhibiting Xa activity. LMWH therapy usually does not require aPTT monitoring but patients with chronic renal failure may need monitoring by measuring factor Xa activity. LMWHs are given subcutaneously.

Advantages of LMWHs

1. They have higher SC bioavailability as compared to conventional heparin (UFH).
2. They have a longer duration of action (longer plasma half life).
3. They do not routinely require aPTT monitoring.
4. There is a lower incidence of thrombocytopaenia.
5. Better patient compliance as there is no need for blood tests.
6. Less bound to plasma proteins.

Heparinoids

Lepirudin: It is a recombinant hirudin. It directly inhibits thrombin and is used as an anti-coagulant in patients with heparin induced thrombocytopaenia (HIT). It is administered intravenously.

Danaparoid: It has mainly inhibits Xa activity. It is for prophylaxis and intravenously for treatment of post operative deep vein thrombosis.

Oral Anti-Coagulants

Mechanism of Action

Clotting factors II, VII, IX and X are synthesized in liver as inactive proteins, where vitamin K acts as a cofactor. Warfarin is a coumarin derivative and has a structure similar to that of vitamin K. Hence, warfarin acts as a competitive antagonist of vitamin K and interferes/inhibits the synthesis of vitamin K dependent factors II, VII, IX and X by inhibiting epoxide reductase enzyme and thus produces anti-coagulant effect. Monitoring of therapy is done by estimation of prothrombin time (PT) of blood. They do not alter bleeding time. There is always a delay in the onset of anti-coagulant effect because the levels of clotting factors already in plasma decline slowly over a period of 1–3 days.

Pharmacokinetics

Commercial warfarin is a racemic mixture of R (+) and S (-) warfarin. S (-) form is more potent. Warfarin is almost completely absorbed after oral administration; oral bioavailability is almost 100%. Food interferes with the absorption of warfarin. It is highly bound to plasma proteins (99%), freely crosses the placental barrier, is metabolized in the liver by glucuronide conjugation and the inactive metabolites are excreted in urine and stool. It has a long half-life of about 40 hours, and the duration of action is 3-6 days.

Adverse Effects

1. *Bleeding:* Vitamin K can be used to treat the over dosage toxicity of oral anti-coagulants.
2. Teratogenic effect.
3. Skin necrosis.
4. Other rare side effect includes diarrhea, alopecia, urticaria, dermatitis, abdominal cramps and anorexia.

Drug Interactions

1. Barbiturates/carbamazepine/rifampicin/griseofulvin: They all are enzyme inducers and increase metabolic clearance of oral anti-coagulants and hence decrease the anti-coagulant effect.
2. Alcohol, Chloramphenicol, Isoniazid, Imidazoles and Disufiram are enzyme inhibitors; thus decrease metabolic clearance of warfarin and hence increase the anti-coagulant effect.
3. Aspirin and other NSAIDs (have an anti-platelet effect) and cotrimoxazole displace warfarin from the plasma protein binding site, thus potentiate the warfarin effect.
4. Liquid paraffin potentiates the activity of warfarin by reducing absorption of vitamin K.

Therapeutic Uses of Anticoagulants

1. Deep vein thrombosis and pulmonary embolism (treatment and prophylaxis).
2. Myocardial infarction, Unstable angina.
3. Atrial fibrillation.

4. Thromboembolism, Disseminated intravascular coagulation.
5. Rheumatic heart disease.
6. Cerebrovascular disease.

Contraindications

1. Bleeding disorders.
2. Severe hypertension.
3. Tuberculosis.
4. Pregnancy (warfarin is contraindicated).
5. Chronic alcoholics.
6. With aspirin (should be used cautiously).

FIBRINOLYTICS (THROMBOLYTICS)

These drugs are used to dissolve the thrombi in blood vessels, mainly coronary arteries. Fibrinolytics promote the conversion of plasminogen to plasmin. Plasmin degrades fibrin and thus rapidly dissolves the blood clot. As compared to arterial thrombi, venous thrombi are lysed more easily. Various fibrinolytic agents are:

1. **Streptokinase**
   It is a protein derived from beta hemolytic streptococci. It has an affinity for fibrin bound plasminogen on the thrombus. Streptokinase binds with circulating plasminogen to form a complex that activates plasminogen to plamsin. Streptokinase is antigenic, pyrogenic and destroyed by circulating anti-streptococcal antibodies. It is given by I.V. infusion. Adverse effects are: hypotension, allergic reactions like fever, chills and skin rashes and rarely anaphylactoid reaction.
2. **Urokinase**
   It is an enzyme isolated from human fetal kidney cell cultures. It directly activates plasminogen to plasmin. It has less affinity for fibrin. Urokinase is non-antigenic, not destroyed by antibodies. It is administered initially as I.V. bolus, followed by I.V. infusion. Bleeding can occur but hypotension and allergic reactions are rare.
3. **Altepase (Tissue plaminogen activator t-PA)**
   It is derived from recombinant DNA technology. It has low affinity for circulating free plasminogen and selectively activates plasminogen that is bound to fibrin and avoids the activation of circulating plasminogen. It is superior to streptokinase and urokinase in dissolving old clots. Alteplase is non-antigenic, non-

pyogenic, not destroyed by antibodies, rapidly acting, more potent, more effective and more expensive. It is administered initially as IV bolus, followed by IV infusion. Bleeding is less with t-PA; no allergic reactions.

4. **Antistreplase:** It is a combination of streptokinase and plasmiogen, have improved pharmacokinetic ($t_{½}$ is > 90 min).
5. **Reteplase:** It is also a recombinant t PA and has longer plasma half life.
6. **Tenecteplase:** It is genetically engineered mutant form of alteplase with longer plasma half life.

Use of Fibrinolytics

1. **Acute MI:** The main aim of fibrinolytic therapy is to restore the coronary artery patency. These drugs dissolve the clot by promoting the conversion of plasminogen to plasmin. Thrombolytic therapy is more effective if they are administered within 6–12 hours of onset of symptoms.
2. **Deep vein thrombosis.**
3. **Pulmonary embolism.**

Contraindications include recent trauma, surgery, abortion, stroke, severe hypertension, diabetes, liver damage, peptic ulcer and bleeding disorders.

Anti-Fibrinolytics

Anti-fibrinolytic blocks the conversion of plasminogen to plasmin by binding with lysine and thus inhibits the fibrinolytic activity. These are:

- Epsilon amino caproic acid (EACA).
- Tranexaemic acid; and
- Aprotinin.

They are used in:

1. Overdose of fibrinolytics.
2. To prevent recurrence of sub-arachnoid and G.I. hemorrhage, menorrhagia.
3. After cardiopulmonary bypass surgery.

ANTI-PLATELET DRUGS (ANTI-THROMBOTIC DRUGS)

Activation and subsequent aggregation of platelets is a major component of arterial thrombus. This may initiate venous thrombosis. Drugs that inhibit platelet aggregation are called anti-platelet drugs.

Classification

1. **TXA_2 synthesis inhibitor:** Aspirin (low dose).
2. **Phosphodiesterase inhibitor:** Dipyridamole.
3. **Thienopyridine derivatives:** Ticlopidine and Clopidogrel.
4. **Glycoprotein (GP)-II_b/III_a**-antibodies (Abciximab) and receptor antagonist (Eptifibatide and Tirofiban).
5. **Others:** Epoprostenol (PGI_2).

Aspirin (TXA_2 Synthesis Inhibitor)

Low dose aspirin (50–325 mg) irreversibly acetylates platelet COX-I and reduces the production of TXA_2, which is a platelet aggregation stimulant and vasoconstrictor. The anti-platelet effect lasts for the life time of the platelets, *i.e.*, 7–10 days thus the activity is restored only by the formation of new platelets.

Dipyridamole (Phosphodiesterase Inhibitor)

It is a coronary vasodilator. It inhibits phosphodiesterase and increases the concentration of cyclic adenosine monophosphate (cAMP) levels which inhibit platelet adhesion and aggregation. It is occasionally used in combination with warfarin during postoperative period in patients with prosthetic heart valves.

Ticlopidine and Clopidogrel

They are prodrugs and structurally related. They inhibit adenosine diphosphate (ADP)-mediated platelet aggregation. There is no effect on platelet TXA_2, but bleeding time is prolonged. They permanently inhibits the P_2Y_{12} receptor, so, has longer duration of anti-platelet effect. The most common side effects are nausea, vomiting, diarrhea, neutropaenia, agranulocytosis, thrombocytopaenia and GI bleeding. **Clopidogrel** is a congener of ticlopidine and safer than ticlopidine. They produce synergistic effect when combined with aspirin or $GPII_b/III_a$ antagonists.

Abciximab, Eptifibatide and Tirofiban

They block the receptors for fibrinogen and von Willebrand factor (vWF) on platelet surface and thus prevent the final step in the process of platelet aggregation.

Abciximab is a chiramic monoclonal antibody which binds to $GPII_b/III_a$ **Eptifibatide** is a cyclic hepta peptide and synthetic drug which is more specific for $GPII_b/III_a$. **Tirofiban** is a nonpeptide, potent GPIIb/III receptor antagonist. These drugs are administered parenterally and are used in percutaneous coronary intervention, unstable angina and acute MI. The main side effect of these drugs is bleeding.

Epoprostenol

It causes vasodilatation and inhibits platelet aggregation. It is used during renal dialysis to inhibit platelet aggregation, but it has a short duration of action (<3 minutes).

Uses

1. Acute MI.
2. Unstable angina.
3. Angioplastic coronary interventions (coronary bypass implants).
4. Prosthetic heart valves and AV shunts.
5. Transient ischemic attack.
6. Cerebrovascular disease.

MULTIPLE CHOICE QUESTIONS

Q. 1 All of the following drugs act by releasing nitric oxide *except:*

(A) Glyceryl trinitrate (B) Sodium nitroprusside
(C) Hydralazine (D) Fenoldopam

Q. 2 Which anti-hypertensive agent can be used during pregnancy?

(A) Spironolactone (B) Labetalol
(C) ACE inhibitor (D) Sodium nitroprusside

Q. 3 Digoxin toxicity is precipitated by all *except:*

(A) Electrolyte disturbance (B) Acute myocardial infarction
(C) Hepatic disease (D) Renal disease

Q. 4 The most significant adverse effect of angiotensin converting enzyme inhibitors (ACEIs) is:

(A) Hypotension (B) Hypercalcaemia
(C) Hypokalemia (D) Hypocalcaemia

Q. 5 All of the following are the indications of angiotensin converting enzyme inhibitors (ACEIs) *except:*

(A) Hypertension
(B) Myocardial infarction
(C) Left ventricular dysfunction
(D) Pheochromocytoma

Q. 6 Aldosterone antagonists (spironolactone) are useful in the treatment of all *except:*

(A) Hypertension (B) Gynecomastia
(C) Hyperaldosteronism (D) Congestive heart failure

Q. 7 Which of the following statement is not true regarding hydralazine?

(A) It causes direct relaxation of blood vessels
(B) It causes dilatation of both arteries and veins
(C) Postural hypotension is not a common problem
(D) It causes lupus syndrome

Q. 8 Which anti-hypertensive is contraindicated during pregnancy?

(A) Enalapril (B) Methyldopa
(C) Nifedipine (D) Labetalol

---

1 (D) 2 (B) 3 (C) 4 (A) 5 (D) 6 (B) 7 (B) 8 (A)

Q. 9 All of the following are useful IV therapy for hypertensive emergency *except:*

(A) Fenoldopam (B) Esmolol
(C) Enalapril (D) Nifedipine

Q. 10 Which statement is not true about clonidine?

(A) It causes reduction in central sympathetic outflow
(B) It increase LDL cholesterol on prolonged use
(C) Sedation and contact dermatitis are common side effect
(D) It can be used in prophylaxis of migraine

Q. 11 Digoxin is contraindicated in:

(A) Supraventricular tachycardia
(B) Atrial fibrillation
(C) Congestive heart failure
(D) Hypertrophic obstructive cardiomyopathy

Q. 12 The true statement regarding losartan is:

(A) It is a competitive angiotensin receptor antagonist
(B) It has a short acting metabolite
(C) It is associated with cough
(D) It causes hyperuricemia

Q. 13 The mechanism of action of sodium nitroprusside is:

(A) It increases cAMP
(B) It is K^+ channel opener
(C) It is calcium channel blocker
(D) It increases guanylyl cyclase (cGMP)

Q. 14 Digoxin is not a drug of choice in:

(A) Atrial flutter
(B) Atrial fibrillation
(C) Paroxysmal supraventricular tachycardia
(D) High output failure

Q. 15 The antihypertensive agent used in elderly diabetic patient with bilateral renal artery stenosis is:

(A) Enalapril (B) Verapamil
(C) Beta blocker (D) Thiazide diuretic

---

9 (C) 10 (B) 11 (D) 12 (A) 13 (D) 14 (D) 15 (B)

Q. 16 Coronary steal phenomenon is caused by:

(A) Diltiazem (B) Propranolol
(C) Verapamil (D) Dipyridamole

Q. 17 The true statement about isosorbide mononitrate is:

(A) It does not undergo first pass metabolism
(B) It has shorter duration of action than isosorbide dinitrate
(C) It has rapid onset of action
(D) It is preferred nitrate in cyanide poisoning

Q. 18 Most suitable anti-hypertensive agent in children with malignant hypertension is:

(A) Sodium nitroprusside
(B) Frusemide
(C) Sublingual nifedipine
(D) Enalapril

Q. 19 All are true about statins *except:*

(A) It inhibits HMG CoA reductase
(B) It decreases number of LDL receptors
(C) It decreases hepatic cholesterol synthesis
(D) It decreases VLDL

Q. 20 True statement about nitrates is:

(A) They release nitric oxide (NO)
(B) They increase AV conduction
(C) They increase cardiac output
(D) They have low first pass metabolism

Q. 21 All of the following anti-arrhythmic drugs causes prolonged effective refractory period (ERP) *except:*

(A) Mexiletine (B) Quinidine
(C) Procainamide (D) Amiodaron

Q. 22 In congestive cardiac failure nitrates are used because:

(A) They decrease preload
(B) They have direct inotropic action
(C) They causes coronary vasodilatation
(D) They decrease afterload

---

16 (D) 17 (A) 18 (A) 19 (B) 20 (A) 21 (A) 22 (A)

Q. 23 Which of the following anti-hypertensive drug is not having any central effect?

(A) Clonidine (B) Reserpine
(C) Propranolol (D) Indapamide

Q. 24 Mechanism of action of digitalis in atrial fibrillation is:

(A) It increase AV node refractoriness
(B) By blocking Na^{+} - K^{+} ATPase pump
(C) It decrease AV node refractoriness
(D) It decreases effective refractory period (ERP) of AV node

Q. 25 Nifedipine and beta blocker are given together in heart block:

(A) To decrease pedal edema due to nifedipine
(B) To overcome increased sympathetic activity of nifedipine
(C) Due to anti-CHF action of propranolol
(D) Due to anti-arrhythmic effect of nifedipine

Q. 26 All are true about calcium channel blocker *except:*

(A) Diltiazem does not cause tachycardia
(B) Verapamil is more effective in ventricular arrhythmia
(C) Nifedipine has mild natriuretic action
(D) Nimlodipine cross blood brain barrier (BBB)

Q. 27 All of the following are predominant arteriolar dilator *except:*

(A) Dizoxide (B) Minoxidil
(C) Hydralazine (D) Sodium nitroprusside

Q. 28 The ACEIs differs than Aldosterone Receptor Antagonists (ARAs) in all manner *except:*

(A) ARAs has no effect on bradykinin
(B) ARAs are more specific for angiotensin II enzyme
(C) ARAs increases circulating angiotensin II levels
(D) ACEIs cause total elimination of angiotensin II

Q. 29 Which nitrate is used in esophageal spasm?

(A) Glyceryl trinitrate
(B) Amyl nitrate
(C) Isosorbide dinitrate
(D) Isosorbide mononitrate

---

23 (D) 24 (A) 25 (B) 26 (B) 27 (D) 28 (D) 29 (A)

Q. 30 Which calcium channel blocker (CCB) release nitric oxide (NO) from the endothelium?

(A) Nitrendipine
(B) Amlodipine
(C) Felodipine
(D) Nifedipine

Q. 31 Which drug is preferred when a patient with hyperthyroidism develop atrial fibrillation?

(A) Verapamil
(B) Propranolol
(C) Digitalis
(D) Tocainide

Q. 32 A drug that can cause renal damage in the fetus if given during pregnancy is:

(A) Angiotensin converting enzyme inhibitors (ACEIs)
(B) Diazoxide
(C) Hydralazine
(D) Fenoldopam

Q. 33 All drugs can precipitate angina *except:*

(A) Amphetamine
(B) Terbutaline
(C) Isoprenaline
(D) Metoprolol

Q. 34 Which calcium channel blocker (CCB) is preferred in patients having sub-arachnoid hemorrhage?

(A) Nimlodipine (B) Amlodipine
(C) Nicardipine (D) Lacidipine

Q. 35 The drug least useful in heart failure is?

(A) Digitalis (B) Diltiazem (CCB)
(C) Beta receptor agonist (D) Diuretics

Q. 36 Which of the following drugs does not reduce mortality in chronic congestive heart failure?

(A) Carvedilol (B) Digoxin
(C) Enalapril (D) Spironolactone

---

30 (A) 31 (B) 32 (A) 33 (D) 34 (A) 35 (B) 36 (B)

Q. 37 Most relevant statement about procainamide is:

(A) It may worsen or precipitate hyperthyroidism
(B) It is not effective for atrial arrhythmias
(C) It prolongs the AP and may precipitate torsade de pointes arrhythmia
(D) It commonly induces headache and tinnitus

Q. 38 Which of the following drug is not suitable for chronic oral therapy in arrhythmias?

(A) Amiodarone (B) Quinidine
(C) Verapamil (D) Esmolol

Q. 39 All are recognized adverse effects of quinidine *except:*

(A) Cinchonism (B) Diarrhea
(C) Thrombocytopenia (D) Lupus erythematosus

Q. 40 Which of the following has longest plasma half life as anti-arrhythmic agent?

(A) Amiodarone (B) Flecainide
(C) Disopyramide (D) Mexiletine

Q. 41 When used for prolonged period thiazide shows the following properties *except:*

(A) Decreased urinary excretion of calcium
(B) Elevation of blood cholesterol and blood glucose
(C) Elevation of plasma uric acid
(D) Ototoxicity

Q. 42 The most useful diuretic in the treatment of pulmonary edema is:

(A) Acetazolamide (B) Furosemide
(C) Mannitol (D) Hydrochlorthiazide

Q. 43 Most common adverse effect of acetazolamide is:

(A) Paresthesia
(B) Metabolic alkalosis
(C) Urinary acidosis
(D) Hyperkalemia

---

37 (C) 38 (D) 39 (D) 40 (A) 41 (D) 42 (B) 43 (A)

Q. 44 Which of the following is the drug of choice for syndrome of inappropriate secretion of anti-diuretic hormone (SIADH)?

(A) Demeclocycline
(B) Vasopressin
(C) Thiazide
(D) Chlorpropamide

Q. 45 Which of the following anti-coagulant can be used during pregnancy?

(A) Warfarin
(B) Heparin
(C) Phenindione
(D) Acenocoumerin

Q. 46 All tests are useful to monitor heparin therapy *except:*

(A) Clotting time
(B) PTT
(C) Thrombin time
(D) Bleeding time

Q. 47 Which of the following anti-thrombotic agent does not inhibit platelet prostaglandin formation?

(A) Ticlopidine (B) Dazoxiben
(C) Aspirin (D) Sulphinpyrazone

Q. 48 Excessive bleeding by warfarin can be reversed by all:

(A) Vitamin K_1 (B) Vitamin K_3
(C) Protamine (D) Sodium citrate

Q. 49 All are the long term adverse effects of heparin *except:*

(A) Alopecia (B) Reduction in AT III
(C) Thrombocytopenia (D) Osteoporosis

Q. 50 The mechanism of action of heparin is:

(A) Direct inhibition of prothrombin to thrombin conversion
(B) Facilitation of AT III mediated inhibition of a factor X_a
(C) Activation of AT III to inhibit factor IX and XI
(D) Inhibition of factor XII_a and XIII_a

---

44 (A) 45 (B) 46 (D) 47 (A) 48 (A) 49 (B) 50 (B)

Q. 51 Anti-coagulants are indicated in:

(A) Deep vein thrombosis
(B) Buerger's disease
(C) Stroke due to cerebral thrombosis
(D) All of the above

Q. 52 Which fibrinolytic is antigenic?

(A) Streptokinase (B) Urokinase
(C) Alteplase (D) Reteplase

Q. 53 All are the important complications of streptokinase *except:*

(A) Hypotension (B) Bleeding
(C) Fever (D) Anaphylaxis

Q. 54 Which of the following drug act without altering levels of TXA_2 or prostacyclin?

(A) Aspirin (B) Sulphinpyrazone
(C) Dipyridamole (D) Clofibrate

Q. 55 As a plasma expander, dextran has the following advantages *except:*

(A) It exerts oncotic pressure similar to plasma proteins
(B) It keeps plasma volume expanded for about 24 hours
(C) It is non-pyrogenic
(D) It does not interfere with grouping and cross matching of blood

Q. 56 Plasma expanders are contraindicated in following condition:

(A) Severe burn
(B) Hypovolumic shock
(C) Septic shock
(D) Anaemia

Q. 57 Nesiritide is a:

(A) Brain natriuretic peptide analogue
(B) Endothelin R-antagonist
(C) Gp IIb/IIIa antagonist
(D) TNF-alpha-antagonist

---

51 (A) 52 (A) 53 (B) 54 (C) 55 (D) 56 (D) 57 (A)

Q. 58 Which anti-hypertensive agent is contraindicated during pregnancy?

(A) Enalapril (B) Methyl dopa
(C) Nifedipine (D) Labetalol

Q. 59 The drug used in idiopathic hypercalciuria is:

(A) Loop diuretics
(B) Carbonic anhydrase inhibitors
(C) Thiazide diuretics
(D) Potassium-sparing diuretics

Q. 60 The drug of choice in ventricular arrhythmia following myocardial infarction is:

(A) Dobutamine (B) Digitalis
(C) Quinidine (D) Lidocaine

Q. 61 Angiotensin converting enzyme inhibitors (ACEI) should not be given concurrently with which of the following group?

(A) Potassium sparing diuretics
(B) Thiazide diuretics
(C) Beta adrenergic blockers
(D) Calcium channel blockers

Q. 62 Which of the following drug is used for the termination of acute attack of paroxysmal supraventricular tachycardia (PSVT)?

(A) Verapamil (B) Digitoxin
(C) Sotalol (D) Quinidine

Q. 63 Which of the following advantage is possessed by beta adrenergic blocking drugs?

(A) They do not cause postural hypotension
(B) They show high anti-hypertensive efficacy when used alone
(C) They can be used in combination with other anti-hypertensive drug
(D) They can be used in elderly

Q. 64 Which of the following drug inhibit HMG-CoA reductase?

(A) Nicotinic acid (B) Rosuvastatin
(C) Cholestyramine (D) Gemifibrozil

---

58 (A) 59 (C) 60 (D) 61 (A) 62 (A) 63 (A) 64 (B)

Q. 65 Anti-arrhythmic drug that can cause fatal pulmonary fibrosis is:

(A) Quinidine (B) Amiodarone
(C) Mexiletine (D) Flecainide

Q. 66 Low molecular weight heparin (LMWH) differs from standard heparin in all of the following respect *except:*

(A) It has equal or greater efficacy
(B) It causes lower incidence of bleeding
(C) It is to be given more frequently
(D) Bioavailability is increased from S.C. injection site

Q. 67 The calcium channel blocker which is particularly effective in dilating cerebral blood vessels is:

(A) Amlodipine (B) Nicardipine
(C) Nimodipine (D) Felodipine

Q. 68 The drug which possesses both diuretic and vasodilator property is:

(A) Chlorthiazide (B) Chlorthalidone
(C) Amiloride (D) Indapamide

---

65 (B) 66 (C) 67 (C) 68 (D)

ANSWERS

Ans. 1 **(D)** Nitrates, hydralazine, sodium nitroprusside and fenoldopam are vasodilators. Hydralazine is arteriolar vasodilator which depends in part of the presence of an intact endothelium. So besides activating K^+ channels, it may generate nitric oxide and stimulation of cGMP. Sodium nitroprusside is arteriolar as well as venodilator. It also activate guanylyl cyclase either directly or through release of nitric oxide (NO). Thus, there is increase in the intracellular levels of cGMP which provides vascular smooth muscle relaxation. Nitrates act through nitrate receptor, cause increase in cGMP and causes smooth muscle relaxation. Fenoldopam is a new peripheral dopamine receptor (D_1) agonist and useful in the treatment of hypertensive emergency associated with impaired renal function.

Ans. 2 **(B)** Centrally acting alpha adrenergic agonist alpha-methyl dopa is used during pregnancy (PIH). It is an FDA category B drug. Other drugs with reasonable safety (category C) include labetalol (alpha$_1$ selective, beta-non selective adrenergic antagonist) and nifedipine (calcium channel blocker). In case of pre-eclampsia, if blood pressure is not controlled, hydralazine (IV/IM) or labetalol (IV) can be given in hospitalized patient. All other three are teratogenic/not safe to be used during pregnancy.

Ans. 3 **(C)** Digoxin is predominantly eliminated by renal excretion while digitoxin is eliminated by hepatic metabolism. So the toxicity is not precipitated by hepatic disease. But the dose adjustment is required in elderly patients due to hepato-renal dysfunction. Other contraindications of digoxin therapy are hypokalemia, children below 10 years of age, myocardial infarction (except when heart failure is associated with atrial flutter or fibrillation), hypothyroidism (slower elimination), myocarditis and WPW syndrome (may enhance transmission through accessory pathway).

Ans. 4 **(A)** Hypotension, particularly in sodium depleted patients (on loop diuretics or on salt restriction) occurs after the first dose of ACEI. Other common adverse effects are dry cough (due to accumulation of bradykinin), renal failure, hyperkalemia, angioneurotic edema altered taste and allergic rash (with captopril). ACEI are not teratogenic but causes fetal malformation and death due to hypotension when given during II or III trimester, so contraindicated during pregnancy.

Ans. 5 (D) ACEI are used to treat hypertension, to decrease morbidity and mortality in heart failure and left ventricular dysfunction after myocardial infarction. They are also useful in patients with diabetic nephropathy as they decrease proteinuria and stabilize renal function. Phenoxybenzamine + propranolol or labetalol are drug of choice in pheochromocytoma but not ACEI.

Ans. 6 (B) Spironolactone, a aldosterone antagonist act on distal part and collecting tubule where 3% NaCl is absorbed. It is used in all conditioned mentioned except of gynaecomastia, which is rather an adverse effect of spironolactone.

Ans. 7 (B) Hydralazine is an arteriolar dilator with selective decrease in vascular resistance in the coronary, cerebral and renal circulations. Because of preferential dilation of arterioles over veins, postural hypotension is not a problem. The common adverse effects include headache, dizziness, angina, myocardial ischemia (due to increased O_2 demand induced by the baro receptor reflex which stimulates sympathetic nervous system). So not advisable in hypertensive patients with coronary artery disease. It also causes drug induced lupus syndrome and poly neuropathy which responds to pyridoxine.

Ans. 8 (A) ACEIs e.g. enalapril, lisinopril etc are contraindicated during pregnancy.

Ans. 9 (C) The drugs used in hypertensive emergency are sodium nitroprusside (IV infusion), labetalol, esmolol, fenoldopam and phentolamine (associated with pheochromocytoma). Diazoxide, hydralazine (PIH) and diuretics are also useful in hypertensive emergencies. ACEI are given orally so not very useful in hypertensive emergencies.

Ans. 10 (B) Clonidine is an $alpha_2$ receptor agonist which decreases sympathetic outflow. It does not increase the LDL levels. Its adverse effects include rebound hypertension, dry mouth, sedation, nasal stiffness, impotence, constipation and contact dermatitis. It can be used in moderate hypertension, to control diarrhea in diabetic patients, migraine, to manage withdrawal symptoms (nicotine, alcohol and opiates) and in management of menopausal hot flushes.

Ans. 11 (D) Therapeutic uses of the digitalis (digoxin) include congestive heart failure (CHF), PSVT, AF, atrial fibrillation and dilated heart. It is contraindicated in myocarditis or grossly damaged myocardium because of the risk of developing arrhythmias (also see Ans 3).

Ans. 12 (A) Losartan, Valsartan, Telmisartan, Irbesartan etc are orally active, potent and specific competitive antagonist of angiotensin AT_1 receptors. The physiological effect of angiotensin II is blocked by ARAs. They cause vasodilatation by activating AT_2 receptors. They are effective anti-hypertensive even in patients with normal or low activity of rennin-angiotensin system. Irbesartan, candersartan and telmisartan are long acting and more effective ARTs. Losartan is safe and very effective in the treatment of portal hypertension with cirrhosis of liver.

Ans. 13 (D) Sodium nitroprusside increases intracellular levels of cGMP which provides vascular smooth muscle relaxation (see also Ans 1).

Ans. 14 (D) Digitalis (digoxin) is not a drug of choice in high output failure (thyrotoxicosis, anaemia, A.V. shunt).

Ans. 15 (B) CCBs are preferred in these patients. Beta-blockers are contraindicated. Thiazides also cause hyperlipidemia and increase BSL. Verapamil and other CCB (long acting) do not impair renal perfusion, reduces albuminuria and slowing disease progression in hypertensive / diabetic nephropathy.

Ans. 16 (D) After myocardial insult, a fall in PO_2 causes hypoxia which stimulates production of lactic acid, adenosine and PGI_2. All of these cause vasodilatation around the ischemic tissue. If other branch of coronary artery is unobstructed and if a powerful arteriolar dilator e.g. dipyridamole is used, the arterioles of the normal vessels are also dilated and increases blood flow in already well perfuse area (which is not needed). This is known as steal phenomenon. This further increases the anginal pain. Those drugs which dilates large arteries and veins are more effectively (nitrates) reduces the pain of angina than those drugs which causes dilatation of resistant vessels.

Ans. 17 (A) Isosorbide 5-mononitrate, a long acting nitrate has excellent bioavailability (100%) as it does not undergo significant first pass metabolism. It has delayed onset of action and it is not used as sublingual preparation. Sodium nitrate is preferred in cyanide poisoning.

Ans. 18 (A) Sodium nitroprusside is drug of choice in malignant hypertension.

Ans. 19 (B) Statins competitively inhibits the HMG CoA reductase enzyme and deplete intracellular supply of cholesterol by inhibiting its biosynthesis. Thus up regulation of LDL receptors occurs and thus decreases LDL levels. Decrease VLDL and moderate reduction in TG levels is also observed.

Ans. 20 (A) Nitrates act on nitrates receptors in vascular smooth muscles which reduce nitrates to nitric acid (NO) and nitrites. They have high first pass metabolism (except isosorbide mononitrates) as they are inactivated by glutathione organic nitrate reductase. They reduce left ventricular end diastolic pressure, decreases preload and oxygen demand by decreasing venous return.

Ans. 21 (A) Quinidine, procainamide, amiodarone and disopyramide are of class Ia anti-arrhythmic drug which slow the rate of rise of 'O' phase of AP, increase ERP and prolong the APD. The drugs of class Ib e.g. Lidocaine, phenytoin, mexiletine etc. decreases ERP. Class Ic drugs e.g. elecainide, encainide, etc also decreases the rate of 'O' depolarization with minimal effect on ERP.

Ans. 22 (A) Nitrates are useful in CHF with dyspnoea, as they reduce the filling pressure, preload and pulmonary congestion.

Ans. 23 (D) Indapamide is a thiazide diuretic. It is long acting and possesses some intrinsic vasodilator activity.

Ans. 24 (A) Digitalis decreases conduction velocity and increase ERP of AV node by direct vagomimetic and anti-adrenergic action. Because of this many AV atrial impulse impinge on it, while it is still refractory. Thus any influence which increases rate of AF, by itself, reduces ventricular rate.

Ans. 25 (B) Nifedipine causes reflex sympathetic stimulation of heart which causes tachycardia, increased contractility and cardiac output. It causes palpitation and other cardiac effect and high mortality among MI patients. Beta-blockers are combined with nifedipine to minimize sympathetic stimulation and adverse effects.

Ans. 26 (B) Diltiazem is less potent vasodilator, but have depressant action on SA node and AV conduction with little change or decrease in HR. Verapamil has direct cardiodepressant effect and is preferred drug in PSVT, AF and AFl. But for rapid control of ventricular rate diltiazem is preferred. Nifedipine has natriuretic action but significant diuresis does not occurs. Nimlodipine is short acting DHP which penetrates BBB.

Ans. 27 (D) Diazoxide, minoxidil, hydralazine are arteriolar while sodium nitropruside is both arteriolar and venodilator. Minoxidil is orally effective. These drugs (arteriolar dilator) activates K^+ channel opening, increases K^+ conductance and hyperpolarization which cause relaxation of vascular smooth muscles. They have no effect on capacitance vessels and not inhibit reflex sympathetic activity. Usually, they are combined with diuretics.

Ans. 28 (D) ARAs differs from ACEI in all ways as mentioned. ACEIs may not suffice for the total elimination of angiotensin II because of adaption of alternate pathway, while in contrast, ARAs are blocking all the effects regardless of any biochemical pathway.

Ans. 29 (A) Sublingual glycerol trinitrate, taken before a meal promptly relieves pain due to esophageal spasm.

Ans. 30 (A) Nitrendipine, a DHP calcium channel blocker having oral bioavailability of 10-30% shown to release NO from the endothelium and inhibit cAMP phosphodiesterase, which may be the additional mechanisms of vasodilator action.

Ans. 31 (B) As in hyperthyroidism, sympathetic overactivity causes tachycardia and there is increase in beta-receptor activity, so beta-blocker, propranolol is drug of choice.

Ans. 32 (A) All ACEIs can cause renal damage in patients with pre-existing renal vascular disease and in the developing fetus.

Ans. 33 (D) Drugs that causes hypertension or tachycardia directly or reflexly (amphetamine, turbutaline, isoprenaline) tend to precipitate angina in individuals with coronary obstruction unless cardiac work is greatly reduced. Metoprolol does not precipitate attack of angina.

Ans. 34 (A) Nimlodipine is highly lipid soluble, showing affinity and selectivity for cerebral blood vessels and appears to reduce morbidity following sub arachnoid hemorrhage.

Ans. 35 (B) The drugs used in heart failure are positive inotropics (e.g. cardiac glycosides digitalis) PD inhibitors (inamrinone etc), beta-adrenergic agonist (dopamine and dobutamine), diuretics, ACEI, cardioselective beta-antagonist, and vasodilators (Nestritidie, hydralazine). CCB although reduces afterload, but they cause too much cardiac depression, so of no use in heart failure.

Ans. 36 (B) All drugs listed have been shown to reduce mortality except cardiac glycosides, which reduces symptoms but not mortality.

Ans. 37 (C) Procainamide is having actions similar to quinidine, has shorter duration of action and less vagolytic effect. Hypersensitivity reactions are common and include drug fever, agranulocytosis and lupus erythematosus syndrome. Its metabolite N-acetyl procainamide has class III anti-arrhythmic property (prolongs ERP). It should be avoided in patients with AV block.

Ans. 38 (D) Esmolol is class II anti-arrhythmic which increases ERP by decreasing conduction. Esmolol is given by IV infusion as it has very short half life (9 min) and used to control abnormal ventricular response to atrial fibrillation or flutter during or after surgery. Other beta-blockers, propranolol, metoprolol and acebutolol can be used orally. Beta-blockers can also prevent recurrent infarction and sudden death in patients recovering from acute MI.

Ans. 39 (D) The common adverse effects of quinidine are diarrhea, thrombocytopenia and quinidine syncope. Large doses of quinidine can produce cinchonism. Lupus erythematosus is side effect of procainamide. Quinidine also has atropine like effect, so seldom used now.

Ans. 40 (A) Amiodarone is having long plasma half life among all.

Ans. 41 (D) Adverse effects of thiazide diuretics includes hypokalemia, hypercalcaemia, hyperurecemia, hypochloraemic, alkalosis, hyperglycemia hyperlipidaemia. Otoxicity can be caused by loop diuretics (more with ethacrynic acid).

Ans. 42 (B) The most common indication of loop diuretics, include edematous conditions (*e.g.* CCF, renal disease nephrotic syndrome) and cirrhosis of liver. Mannitol, an osmotic diuretic is used to treat acutely raised intracranial (cerebral edema) and IOP (glaucoma). It has no effect on kidney (no diuretic effect).

Ans. 43 (A) Acetazolamide is a carbonic anhydrase inhibitor, rarely used now as diuretic. It is used for alkalinization of urine to treat urate calculi, and cysteinuria (in patients with leukemia/lymphoma receiving chemotherapy) and in mountain sickness. The common adverse effects are refractoriness, paraesthesia hyperchlorimic acidosis and hypokalemia.

Ans. 44 (A) Demeclocyclin, a tetracycline derivative and lithium can be used in SIADH, as they have an additional activity of blocking ADH receptors but not used due to their toxicities. So the restricted water intake is the only remedy for the treatment of SIADH.

Ans. 45 (B) Heparin is the safest to be used during pregnancy as it does not cross placental barrier.

Ans. 46 (D) The dose of the heparin is so adjusted that the whole blood clotting time is raised to 2–3 times more than normal or activated partial thromboplastin time is raised to 1½–2 times to normal value.

Ans. 47 (A) Ticlodipine prevents fibrinogen binding to platelets without modifying $GPII_b/III_a$ receptors. There is no effect on platelet TXA_2, but bleeding time is prolonged and platelet survival in extracorporeal circulation is increased. So it acts synergistically with aspirin.

Ans. 48 (A) Bleeding due to oral anticoagulant is treated by withholding anti-coagulant, fresh blood transfusion which supplies clotting factors. Vitamin K_1 which is a specific antidote can be used, but it takes 6–24 hours to re-synthesize and release of clotting factors.

Ans. 49 (B) The common adverse effects of heparin are bleeding, thrombocytopenia, transient and reversible alopecia, osteoporosis and hypersensitivity reaction (see also Ans. 50).

Ans. 50 (B) Heparin is a powerful anti-coagulant it act by activating anti-thrombin III (AT III) which binds to clotting factors

(X_a, II_a, IX_a, XII_a and XIII_a) and inactivates them (mainly inhibit X_a factors as well as thrombin).

Ans. 51 (A) Indication of anti-coagulants are deep vein thrombosis, post MI, unstable angina, rheumatic heart disease (AF), cerebro-vascular disease, vascular surgery etc.

Ans. 52 (A) Streptokinase is antigenic and cause hypersensitive reaction and anaphylaxis.

Ans. 53 (B) Repeated doses of streptokinase are less effective due to formation of antibodies. Fever, hypotension arrhythmias and anaphylaxis are reported with streptokinase (not bleeding).

Ans. 54 (C) Dipyridamole is a vasodilator. It inhibits phosphodiesterase and blocks uptake of adenosine (to increase platelet cAMP) which potentiates PGI_2 and interfere with aggregation without altering the level of TXA_2 or PGI_2.

Ans. 55 (D) Dextrans, human albumin, degraded gelatin polymer, hydroxyethyl starch (Hetasearch) and polyvinylpyrrolidone are plasma expanders. Dextran may interfere with blood grouping and cross-match. They may be antigenic and interfere with coagulation and platelet function. Degraded gelatin polymer is non-antigenic and does not interfere with blood grouping and cross- matching but it is more expensive.

Ans. 56 (D) Plasma expanders are the substitute for plasma in severe burns and extensive tissue damage, shock etc. It can be used as a temporary measure in case of whole blood loss but cannot be used in anaemia as they do not have oxygen carrying capacity, so have no role in anaemia.

Ans. 57 (A) It is a recombinant form of human B type natriuretic peptide and used in acute heart failure. It increases cGMP in vascular smooth muscles, similar to that of nitrates. They reduce venous as well as arteriolar tone and have short plasma half life (18 minutes).

Ans. 58 (A) ACE inhibitors *e.g.* Enalapril, lisinopril etc. are known teratogenic drugs and hence contraindicated during pregnancy. Methyldopa is the safest drug to be used during pregnancy.

Ans. 59 (C) Thiazide diuretics decreases excretion of calcium and thus can be used for this condition. Loop diuretics stimulate tubular calcium excretion and can be used to treat hypercalcemia. Carbonic anhydrase inhibitors, potassium-sparing diuretics do not have a significant role on calcium balance.

Ans. 60 (D) Lidocaine is the best agent for ventricular arrhythmias associated with MI. It has little effect on atrial function. All other agents induce tachyarrhythmia.

Ans. 61 (A) ACEI should not be combined with potassium sparing diuretics. There is increased in plasma K^+ level and plasma renin and angiotensin-I are increased as a compensatory measure which can cause hyperkalemia. More pronounced or dangerous hyperkalemia may occur when ACEI are used with potassium sparing diuretics.

Ans. 62 (A) Vagal maneuvers may abort an acute attack of PSVT, which include carotid sinus massage valsalva or gagging. If this fails IV verapamil (5–10 mg) or diltiazam (0.25–0.35 mg/kg) terminates the tachycardia in few minutes in 90% of cases. Digitoxin is not useful in terminating acute attack. Quinidine on other hand in view of large number of side effects and drug interactions is not an ideal drug nowadays. Sotalol, currently used in maintenance of sinus rhythm after cardioversion for atrial fibrillation.

Ans. 63 (A) The main advantage of beta-blockers are they do not cause postural hypotension. Also they have low incidence of side effects, low cost and once a day regimen is used. They are preferred drug in young non-obese hypertensive. But they cannot be used with verapamil/diltiazem, as it causes marked bradycardia and AV block. Beta-blocker is inferior to low doses thiazide or ACEI in preventing stroke.

Ans. 64 (B) Rosuvastatin, a statin, is an HMG-CoA reductase inhibitor which converts HMG-CoA to mevalonic acid and therefore depletes the intracellular supply of cholesterol by inhibiting its synthesis. Nicotinic acid is inhibitor of VLDL secretion. Gemifibrozil is activator of lipoprotein lipase and cholestyramine is a bile acid binding resin.

Ans. 65 (B) Amiodarone is class III anti-arrhythmic drug useful in preventing and treating both supraventricular and ventricular tachyarrhythmia even in those with poor L.V. function. It causes dose dependent adverse effects which includes photosensitivity, abdominal pain hypersensitivity, pneumonitis and pulmonary fibrosis.

Ans. 66 (C) Advantages of low molecular weight heparin are they have better bioavailability, long half life, weak interaction with platelets as it inhibit factor X_a and minimum effect on II_a and less chances of thrombocytopenia.

Ans. 67 (C) Nimodipine is related to nifedipine but have a preferential vasodilating action on the cerebral arteries and its use is confined to the prevention of vascular spasm following subarachnoid hemorrhage.

Ans. 68 (D) Indapamide, a non-thiazide diuretic, a potent diuretic have 95% oral bioavailability. It has long half life ($t_{½}$ 15 hours). It has direct vasodilator activity with the result that cardiac output is not changed or may increase slightly.

CHEMOTHERAPY OF MICROBIAL DISEASES

GENERAL CONSIDERATION

Introduction

The development of anti-microbial drugs is one of the important advances of modern medicine. **Chemotherapy** can be defined as treatment of systemic/topical infection by the use of chemicals to destroy micro-organisms without damaging the host tissues. Anti-microbial agents are substances produced by micro-organisms (which suppress the growth or destroy other micro-organisms) as well as drugs synthesized in laboratory.

Classification

(A) Based on their mechanisms of action

They may:

1. **Inhibit cell wall synthesis:** Penicillins, Cephalosporins, Vancomycin, Bacitracin, Cycloserine, Monobactams, Carbapenems–They inhibit bacterial cell wall synthesis by inhibiting the peptidoglycan (the building blocks) synthesis in bacterial cell wall. The formation of an imperfect cell wall leads to an osmotic drive of the fluid from outside of the environment to inside of the hypertonic fluid of the bacteria. As a result, the bacteria swell and burst to die.
2. **Damage cell membranes and causing leakage and alteration of cell membrane integrity:** Polymyxins, Colistin, Amphotericin B, Nystatin, Chlorhexidine and Cetrimide–They function as cationic detergents and disrupt the bacterial cell membrane osmotic integrity. This ends up in the leakage of intracellular constituents and the death of bacteria.

3. **Bind to ribosome and inhibit protein synthesis:** Chloramphenicol, Tetracyclines, Erythromycin, Aminoglycosides, Clindamycin, Linezolid–Ribosomes are involved in the protein synthesis of the bacteria. Ribosomes are different in eukaryotes and prokaryotes. The bacterial ribosome consist of a 50S and 30S subunit which when combined, form 70S subunit while in the mammalian ribosomes the 60S and 40S subunits combine to form 80 subunits. Aminoglycosides group of antibiotics and tetracyclines bind to 30S ribosomal units of the bacteria and prevent its protein synthesis. Macrolide group of antibiotics (erythromycin group) inhibit bacterial protein synthesis by binding reversibly to the 50S ribosomal unit.
4. **Inhibit DNA gyrase:** Fluoroquinolones.
5. **Inhibit DNA function:** DNA dependent RNA polymerase: Rifampicin, Anti-protozoal, Antiviral drugs.
6. **Interfere with metabolic steps:** Anti-metabolite action Sulfonamides, Sulfones, Trimethoprim, Pyrimethamine: By inhibiting synthesis of folic acid.

(B) Based on type of action

1. **Bacteriostatic** agents that suppress the growth of bacteria *e.g.* Sulfonamides, Tetracyclines.
2. **Bactericidal** agents that kill the bacteria, *e.g.,* Penicillins, Cephalosporins, Aminoglycosides.

Some drugs may be bacteriostatic at low doses and bactericidal at higher doses, *e.g.,* erythromycin. Some drugs may be bacteriostatic to some microorganisms and 'cidal' to others, *e.g.,* chloramphenicol is bactericidal to H. influenzae, S. pneumoniae and N. meningitides, while it is bacteriostatic to other microorganisms.

(C) Based on spectrum of activity

(a) **Narrow spectrum,** *e.g.*, Penicillins, Erythromycin, Streptomycin.

(b) **Broad spectrum:** Tetracyclines, Chloramphenicol.

Factors that influence the successful chemotherapy of an infection are:

- *Site:* The drug should reach to the site of infection.
- *Concentration:* It should attain adequate concentration at the site.

- *Host defense:* Active host defense reduce the antibiotic requirement.
- *Sensitivity:* The microorganism should be sensitive to the antimicrobial agent.

Resistance to Anti-Microbial Agents

Unresponsiveness of micro-organism to an anti-microbial agent is termed as drug resistance. It may be:

Natural resistance: The organisms have never responded to the antimicrobial. It may be due to the absence of the particular enzyme or target site affected by the drug, *e.g.*, gram negative bacilli are not sensitive to penicillin G (as they have thick cell wall).

Acquired resistance: The microbes which were previously sensitive to the antimicrobial agents become resistant to it. This type of resistance develops due to:

(a) Mutation is a genetic change that in the DNA structure and occurs spontaneously. When the sensitive organisms are destroyed during the therapy with the antibiotic, the resistant ones freely multiply and cause resistance to AMA. Mutation may take place in a single step (*e.g.*, Staphylococcus aureus to rifampicin) or multiple steps where several gene modifications are made, *e.g.*, gonococci to penicillin G.

(b) Transfer of genetic material: Many bacteria contain extra chromosomal genetic material that can replicate independently in the cytoplasm. They are called plasmids. These carry genes coding for resistance to antibiotics called R factors. These R factors are transferred from one R-plasmid to other plasmid and spread resistance. This transfer takes place by:

1. *Conjugation* is the most important mode of spread of resistance. The R factor is transferred from cell to cell by direct contact through a sex pilus or bridge and the process is known as conjugation.
2. *Transduction:* Plasmid DNA is enclosed in a bacteriophage, is transferred to another bacterium of the same species, *e.g.*, transfer between stains of streptococci and stains of staphylococci.
3. *Transformation:* Resistant bacteria may release genetic material (DNA) into the medium, which is taken up by other

bacteria. The new DNA is then incorporated into the genome, which become resistant.

4. *Transposon* are DNA segments that cannot self replicate but can self transfer between plasmids to or from plasmid to chromosome, thus transfer of resistance.

(c) By biochemical mechanism

1. Production of enzymes that inactivate the drug, *e.g.*, beta-lactamase by staphylococci.
2. Decreased accumulation of the drug in the bacterium, *e.g.*, resistance to tetracyclines by gram positive and gram negative bacteria, *e.g.*, chloramphenicol aminoglycosides.
3. *Altered target for the drug:* The binding site may be altered on the ribosomes, *e.g.*, binding sites for aminoglycosides, macrolides, clindamycin.
4. *Altered metabolic pathway:* Bacteria may produce folic acid by an alternative pathway, *e.g.,* Sulfonamides.
5. *By quorum sensing:* Microbes communicate with each other and exchange signaling chemicals and allow to co-ordinate gene expression.

Cross Resistance: When a microorganism develops resistance to one drug, it is also resistant to other drugs, which are chemically related drugs of the same group, even when not exposed to it.

Prevention of Resistance to Antimicrobials (AMA)

Development of resistance to drugs can be avoided to some extent by the following measures:

- AMA should be used only when necessary.
- Selection of the appropriate AMA is absolutely important.
- Correct dose and duration of treatment should be followed.
- Combination of drugs should be used, as in tuberculosis to delay the development of resistance.

A combination of antimicrobial agents is indicated in certain specific situations. The combination serves one of the following purposes:

1. To obtain synergism in following condition:

- *Bacterial endocarditis:* Penicillin + streptomycin/gentamicin are synergistic.
- *Pseudomonas infections:* Carbenicillin + gentamicin.

- Pneumocystis carinii pneumonia. Trimethoprim+sulfamethoxazole.
- Beta-lactamase producing organisms like H. influenzae Amoxicillin + Clavulinic acid.
- Tuberculosis INH + rifampicin.

2. **Treatment of mixed infections:** Intra-abdominal infections, genitourinary infections and traumatic wound infections are often having mixed infections and aerobic and anaerobic organisms may be involved. Two or more antimicrobials can be used (to broaden the spectrum of AMA) depending on the culture and sensitivity report.
3. **Initial treatment of severe infections:** Drugs covering both gram positive and gram negative pathogens may be used initially till the culture report is available, *e.g.*, penicillin + aminoglycoside; cephalosporin + aminoglycoside. If anaerobes are likely to be present, metronidazole may be added.
4. **To prevent the emergence of resistance:** In the treatment of tuberculosis and leprosy multi-drug therapy is given.
5. **To reduce the adverse effects:** The doses needed may be lower when a combination is used, *e.g.*, Amphotericin B + flucytosine in cryptococcal meningitis.

Disadvantages of Antimicrobial Combination

1. *Risk of toxicity from each agent:* Toxicity of one drug may be enhanced by another, *e.g.*, Vancomycin + ammoglycoside may cause severe renal toxicity.
2. Resistant strains may multiply by wrong selection of AMA.
3. Increased cost of therapy.
4. Increased chance of super infection.

Chemoprophylaxis

Chemoprophylaxis is recommended in the following situations:

1. **To protect healthy persons,** *e.g.*:
   - Penicillin G for gonorrhea, rheumatic fever.
   - For preventing meningococcal infection in healthy children during an epidemic rifampicin or sulfonamides.
   - *Anti-malarial drugs:* In healthy individuals visiting an endemic area.

2. **To prevent infection in high risk patients:**
   - In patients with contaminated or exposed wounds as in road accidents.
   - Catheterisation of urinary tract norfloxacin is used.
   - In burns to prevent colonization by bacteria.
3. **Surgical prophylaxis.**
4. **In close contacts:** Chemoprophylaxis is recommended particularly in children when infectious cases of leprosy or tuberculosis are in close contact.
5. To prevent postpartum infections in the mother after normal delivery, to prevent infection in unconscious patients.

Minimum Inhibitory Concentration (MIC): The MIC is the lowest antibiotic concentration that prevents the visible growth of microorganism after a 24 hour incubation period with a standard organism inoculation using serial dilutions of the AMA. It has certain inherent limitations as it is an in vitro measure and tells nothing about the true antibiotic activity at the locus of infection.

Post-Antibiotic Effect (PAE)

A persistent suppression of bacterial growth after a brief exposure of an antimicrobial agent is known as post-antibiotic effect. It is observed even when the concentration of antibacterial agent is well below MIC. It reflects the time required for the bacteria to return to normal growth. The longer the time the bacteria needs for return to logarithmic growth, the greater is the PAE of that antibiotic specially those which act by inhibiting bacterial protein/DNA synthesis, *e.g.*, aminoglycosides, fluoroquinolone, tetracycline etc.

Superinfection

This refers to the appearance of a new infection as a result of anti-microbial therapy. Use of AMA markedly reduces flora (indigenous bacterial flora present in GIT and oral cavity) allowing invasion by opportunistic organisms such as proteus, resistant staphylococci and pseudomonas etc. This is termed as superinfection, which is manifested as antibiotic induced diarrhea and colitis. This is more common in immunocompromised patients and when host defense is poor.

Probiotics

Probiotics are products containing viable, non-pathogenic micro-organisms administered orally to alter the intestinal microflora. Lactobacillus, Bifido bacterium, Streptococcus salivarius, some enterococci and saccharomyces boulardii are some of the presently tried probiotics.

Problems arising while using AMA: These are toxicities (local and systemic), resistance, tolerance, hypersensitive reactions, super infection, nutritional deficiencies, masking of infections etc.

SULFONAMIDES, COTRIMOXAZOLE AND QUINOLONES

Sulfonamides

Sulfonamides were the first effective anti-bacterial agents to be used systemically. They are synthetic agents that contain a sulfonamide group.

Anti-bacterial spectrum: Sulfonamides inhibit gram positive and some gram negative bacteria, Nocardia, Chlamydia, Plasmodium falciparum Toxoplasma gondii and actinomyces. Anaerobic bacteria show resistance to sulfonamides.

Mechanism of Action

Bacteria synthesize their own folic acid from para amino benzoic acid (PABA) with the help of the enzyme folic acid synthetase. Sulfonamides are structurally similar to PABA and competitively inhibit the enzyme folic acid synthetase. This results in folic acid deficiency and injury to the bacterial cell.

Human cells are not affected because they require preformed folic acid supplied from the diet and cannot synthesize folic acid by themselves. Sulfonamides are bacteriostatic but bactericidal concentration achieved in urine.

Presence of pus, blood and tissue breakdown products make sulfonamides ineffective as these are rich in PABA.

Bacteria, *e.g.*, gonococci, pneumococci, S. aureus etc and anaerobes acquire resistance to sulfonamides. This is due to mutation which results into:

1. Overproduction of PABA.
2. Bacteria used alternative metabolic pathway for folic acid synthesis.
3. Low permeability to sulfonamides to bacteria.

Classification

Sulfonamides may be classified on the basis of the rapidity with which they are absorbed and excreted. Accordingly, they are:

1. *Agents absorbed and excreted rapidly (short acting):* Sulfasoxazole, Sulfadiazine, Sulfamethizole.
2. *Intermediate acting:* Sulfamethoxazole, Sulfamoxole.
3. *Long acting:* Sulfamethopyrizine, Sulfadoxine
4. *Poorly absorbed:* Sulfasalazine, Olsalazine, Balsalazine.
5. *Topical:* Sulfacetamide, Mefenide Silver Sulfadiazine.

Pharmacokinetics: Sulfonamides are well-absorbed. They are extensively bound to plasma proteins (differ in extent of protein binding hence short or long acting).

They are well distributed to all tissues. They are metabolized in the liver by acetylation. They are mainly excreted in urine. The more lipid soluble drugs are reabsorbed and have longer duration of action. Bound sulfonamide has less bacteriostatic activity and not useful in acute infections. Because of relatively high solubility in the urine, incidences of hematuria or crystalluria is very less with sulfisoxazole.

Adverse Effects

1. Renal irritation, haematuria, albuminuria and crystalluria due to precipitation of the drug in acidic urine. This can be avoided by intake of large volumes of fluids and by alkalinization of the urine.
2. Hypersensitivity reactions like rashes, fever, Stevens-Johnson syndrome and rarely exfoliative dermatitis, eosinophilia can occur.
3. *GIT:* Anorexia, nausea and abdominal pain.
4. Haemolytic anaemia is rare and develops in patients with G6-PD deficiency.
5. *Kernicterus:* Sulfonamides displace bilirubin from the binding sites which crosses the BBB and may cause kernicterus in the newborn. Hence sulfonamides are contraindicated in pregnancy and in infants.
6. *CNS toxicity:* Confusion, depression, ataxia, fatigue.

Uses

Because of the development of resistance and availability of better antimicrobials, sulfonamides are not commonly used now except in a few cases, *e.g.*:

1. *Nocardiosis* (pulmonary lesions or brain abscess).
2. *Urinary tract infection/Prostatitis.*
3. *Malaria:* Sulfadoxine is used with pyrimethamine in chloroquine resistant malaria, toxoplasmosis.

4. *Prophylactic use:* In streptococcal pharyngitis in rheumatic fever.
5. *Topical:* Sulfacetamide eye drops in bacterial conjunctivitis; silver sulfadiazine in burns to prevent infection and sulfasalazine in ulcerative colitis.

Cotrimoxazole

The combination of trimethoprim and sulfamethoxazole is cotrimoxazole.

Mechanism of action: Sulfonamides inhibit the conversion of PABA to dihydrofolic acid (DHF) and trimethoprim inhibits dihydrofolate reductase and thus prevents the reduction of DHF to tetrahydrofolic acid (THF). The two drugs thus block sequential steps in folic acid synthesis and the combination is bactericidal and resistance to this combination develops less frequently. The ratio of trimethoprim: sulfamethoxazole used is 1:5 to attain the right plasma concentration. Sulfamethoxazole has similar pharmacokinetic as of trimethoprim (same $t_{1/2}$ 10 hours). Trimethoprim has large volume of distribution.

Anti-bacterial spectrum: Cotrimoxazole is effective against Staph. aureus, Streptococci, Meningococci, C. diphtheriae, E. coli, Proteus, H. influenzae, Salmonella and Shigella. Bacteria may acquire resistance by mutation or by acquisition of a plasmid coding for an altered DHFR.

Adverse Effects

- Nausea, vomiting, headache, glossitis, stomatitis and allergic skin rashes are relatively common.
- Megaloblastic anaemia and granulocytopenia are rare.
- Patients with renal disease may develop uraemia.

Uses

1. Urinary tract infection/prostatis.
2. Respiratory tract infections.
3. Bacterial gastroenteritis.
4. Typhoid: Ciprofloxacin is preferred.
5. Pneumocystis carinii infection.
6. Chancroid, gonorrhea.

Iclaprim: It is a trimethoprim analogue effective against skin and soft tissue infections caused by methicillin resistant staph. aureus (MRSA).

Quinolones

Nalidixic Acid

Nalidixic acid is bactericidal against various organisms, *e.g.*, E. coli, Shigella, Proteus and Klebsiella. Nalidixic acid is well absorbed orally. It attains high concentrations in the urine. **Adverse effects** include hemolytic anaemia, allergic reactions, headache, myalgia, drowsiness and convulsion. Nalidixic acid was used in uncomplicated UTI and diarrhea due to E. coli, Shigella and Proteus, but because of its toxicity, FQ are now preferred.

Fluoroquinolones (FQ)

The quinolones, when fluorinated, obtain compounds with a wider spectrum of activity, fewer side effects, lesser chance of resistance and better tissue penetration. These include norfloxacin, ciprofloxacin, pefloxacin, ofloxacin, lomefloxacin and sparfloxacin. The newer agents include trovafloxacin, gatifloxacin, moxifloxacin, purlifloxacin, gemifloxacin, finafloxacin and alatrofloxacin.

Mechanism of Action

Fluoroquinolones are bactericidal. They enter in the cells by passive diffusion and inhibit the bacterial enzyme DNA gyrase (topoisomerase II) which is required for DNA replication and transcription. They also inhibit topoisomerase IV. They also causes filamentation, vacuole formation and degradation of chromosomal DNA.

Anti-bacterial spectrum: Gonococci, meningococci, H. influenzae, E. coli, salmonella, shigella, enterobacteria, H. pylori, staphylococci, chlamydiae, mycoplasma and mycobacterium are susceptible. Some of the newer fluoroquinolones are effective against some anaerobic organisms and Streptococcus pneumonae.

Resistance is comparatively not very frequent due to the unique mechanism of action but several strains of E. coli, Staphylococci, Pseudomonas and Serratia have now developed resistance due to modification of porin channels, development of efflux mechanism and mutation topoisomerase.

Pharmacokinetics: Fluoroquinolones are well absorbed and widely distributed. Food and antacids interfere with absorption; pefloxacin and ofloxacin cross the BBB. All FQs are metabolized by hepatic microsomal enzymes and FQs are (ciprofloxacin) microsornal enzyme inhibitors. These drugs (levofloxacin, lomefloxacina and ofloxacin) are excreted by the kidneys. Hence dose should be reduced in renal failure.

Adverse Reactions: Nausea, vomiting, abdominal discomfort, photosensitivity, diarrhea and rashes may be seen. Fluoroquinolones damage the growing cartilage resulting in arthropathy and are therefore contraindicated up to 18 years of age. In patients receiving NSAIDs, fluoroquinolones can sometimes precipitate seizures. Sparfloxacin and moxifloxacin can prolong QT interval in patients on anti-arrhythmic drugs.

Uses

1. Complicated urinary tract infection, prostatitis, cervicitis.
2. Typhoid.
3. Diarrhoea due to shigella.
4. Gonorrhoea, chancroid.
5. Respiratory tract infections (M. avium infection), anthrax.
6. Bone, joint, soft tissue and intra-abdominal infections.
7. *Tuberculosis:* Ciprofloxacin is one of the drugs in multi-drug regimens used for resistant tuberculosis and in leprosy.
8. *Eye infection:* Ciprofloxacin and ofloxacin may be used topically in the treatment of eye infections.
9. *Pefloxacin accumulates in CSF:* used in meningitis due to gram negative organisms.

BETA LACTAM ANTIBIOTICS

The beta lactam antibiotics have a beta lactam ring which is essential for their anti-bacterial activity. Penicillins, Cephalosporins, Monobactams and Carbapenems are beta lactam antibiotics.

Mechanism of action: The beta lactam antibiotics act by inhibiting the cell wall synthesis in the bacteria. Peptidoglycan, a complex polymer is an important component of the cell wall. It consists of glycan chains which are cross-linked by peptide chains which do not allow bacteria to swell up and prevents its death and lysis. The synthesis of this peptidoglycan requires enzymes called transpeptidases. The process of transpeptidation is catalyzed by penicillin binding protein (PBP). Beta lactam antibiotics inhibit these PBP and transpeptidases and thus inhibit the synthesis of the peptidoglycan, resulting in the formation of cell wall deficient bacteria. Such bacteria undergo lysis. Thus penicillin is bactericidal and lethal in the multiplying phase of bacteria. They do not have effect on host cells as they are lacking PBP.

Classification

I. Narrow spectrum penicillins

A. Beta lactamase sensitive (Natural penicillin)

a. *Acid labile:* Penicillin G, Procaine Penicillin, Benzathine penicillin.

b. *Acid stable:* Penicillin V.

B. Beta lactamase resistance (Anti staphylococcal penicillin)

a. *Acid labile:* Methicillin (IM/IV), Nafcillin (IM/IV).

b. *Acid stable:* Cloxacillin, Dicloxacillin, Flucloxacin (oral).

II. Extended spectrum penicillins (All are sensitive to beta lactamase degradation)

a. *Acid stable (Aminopenicillin):* Ampicillin, Amoxycillin, Talampicillin.

b. *Acid labile (Anti-pseudomonal penicillins):* Ticarcillin, Carbenicillin, Piperacilline, Mezlocillin, Azlocillin.

Natural Penicillins

Penicillin G (Benzyl Penicillin)

Penicillin G is the most potent AMA and is effective against gram positive cocci and bacilli, *e.g.*, streptococci, pneumococci, gonococci, meningococci. B. anthracis, C. diphtheriae, Clostridia and Spirochetes are also highly sensitive. They are not effective against gram negative organism, as peptidoglycan layer is very thin and present in between the two layers of lipo polysaccharide with small porin channels. So, penicillins cannot diffuse through this.

Penicillin Resistance

Many organisms like staphylococci produce an enzyme penicillinase (beta lactamase) which opens the beta lactam ring and inactivates penicillins. Altered target proteins on the bacteria cell which reduces affinity for penicillins and production of an efflux pump which ejects antibiotic back across the cell membrane before it binds with PBP (*e.g.*, nafcillin) also lead to resistance.

Pharmacokinetics: PnG is destroyed by gastric juice; food interferes with its absorption. Though it does not readily cross the BBB but in the presence of inflammation of meninges, therapeutic concentration is attained in the CSF. It is excreted by the kidneys. Probenecid blocks the renal tubular secretion of penicillin and thereby prolongs its duration of action.

Adverse Effects

1. *Hypersensitivity:* Manifestations range from skin rashes, urticaria, fever, bronchospasm, serum sickness and rarely exfoliative dermatitis and anaphylaxis. There is cross-sensitivity among different penicillins.
2. *Jarisch Herxheimer reaction.*
3. *Local:* Pain at the site of injection, thrombophlebitis on IV injection.
4. *CNS:* Large doses of PnG (IV) may produce confusion, muscle twitching, convulsions and coma.

Uses

1. Gram positive cocci, *e.g.*, Pneumococcal, Streptococcal, Meningococcal, Staphylococcal infections.
2. Syphilis.
3. Diphtheria.
4. Anaerobic infections.
5. Actinomycosis.
6. Tetanus and gas gangrene.
7. PnG is the agent of choice for infections like anthrax, trench mouth, rat bite fever and listeria infections.
8. Prophylactic uses:
   a. *Rheumatic fever:* Benzathine penicillin 1.2 MU every month prevents colonization by streptococci and thereby decreases the recurrences of rheumatic fever and valvular heart disease.
   b. *Gonorrhoea and syphilis:* when treated with penicillin within 12 hours of exposure.
   c. *Bacterial endocarditis.*

Disadvantages of Natural Penicillin: They:

1. Are not effective orally.
2. Have a narrow spectrum of activity.
3. Are susceptible to beta lactamase.
4. Can cause hypersensitivity.

Semi-Synthetic Penicillins

a. *Acid resistant penicillins:* Penicillin V is acid stable and can be given orally. It is used only in mild streptococcal pharyngitis, sinusitis and trench mouth.

b. *Penicillinase resistant penicillins* are resistant to hydrolysis by penicillinase produced by bacteria and are less effective than PnG. They are the drugs of choice for infections with penicillinase producing staphylococci.

c. *Extended spectrum penicillins:* They all are sensitive to beta lactamase.

   i. They cover a wider antibacterial spectrum including many gram negative bacilli. They are orally effective. Streptococci, meningococci, penumococci, H. influenzae, E. coli, Proteus, Salmonella, Shigella but not against Pseudomonas, Klebsiella and other gram negative aerobes.

   ii. Ampicillin is well absorbed orally; food interfere its absorption. It is excreted mainly through kidneys. Diarrhea due to irritation of the gut by the unabsorbed drug is the most common adverse effect with ampicillin. Amoxicillin is better absorbed orally, so causes no/less diarrheas. Food does not interfere with the absorption of amoxicillin.

Uses

1. Respiratory, tract infections.
2. Urinary tract infections.
3. Meningitis.
4. Typhoid.
5. Septicemia due to gram negative organisms.
6. Dental infections.

d. *Anti pseudomonal penicillins:*Carbenicillin is effective in Pseudomonas aeruginosa and Proteus infections. Carbenicillin is given parenterally while carbenicillin indanyl is effective orally. Ticarcillin has better activity against P. aeruginosa. Carbenicillin may cause edema CCF and bleeding due to abnormal platelet aggregation. Azlocillin, mezlocillin and piperacillin are all administered intravenously and are used for the serious infections due to Pseudomonas, Proteus or Klebseilla.

Beta Lactamase Inhibitors

Beta lactamase inhibitors bind to and inactivate beta lactamases. Thus, they prevent the destruction of the beta lactam antibiotics. Beta lactamase inhibitors are clavulanic acid, sulbactam and tazobactam. Clavulanic acid is called "suicide inhibitor" as it gets inactivated after binding to the enzyme. In addition, they also inhibit organisms like beta lactamase producing staphylococci, gonococci, E. coli, H. influenza, Moraxella and MRSA. The combination is used for mixed aerobic-anaerobic infections. They require dose adjustment in renal dysfunction.

They are available in fixed dose combinations.

- Clavulanic acid + Amoxicillin – Oral.
- Clavulanic acid + Ticarcillin – IV.
- Sulbactam + Ampicillin – IV/IM.
- Tazobactam + Piperacillin – IV/IM.

Cephalosporins

Cephalosporins are semi-synthetic antibiotics with a beta lactam ring related to penicillins. They have a wider spectrum of activity than penicillins.

Mechanism of actions is similar to penicillins.

Classification

First generation	:	Parenteral – Cephradine, Cefazolin. Oral – Cephalexin, Cefadroxil.
Second generation	:	Parenteral – Cefamandole, Cefuroxime, Cefotetan, Cefoxitin. Oral – Cefaclor, Cefuroxime, Cefprozil.
Third generation	:	Parenteral – Cefotaxime, Ceftrioxone, Cefoperazone, Ceftizoxime, Ceftazidime. Oral – Cefixime, Cefpodoxime Proxetil, Cefdinir, Ceftibuten, Cefditoren.
Fourth generation	:	Parenteral – Cefepime, Cefpirome, Cefozopran.
Fifth generation	:	Parenteral – Ceftobiprole and Ceftaroline.

First Generation Cephalosporins

First generation cephalosporins are very effective against gram positive organisms. Cephalothin is resistant to penicillinase, Cefazolin has a longer plasma $t_{½}$. Cephalexin is used orally for minor infections. They do not cross BBB. They are effective against gram positive cocci, moderate to gram negative cocci and anaerobic gram positive cocci. They are not useful in serious infections.

Second Generation Cephalosporins

Second generation cephalosporins are more active against some gram negative organisms, as compared to first generation. H. influenzae, E. coli, Proteus and Klebsiella are inhibited. Except cefaclor, they are resistant to beta lactamases; attains good CSF concentration and are useful in meningitis. They are excreted unchanged in urine. There use is declined as third and fourth generations are more effective against gram negative infections.

Third Generation Cephalosporins

Third generation cephalosporins are highly resistant to beta lactamases; have good activity against gram negative organisms including Citrobacter, Serratia, Enterobacteriaceae Pseudomonas aeruginosa, N. gonorrhoeae and beta lactamase producing H. influenzae; but they have weak activity against gram positive cocci. Many cross BBB and are useful in meningitis and other serious infections. Ceftrioxone has a long $t_{½}$ and high brotein binding. It is excreted mainly through biliary tract (also cefperazone) and no dosage adjustment is needed in renal insufficiency.

Fourth Generation Cephalosporins

Fourth generation cephalosporins Cefepime and Cefpirome are active against a variety of gram positive and gram negative organisms including streptococci, staphylococci, meningococci, gonococci, some enterococci, enterobacteriacae, H. influenzae and Pseudomonas aeruginosa. Both are excreted almost completely through the kidneys.

The fourth generation agents are used in hospital acquired pneumonia, septicemia, nosocomial and other serious infections of the skin, respiratory and urinary tract as well as infections in immunocompromised patients.

Fifth Generation Cephalosporins

They inhibit PBP-2 a produced by MRSA so effective against MRSA, penicillin resistant strepto penumoniae and enterococci.

Adverse Reactions of Cephalosporins

1. Hypersensitivity reactions.
2. Nephrotoxicity.
3. Super infection, Pseudomembranous colitis and diarrhoea.
4. Bleeding is due to hypoprothrombinaemia and low WBC count.
5. Pseudolithiasis (gallbladder sludge) with ceftriaxone.
6. Pain at the injection site
7. Disulfiram like reaction with alcohol is reported with some cephalosporins (Cefperazone).

Combination of cephalosporins with clavulanic acid and sulbactam are also available which have extended spectrum.

Uses of Cephalosporins

1. *Gram negative infections:* Third generation agent is used.
2. *Surgical prophylaxis:* Cefazolin is preferred.
3. *Gonorrhoea:* Ceftriaxone is the drug of choice.
4. *Meningitis:* Cefotaxime or ceftrioxone may be used.
5. *Mixed aerobic anaerobic infections* (Hospital acquired infection).
6. *Typhoid:* As an alternative to ciprofloxacin, ceftriaxone and cefoperazone are used.
7. *Nosocomial infections.*

Carbapenems

Carbapenems contain a beta lactam ring fused with a five-member penem ring. Carbapenems include Imipenem, Meropenem, Ertapenem, Doripenem, Faropenem, Razupenem.

Carbapenems have a wide anti-bacterial spectrum and inhibit various gram positive, gram negative organisms and anaerobes including streptococci, staphylococci, enterococci, listeria, enterobacteriacae, Pseudomonas and B. fragilis. Razupenem has high activity against multi-drug resistant gram positive and gram negative bacteria.

Mechanism of Action

Carbapenems inhibit bacterial cell wall synthesis similar to penicillins. **Imipenem** is not absorbed orally and is administered intravenously; it has good tissue penetrability. Imipenem is inactivated quickly by a dehydropeptidase in the renal tubules. Hence it is always combined with cilastatin, an inhibitor of dehydropeptidase, in order to prolong its plasma half life.

Adverse Effects include nausea, vomiting, diarrhoea and allergic reactions especially in patients allergic to other beta lactam antibiotics. High doses can occasionally cause seizures (with imipenem).

Uses

Imipenem + cilastatin is used in UTI, respiratory, skin, bone, soft tissue, intra abdominal and gynaecological infections. It is used with an aminoglycoside in pseudomonas infections.

Meropenem has the following advantages over imipenem.

- It is not destroyed by renal dehydropeptidase and therefore does not require to be combined with cilastatin.
- Risk of seizures less than with imipenem.

Ertapenem is similar to meropenem except that it is not useful against P. aeruginosa.

Monobactams

Monobactams are monocyclic beta lactams, *i.e.*, they contain a single beta lactam ring. They are Aztreonam, Tigemonam, Carumonam.

Aztreonam: It is active against gram negative bacilli including Pseudomonas aeruginosa but is not effective against gram positive organisms and anaerobes. Aztreonam can be used in patients allergic to penicillins because there is no cross allergy with other beta lactams. It crosses BBB and useful during for the treatment of meningitis caused by gram negative organism.

MACROLIDES AND NEWER ANTIBIOTICS

Macrolides

These are agents having macrocyclic lactone ring with attached sugar. This group includes: Erythromycin, Roxithromycin, Clarithromycin and Azithromycin.

Mechanism of Action

Macrolides inhibit protein synthesis by binding reversibly to the 50S ribosomal subunit of the bacteria and inhibit its protein synthesis. They inhibit the translocation steps, so tRNA with growing peptide chain is not translocated from ribosomes acceptor (A site) to peptidyl site (P-site).

Antibacterial Spectrum

The macrolides are effective against a number of organisms cited below:

1. **Gram positive cocci:** Streptococcus pneumoniae, Strepto-pyogenes and staphylococci.
2. **Gram negative cocci:** N. gonorrhoea and Moraxella catarrhalis.
3. **Gram positive bacilli:** C. diphtheriae and B. anthracis.
4. **Gram negative bacilli:** L. pneumophila, B. pertussis, H. influenzae and H. pylori.
5. **Acid fast bacilli:** Mycobacterium avium complex, M. leprae.
6. **Spirochetes:** Treponema pallidum.
7. **Miscellaneous organisms:** Mycoplasma pneumoniae and Chlamydia trachomatis.

Pharmacokinetics

- *Erythromycin* free base is destroyed by gastric acid and therefore administered orally with an enteric coating that dissolves in duodenum. Food interferes with its absorption.
- *Roxithromycin and clarithromycin* are long acting ($t_{1/2}$ 12 hours), acid stable macrolide.
- *Azithromycin* is more acid stable with wider tissue distribution (except CSF). Therapeutic concentrations are achieved in lung, genital tissue, liver and prostate. Elimination half life is about 68 hours, which permits once daily dosing, and shortening the duration of treatment (3 days). Food interferes with its absorption; hence it is administered either one hour before or 2 hours after meals. It also exhibits significant post-antibiotic effects. Resistance to macrolides results due to either modification of the receptor site on 50S sub unit or due to efflux system.

Therapeutic Uses

1. Respiratory tract infections, *e.g.*, Atypical pneumonia, L. pneumonia, whooping cough due to B. pertussis, eradication of Corynebacterium diphtheriae from pharyngeal carriers. Erythromycin and roxithromycin are more effective.
2. Erythromycin has anti-inflammatory effects so can be used in rheumatoid arthritis, cystic fibrosis, chronic sinusitis and asthma.
3. They are also useful as a penicillin substitute in penicillin allergic individuals with infections caused by Strepto. pyogenes, S. pneumoniae and Staphylococcal infections.
4. Clarithromycin is very effective against Mycobacterium avium complex, H. influenzae and H. pylori. M. avium and M intracellulare. Combination of clarithromycin 500 mg BD+ ethambutol is an effective therapy to suppress the disease.
5. Azithromycin is highly active against Chlamydia and community acquired pneumonia.
6. Spiramycin use is restricted to treat Toxoplasmosis gondil to prevent transmission of infection from mother to fetus.

Adverse Effects

1. Allergic reactions, rashes, fever, eosinophilia and skin eruptions may occur with the use of erythromycin estolate.

2. Cholestatic hepatitis is much more common with erythromycin estolate than with other macrolides.
3. Erythromycin use is also associated with severe epigastric pain which results from stimulation of gastric smooth muscle motilin receptors.
4. All macrolides induce ototoxicity in high doses.

Drug Interactions

1. Erythromycin and clarithromycin inhibit cytochrome P-450 enzyme system which can lead to significant drug interactions. Thus, they can inhibit the metabolism and increase the serum levels of theophylline, warfarin and other drugs.
2. Macrolides decrease digoxin metabolism by inhibiting the microbial flora responsible for degrading digoxin.
3. Concomitant use of macrolides with statin group of anti-hyperlipidaemic agents may increase the incidence of myopathy and rhabdomylosis.

Lincosamides

The lincosamide family of antibiotics includes **lincomycin and clindamycin.** They also bind to 50S ribosomal subunits resulting in inhibition of bacterial protein synthesis (bacteriostatic). **Clindamycin** is highly active against streptococci, pneumococci (except enterococci) and staphylococci (except MRSA). Bacteroides fragilis, Clostridium and anaerobes are also susceptible. It is well absorbed orally. It is 90% protein bound and accumulates in neutrophills and macrophages. It penetrates well in most tissues, including bones and phagocytes but not CSF, brain and eye. It readily crosses placental barrier.

Because of toxicity clindamycin use is restricted in treating serious anaerobic infections, notably due to Bacteroides fragilis and susceptible staphylococcal and streptococcal infections, *e.g.*, liver abscess, lung abscess, staphylococcal bone and joint infections, septicaemia and pelvic inflammatory disease. It is given with aminoglycoside. It is also used in the prophylaxis of endocarditis in penicillin allergic patients. Topically it is used to treat acne.

Adverse Effects

1. In some patients, clindamycin associated diarrhoea and pseudomembranous colitis may develop which may prove fatal.

2. Hypersensitivity reactions including rashes, urticaria and stomatitis can occur.

Lincomycin is not used because of its toxicity.

Ketolides

- The ketolides, of which only Telithromycin is in clinical use, is a semisynthetic derivative of erythromycin and having mechanism of action similar to erythromycin. It has enhanced activity against erythromycin resistant gram positive cocci, gram negative cocci, gram negative bacilli, and to some anaerobes, streptococcus and Bacteroides fragilis.
- It is indicated for macrolide resistant community acquired pneumonia, acute exacerbations of chronic bronchitis, sinusitis and streptococcal pharyngitis. It exhibit longer post-antibiotic effects.
- Adverse effects are mild. No pseudomembranous colitis occurs.

Oxazolidinones

Linezolid, Radezolid, Torezolid

Linezolid is the first orally synthetic new antibiotic. It inhibits bacterial protein synthesis by binding to the 23S fraction of 50S ribosomal subunit near the interface, so having no cross resistance to other drugs. Linezolid is reserved for the treatment of infections caused by multidrug resistant gram positive bacteria (both aerobic and anaerobic) and MRSA. The oral bioavailability of linezolid is 100% and hence dose adjustment is not required when switching from IV to oral and vice versa. Linezolid is not useful against gram negative bacteria. The main adverse effects of linezolid are reversible thrombocytopenia (if used for more than 15 days) and neutropenia. Hence, weekly monitoring of platelet counts is required.

Glycopeptide Antibiotics

Vancomycin, Teicoplanin

Vancomycin is bactericidal, act by inhibiting bacterial cell wall. It is not absorbed orally. When given IV, it is widely distributed, penetrates serous cavities and inflamed meninges. It is highly toxic drug causes nerve deafness, renal damage, fall in B.P. It also causes **"red man syndrome"** due to intense flushing. It is used as surgical prophylactic in MRSA, penicillin resistant pneumococci.

Teicoplanin is more active and less toxic to vancomycin. It is indicated in enterococcal endocarditis.

Polymyxin B being very toxic is rarely used now except topically. It has a bactericidal action on most gram negative bacilli. It is used topically in combination with other drugs, in the treatment of skin, ear and eye infections. **Mupirocin** is used as ointment topically for treatment of impetigo, folliculitis, burns and leg ulcers. It is highly lipid soluble agent which readily penetrates the skin. Hence it is useful in deeper skin infections such as boils, impetigo and pyoderma.

BROAD SPECTRUM ANTIBIOTICS (TETRACYCLINE AND CHLORAMPHENICOL)

Tetracyclines

Mechanism of Action

The susceptible bacteria accumulate the antibiotic by an active transport. Once inside the bacterial cell, tetracyclines inhibit the bacterial protein synthesis by binding to their 30S ribosomal subunit and subsequent attachment of aminoacyl tRNA to the "A" site. As a result, the peptide chain fails to grow. Tetracyclines are bacteriostatic.

Antibacterial Spectrum and Therapeutic Uses

Tetracyclines are drug of first choice for the treatment of cholera, rickettsia infection, chlamydial diseases, atypical pneumonia, lyme disease and relapsing fever (doxycycline is preferred). It is second choice with gentamicin in the treatment of brucellosis, in tularemia, plague, bacteremia and abscess, trachoma, non-specific urethritis and cervicitis. It is also used to treat acne because of their antioxidant effect on the degranulated neutrophils in the acidic contents of sebaceous material.

Minocycline is effectively used in the treatment of swimming pool granuloma.

Demeclocycline inhibits the actions of ADH in the renal tubules and has been used in the treatment of inappropriate (excess) secretion of ADH (SIADH).

Pharmacokinetics

Tetracyclines are variably absorbed with significant difference in bioavailability. Food retards absorption of all tetracyclines, except doxycyclin and minocycline. Dairy products like milk or curd, Ca^{2+}, Mg^{2+}

and Al^{3+} (present in antacids), Fe^{2+} (present in iron preparations) and $NaHCO_3$ (in antacids), significantly impair tetracycline absorption either by chelation or by altering gastric pH. Tetracyclines are widely distributed. They get deposited in teeth and bones. Urinary excretion ranges from 70–75% for tetracycline, oxytetracycline and chlortetracycline; to 30-40% for doxycycline, and 12–18% for minocycline. Hence, in renal impairment only doxycycline and minocycline can be administered with safety without dose adjustment. Doxycycline and minocycline are excreted mainly in bile.

Adverse Effects

1. Nausea, vomiting, epigastric burning and stomatitis.
2. Super infection or pseudo membranous colitis (PMC) can result on prolonged use.
3. Staining of both the deciduous and permanent teeth and retardation of bone growth usually.
4. Hepatotoxicity may occur particularly during pregnancy.
5. The renal toxicity has also been observed with the use of tetracycline preparations after expiry date (Fanconi's syndrome which is characterized by glycosuria, proteinuria and aminoaciduria).
6. Pulmonary eosinophilic syndrome.
7. Minocycline can cause vestibular toxicity.
8. Demeclocycline and doxycycline can induce photosensitivity to sunlight or ultraviolet light.
9. Demeclocycline antagonises renal actions of ADH and can induce nephrogenic diabetes insipidus.

Contraindications of tetracyclines are renal impairment, hepatic insufficiency, pregnancy, lactation and in children below 10 years of age.

Chloramphenicol

It is a broad spectrum antibiotic.

Mechanism of Action

It inhibits bacterial protein synthesis by binding to the 50S ribosomal subunit. It interferes with the interaction between peptidyl transferase and amino acids, thereby inhibiting peptide bond formation. It is bacteriostatic to most pathogens. The drug induced inhibition of mitochondrial protein synthesis, by inhibiting eukaryotic mitochondrial 70S ribosomes, probably is responsible for the associated host toxicity.

Clinical Use

Because of the propensity to induce bone marrow depression and aplasia, use of chloramphenicol is no longer justified in treating minor infections. However, it can be used as an alternative drug for some and a choice of drug for a few infections.

1. For meningitis caused by H. influenzae, N. meningitidis and Strepto. pneumoniae, particularly if the patient is hypersensitive to beta lactams.
2. It is used for the treatment of serious anaerobic infections (pelvic and brain abscess) caused by penicillin resistant B. fragilis. However, clindamycin and metronidazole are more preferred for this purpose.
3. Used topically for treating conjunctivitis and external ear infections.
4. It is second choice drug for treatment of rickettsial infections particularly in children below 10 years of age where tetracyclines are contraindicated.

Adverse Effects

1. Dose related bone marrow depression is characterized by anaemia, leukopenia and thrombocytopenia. Non dose related is idiosyncratic aplastic anaemia,
2. **Grey Baby Syndrome:** Neonates/premature babies cannot adequately conjugate chloramphenicol to form the glucuronide. They also have slow rates of glomerular filtration and tubular secretion. Consequently, high levels of free chloramphenicol may accumulate to cause potentially fatal neonatal toxicity, when given in high doses. This is characterized by abdominal distension, progressive cyanosis (grey body), hypothermia, vomiting, loss of hunger and ultimately cardiovascular collapse and death. So chloramphenicol should not be used in neonates. If at all required, the dose should not exceed to 25 mg/kg/day.
3. Super infection, as seen with tetracyclines.

Drug Interactions

Enzyme inducer decrease the efficacy and chloramphenicol.

1. Paracetamol increases the bioavailability of chloramphenicol by 28%.

2. Chloramphenicol is a potent enzyme inhibitor and inhibits the metabolism of tolbutamide, morphine, chlorpropamide, phenytoin and warfarin. So increases the plasma levels and toxicity.

AMINOGLYCOSIDES

Aminoglycosides are polycations antibiotics with amino sugars in glycoside linkage and are mainly used to treat gram negative infection.

Salient Features of Aminoglycosides

1. Aminoglycosides are highly polar and are not absorbed orally therefore they are given parenterally.
2. They remain distributed extra cellular and penetration into CSF is very poor.
3. They are excreted unchanged and rapidly by the kidneys.
4. They are all bactericidal and their activity is maximum in alkaline medium.
5. They act by inhibiting bacterial protein synthesis.
6. They are mainly effective against gram negative organisms.
7. They produce variable degrees of ototoxicity and nephrotoxicity as high concentration are found in renal cortex and in endolymph and perilymph of inner ear.
8. Bacteria develops resistance to them fairly rapidly.
9. They have synergistic effect when combined with beta lactam AMA.

Antibacterial Spectrum

Aminoglycosides have a narrow spectrum and are effective mainly against gram negative organisms, *e.g.,* E. coli, Proteus, Pseudomonas, Brucella, Salmonella, Shigella and Klebsiella.

Mechanism of Action: It has two steps:

Aminoglycosides penetrate the bacterial cell membrane through aqueous pores and from there they are taken up by an active transport process. This is O_2 dependent process. They bind to 30S ribosomes (SM) and 50S unit (with other agents) and inhibit bacterial protein synthesis. They also cause distortion of mRNA codon recognition so, form abnormal peptide chain. Higher the concentration, greater is the bactericidal effect. Post antibiotic effect remains even after the plasma levels of aminoglycosides fall. Hence, even though they have a short $t_{1/2}$, they can be given once a day.

Resistance to Aminoglycosides is Acquired by

1. Acquisition of inactivating enzymes which is R-factor mediated (by conjugation).
2. Low affinity of ribosomes; acquired by mutation – high level resistance.
3. Decrease in permeability to the antibiotic – low level resistance.

Pharmacokinetics

Aminoglycosides are not absorbed from the gut but when instilled into body cavities or applied over large wounds, they may get rapidly absorbed. Following IM injection peak levels are seen in 60 minutes. They are not bound to plasma proteins and mostly remain in the vasculature. They diffuse into the synovial, pericardial and peritoneal fluid and crosses BBB in presence of inflammation. They crosses placental barrier.

Adverse Effects

1. Ototoxicity is the most important toxicity. Both vestibular and auditory dysfunction can occur depending on the dose and duration. There is progressive, permanent deafness.
2. Nephrotoxicity: Aminoglycosides attain high concentration in the renal cortex and cause damage to the renal tubules. This results in loss of urine concentrating capacity, low GFR and albuminuria.
3. Neuromuscular blockade: Aminoglycosides have curare like effects and block neuromuscular transmission.
4. Local irritation and allergy.

Precautions in Using Aminoglycosides

1. Avoid concurrent use of other ototoxic drugs like loop diuretics, other nephrotoxic drugs like amphotericin B, cephalothin and cisplatin.
2. To be used cautiously in elderly, in renal damage and in combination with skeletal muscle relaxants.
3. Contraindicated in pregnancy because of risk of deafness in the child.
4. Do not mix aminoglycosides with any other drug in the same syringe.

Uses

1. *Tuberculosis* (streptomycin).

2. *Sub acute bacterial endocarditis (SABE):* Combination of streptomycin and penicillin is synergistic in this condition.
3. *Plague, Tularemia and Brucellosis.*

Gentamicin is more potent and has a broader spectrum of action compared to streptomycin. Gentamicin is used in:

1. *Uncomplicated UTI.*
2. *Pneumonia* (gentamicin + penicillin), meningitis (gentamicin + Penicillins), osteomyelitis, peritonitis, septicemia (with a third generation cephalosporin).
3. *Topical:* Gentamicin is used in burns and other infected wounds. Eye drops are used for prevention and treatment of bacterial conjunctivitis.

Tobramycin has better activity against Pseudomonas and is used with anti-pseudomonal penicillin in such infections.

Kanamycin: Due to its toxicity, its use is limited to multi-drug resistant tuberculosis.

Amikacin has widest anti-bacterial spectrum and is used in:

1. Nosocomial infections due to gram negative organisms.
2. *Tuberculosis:* Amikacin is useful in multi-drug resistant tuberculosis in combination with other drugs. It is also used in infections due to atypical mycobacteria in patients with AIDS.

Netilmicin: It is used in serious infections due to gram negative bacilli.

Neomycin: It is not given systemically. It is used topically as ointments, creams and powder for ear, eye infection. Oral use can cause diarrhea, steatorrhoea and malabsorption due to damage to the intestinal villi. It is used:

1. As intestinal anti-septic as neomycin is not absorbed when given orally. It is used to prepare the bowel for surgery, *i.e.*, for preoperative gut sterilization.
2. *Hepatic coma:* Ammonia produced by colonic bacteria is absorbed and converted to urea by the liver and causes severe hepatic failure, as liver is unable to handle this NH_3. Blood NH_3 levels rise resulting in encephalopathy. As neomycin inhibits intestinal flora, NH_3 production falls. Neomycin is given orally for this purpose. Nowadays lactulose is preferred as it is less toxic than neomycin.

CHEMOTHERAPY OF TUBERCULOSIS AND LEPROSY

Tuberculosis

Tuberculosis is primarily caused by Mycobacterium tuberculosis and it is due to inhalation of infected droplet nuclei. Lung is generally the first organ to be affected. Symptoms include low grade fever (99.1°F) in the evening, night sweats, malaise, fatigue, weight loss and a blood streaked productive cough.

M. avium complex (MAC) includes both M. avium and M. intracellulare. MAC is an important and common cause of disseminated tuberculosis type disease in late stages of AIDS.

Unlike other infections, tuberculosis is difficult to treat because:

1. Tubercular bacilli grow very slowly and dividing once in 1–2 day. They may persist for many years in macrophages (dormant) and go on multiplying.
2. Caseation and fibrosis tends to block the blood vessels supplying the necrotic areas, so the penetration of anti-tubercular drugs is very difficult.
3. Development of resistance is very rapid.
4. Non-compliance of the treatment.

Important criterias in the treatment of tuberculosis are: (1) The therapy must contain two or more drugs to avoid development of resistance, (2) the drugs must be taken regularly (strict drug compliance) and (3) the drug therapy must continue for a sufficient duration to achieve adequate therapeutic results.

The first line drugs are superior in efficacy and possess an acceptable limit of toxicity. A three-drug or a four-drug combination is used for a specified period as per WHO prescribed regimens to avoid development of resistance. The second line drugs are used if there is resistance to first line drugs or when the first line drugs are contraindicated for some other reason.

Classification of Anti-Tubercular Drugs

A. *First line essential drugs:* Isoniazid, Rifampicin, Ethambutol and Pyrazinamide.
B. *First line supplement drugs:* Rifabutin, Rifapentine, Streptomycin (kept reserved for specific conditions as first line, has acceptable toxicity).

C. *Second line drugs:* Amikacin, Capreomycin, Ethionamide, Kanamycin, Thiacetazone, PAS, Cycloserine, Fluoroquinolones, Azithromycin, Clarithromycin.

(A) First Line Essential Anti-Tubercular Drugs

Isoniazid (INH)

It is primary anti-tubercular drug. Isoniazid inhibits the synthesis of mycolic acid which is essential components of mycobacterial cell wall. It also suppresses the formation of RNA and DNA. INH, therefore, reduces the lipid content of mycobacterial cell wall. It is primarily tuberculocidal drug which acts on extracellular as well as on intracellular tubercle bacilli (present within macrophages) and is equally active in acidic and alkaline medium. It gets concentrated into the cavity after getting diffuse through caseous material. So, it is a part of all drug regimens.

It is completely and rapidly absorbed orally. It is metabolized in liver, by N-acetyl transferase, to acetyl isoniazid. Genetic variation has been observed in its rate of N acetylation. 30–40% of Indians are usually rapid acetylators. 60–70% of Indians are slow acetylators ($t_{1/2}$ 3 hours). The acetylator status of an individual may influence the nature of INH toxicity but not the therapeutic response.

INH is well tolerated. Peripheral neuritis and hepatotoxicity are the two major, but dose dependent, adverse effects. Peripheral neuritis (paraesthesia, numbness) is more common with slow acetylators because of two reasons: (a) INH induced increase in the excretion of pyridoxine in urine; and (b) INH induced decrease in the peripheral utilization of pyridoxine by inhibiting pyridoxine kinase. This neurotoxicity can be prevented by prophylactic use of vitamin B_6. The risk of hepatitis is higher in fast acetylators (fast metabolism of INH provides high concentrations of hepatotoxic metabolites acetyl isoniazid and acetyl hydrazine). Other adverse effects include allergic reactions, xerostomia, hematological changes and drug induced systemic lupus erythematosus. Aluminum hydroxide (as in antacids) inhibits the absorption of INH. Stimulation of CNS may cause ataxia and muscle twitching.

INH resistance: Some bacilli are inherently resistant to INH. They proliferate rapidly and leads to development of resistance when INH is used alone.

INH inhibits the metabolism of phenytoin, carbamazepine, diazepam and warfarin.

Rifampicin (Rifampin, RMP)

Rifampicin binds strongly to bacterial DNA dependent RNA polymerase and thereby inhibits RNA synthesis of bacteria, leading to suppression of initiation of chain formation. The drug is tuberculocidal for both intracellular and extracellular M. tuberculosis. In addition to M. tuberculosis, rifampicin is also active against M. leprae. It acts on persisters.

It is well-absorbed orally. Rifampicin in combination with other first line anti-tubercular drugs is used for the treatment of all forms of pulmonary and extra pulmonary tuberculosis. Other indications for rifampicin include: treatment of lèprosy in combination with dapsone, meningitis and brucellosis.

Adverse Effects

Hepatitis is the major adverse effect and the risk may be increased in patients with underlying liver disease. Occasional adverse effects include rashes, GI disturbances, dizziness, fatigue, flu-like syndrome and respiratory syndrome associated with shock and collapse. Rifampicin imparts a harmless red orange color to urine and other secretions.

The drug is a potent enzyme inducer. Hence, it accelerates the metabolism of several other drugs such as oral contraceptives and anti-coagulants.

Ethambutol (ETB)

Ethambutol is a synthetic tuberculostatic drug, active against M. tuberculosis, M. kansasi and M. avium intracellulare. Its mechanism of action is not fully understood but it inhibits mycobacterial cell wall synthesis by interfering with mycolic acid and inhibits RNA synthesis. It penetrates RBCs which act as depot from which drug is released.

It is commonly included as a fourth drug along with INH, rifampicin and pyrazinamide in the treatment regimen of tuberculosis. It is also used in combination with other drugs, in the treatment of M avium intracellular infection in AIDS patients.

Ethambutol can cause retrobulbar neuritis, impairing visual acuity and red green color discrimination. It should also be avoided in children below 5 years of age, where it is difficult to assess visual acuity and red green color blindness, Ethambutol decreases renal excretion of urates and may precipitate gouty arthritis.

Pyrazinamide (PZA)

PZA is thought to enter M. tuberculosis by passive diffusion and is converted to its active metabolite pyrazinoic acid which disrupts mycolic acid synthesis needed for cell wall synthesis. PZA is tuberculocidal to M. tuberculosis and is active at low (acidic) pH. PZA is highly effective on intracellular mycobacteria. It is effective uniquely in zones of acute inflammation and against quiescent bacilli within macrophages. It is not very effective in later phase of treatment, when inflammation subsides.

Hepatotoxicity is the major adverse effect occurs in about 15%. Other adverse effects include nausea, vomiting, anorexia, drug fever and malaise. Hyperuricaemia and gouty arthritis may also occur. PZA should be avoided during pregnancy.

(B) First Line Supplement Drugs

Streptomycin (SM)

It was the first drug to exhibit an effective tuberculocidal activity against M. tuberculosis but because of poor penetration, it acts only on extra-cellular tubercular bacilli (CSF penetration is also poor). Streptomycin is less effective than INH or rifampicin and given IM. It is kept in reserve as first line drug in life threatening tuberculosis.

Rifabutin

Rifabutin is a structural analogue of rifampicin. It has all major pharmacological characteristics similar to rifampicin.

It differs from rifampicin in the following features: It is a less potent inducer of cytochrome P-450 enzymes and causes lesser drug interactions, it has better activity than rifampicin, against M. avium complex (MAC). It is not only active against M. tuberculosis but also active against some rifampicin resistant strains of M. leprae. It is well absorbed orally. Plasma half life is very long (45 hours). It can be used in place of rifampicin for the treatment of tuberculosis in HIV infected patients and for prevention and treatment of disseminated MAC infection.

Adverse effects include skin rash, hepatitis and red orange discoloration of urine (like rifampicin).

Rifapentine

Similar to rifampicin, but the potential for drug interaction is low.

(C) Second Line Anti-Tubercular Drugs

Ethionamide, capreomycin, amikacin, cycloserine and para-amino-salicylic acid (PAS) are very rarely used. They are bacteriostatic and highly toxic drugs.

Fluoroquinolones

Fluoroquinolones are important in M. tuberculosis infection especially in multi-drug resistant strains. They are very effective when used as a part of combined regimen in HIV infected patients. Ciprofloxacin, Ofloxacin and Moxafloxacin inhibit 90–95% of the strains of susceptible tubercular bacilli including M. avium complex. Due to good penetration into the cells, these are capable of killing intracellular pathogens, and because of their convenient dosage schedule and good tolerability, these are being increasingly included in combination regimens against multi-drug resistant tuberculosis and MAC infection in AIDS patients.

Macrolides

Clarithromycin and azithromycin are very active against MAC. Clarithromycin is four times more potent than azithromycin against M. avium complex but azithromycin have the greater intracellular penetration. WHO has recommended the Directly Observed Treatment Strategy (DOTS) wherein the anti-tubercular drugs are given under the direct supervision of the medical professional three days a week (Table 6.1).

Table 6.1: RNTCP Guideline 2009

TB category	Initial Phase	Continuous Phase	Total duration of therapy (in months)
I	$2H_3R_3Z_3E_3$	$4H_3R_3$	6
II	$2H_3R_3Z_3E_3S_3 + 1H_3R_3Z_3E_3$	$5H_3R_3E_3$	8
III	$2H_3R_3Z_3$	$4H_3R_3$	6

Category I	New TB patients smear positive, seriously ill (smear negative) and seriously ill (extra-pulmonary TB)
Category II	Sputum smear positive relapse, failure, default
Category III	New sputum smear negative, not seriously ill, new extrapulmonary, not seriously ill

This regimen has an initial intensive phase, which is followed by a continuation phase. Intensive phase lasts for a period of 2 months and is aimed to rapidly kill the bacteria, to minimize the chances for developing resistance and to bring about sputum conversion and symptomatic relief.

The continuation phase lasts for 4 months in which duration the remaining bacilli are eliminated to minimize the chances of relapse.

Tuberculosis During Pregnancy and Breast Feeding: INH, RMP, PZA and even ETB are safe in pregnancy. However, ETB may be added during last trimester of pregnancy, not earlier.

Corticosteroids

They may be used in special circumstances under adequate chemotherapeutic cover, *e.g.*, (a) in AIDS patients with serious illness; (b) in meningeal or renal tuberculosis or pleural effusion to minimize inflammation and exudation; and (c) if hypersensitivity reaction occurs to any anti-tubercular drug; corticosteroids, if used, should be gradually withdrawn when the condition of the patient improves.

Drugs Active Against M. Avium Complex in AIDS Patients

TB infection in HIV positive case is more severe and is a serious problem. The drug regimen is same as but the continuation phase lasts for 7 months instead of 4 months (*i.e.*, total duration is of 2 + 7 = 9 months instead of 6 months).

M. avium, complex infection is also particularly common in HIV infected patients. M. avium complex (MAC) includes two atypical mycobacteria.

M. avium and M. intracellulare. The most common drug regimens are as under:

Clarithromycin/azithromycin (500 mg BD, orally) + ethambutol (15 mg/kg/d) + Ciprofloxacin (750 mg BD, orally) + rifabutin (300 mg OD, orally).

Drug Treatment of Leprosy

Leprosy is a chronic granulomatous infection caused by an acid fast bacilli Mycobacterium lepare. Leprosy may be classified as:

1. Paucibacillary leprosy is non-infectious. Its important features are:
   a. Less than 5 hypoaesthetic skin lesions.
   b. Normal or only partially deficient cell mediated immunity.
   c. Bacilli are rarely found in biopsies.
   d. Lepromin test is positive. (Lepromin is an extract of tissue infected with M. leprae, used in skin test to determine tissue resistance to leprosy).

e. There are prolonged remissions with periodic exacerbations.

2. Multibacillary leprosy is an infectious leprosy. The important features of this type of leprosy are:
   a. More than 5 hypoaesthetic but diffused skin lesions with mucous membrane infiltrations.
   b. Cellular immunity is largely deficient.
   c. Skin and mucous membrane have numerous bacilli.
   d. Lepromin test is negative.
   e. The disease later progresses to anaesthesia of distal parts and wounds.

Classification of Drugs Used in Leprosy

1. *Sulfones:* Dapsone.
2. *Phenazine derivatives:* Clofazimine.
3. *Anti-tubercular drugs:* Rifampicin, Ethionamid.
4. *Antibiotics:* Ofloxacin, Sparfloxacin, Clarithromycin, Minocycline.

Dapsone (Diamino Diphenyl Sulfone, DDS)

It is closely related to sulfonamides and shares a common mechanism of action, *i.e.*, inhibition of bacterial folic acid synthesis. It is leprostatic at low concentration.

Dapsone is usually well tolerated. It may produce hemolytic anaemia and methaemoglobinaemia in persons having G6PD deficiency, cutaneous reactions, *e.g.*, allergic rash, drug eruption phototoxicity also occur. Resistance usually emerges in some patients if dapsone is used as a monotherapy. Therefore, the combination of dapsone with rifampicin and clofazimine is recommended for treatment of leprosy.

During dapsone therapy for lepromatous leprosy and tuberculoid leprosy, some reactive episodes may occur.

Type-1 lepra reaction which is delayed hypersensitivity reactions to M. leprae antigens (Type IV hypersensitivity). It is characterised by cutaneous ulceration, and multiple nerve involvement. Prompt treatment with corticosteroids is necessary to prevent nerve damage.

Type-2 lepra reactions represent a humoral antibody response (Type III hypersensitivity) to dead bacteria. This lepra reaction is of abrupt onset, existing lesions enlarge, become red, inflamed and painful. This reaction can be treated with clofazimine or corticosteroid or thalidomide.

Clofazimine

It binds preferentially to mycobacterial DNA, and inhibits mycobacterial growth. It is leprostatic drug with anti-inflammatory properties. Clofazimine is used for dapsone resistant leprosy or in patients intolerant to dapsone.

Side effects of clofazimine are: red brown discoloration of skin, and abdominal pain with loose stools due to deposition of clofazimine in intestinal mucosa. It should be avoided in pregnancy. Clofazimine is preferred drug in multi-drug therapy of leprosy and is useful in lepra reaction.

Rifampicin

Though it rapidly renders leprosy patients non-contagious but resistance develops after prolonged treatment. Hence it is not used alone but as a component in multi-drug therapy of leprosy, to shorten the duration of treatment.

Ofloxacin and Sparfloxacin

Ofloxacin (400 mg/day orally) or sparfloxacin (400 mg once on first day followed by 200 mg/day) if used as monotherapy have been reported to kill 99.9% of M. leprae in 3 weeks period. These are used as alternative drugs (and not as main drugs) in the treatment of leprosy or to shorten the duration of therapy. Clarithromycin and Minocycline also used in MDT regimen.

WHO Regimen for Leprosy Treatment

Multibacillary (Lepromatous) Leprosy

Dapsone 100 mg daily + Clofazimine 50 mg daily together with 300 mg once a month supervised (*i.e.*, 29 + 1 = 30 days) + Rifampicin 600 mg once a month (supervised) for 12 months.

Paucibacillary (Tuberculoid) Leprosy

Dapsone 100 mg daily + Rifampicin 600 mg once a month (supervised) for 6 months.

ANTI-FUNGAL DRUGS

Fungal infections may be systemic or superficial. This may be consequent to the use of broad spectrum antibiotics, anti-cancer drugs and HIV infections, all of these impair host defense mechanisms.

Classification

1. **Anti-fungal antibiotics:**
   a. *Polyene antibiotics:* Amphotericin B, Nystatin, Hamycin, Natamycin.
   b. *Heterocyclic benzofuran:* Griseofulvin.
2. **Anti-metabolites:** Flucytosine (5 FC).
3. **Azoles:**
   a. *Imidazoles:* Clotrimazole, Econazole, Miconazole, Ketoconazole, Butaconazole, Oxiconazole, Sulconazole, Isoconazole.
   b. *Triazoles:* Fluconazole, Itraconazole, Terconazole, Voriconazole.
4. **Allylamine:** Terbinafine, Pneumocandins.
5. **Other topical agents:** Tolnaftate, Undecylenic acid, Benzoic acid, Salicylic acid, Selenium sulfide, Ciclopirox olamine, Butenafine, Sodium thiosulfate.

Sites of Action: Anti-fungal drugs may act on the fungal cell wall (pneumocandins), cell membrane (polyenes, azoles) or on the nucleus (griseofulvin, flucytosine).

Anti-Fungal Antibiotics

Amphotericin B: It has a wide anti-fungal spectrum. It inhibits the growth of Candida albicans, Histoplasma capsulatum, Cryptococcus neoformans, Coccidioides, Aspergillus and Blastomyces dermatitidis. It is fungistatic at low and fungicidal at high concentrations. Amphoterecin B also has activity against Leishmania.

Mechanism of Action

Amphotericin B binds to ergosterol present in fungal cell membrane and forms pores in the cell membrane. Through these pores, cell contents leak out resulting in cell death. Since amphotericin has greater affinity for the fungal membrane sterol (ergosterol), action is selective for the fungi but it may bind with host cell membrane, though with less affinity. This may cause toxic effects.

Amphotericin is not absorbed orally. It is insoluble in water. Given IV, it is widely distributed in the body and has a long $t_{1/2}$ of 15 days.

Adverse Effects: Fever, chills, muscle spasms, vomiting, dyspnoea, headache and hypotension can be encountered on IV infusion due to release of cytokines. Pain and thrombophlebitis at the site of injection are common. Renal impairment, neurotoxicity and anaemia due to decreased production of erythropoietin and bone marrow depression can also occur. Concurrent administration of other nephrotoxic drugs should be avoided.

Uses

- Amphotericin B is the drug of choice for all life threatening mycotic infections.
- In cystitis due to candida.
- Used to prevent relapse of cryptococcosis and histoplasmosis in patients with AIDS, invasive aspergillosis, blastomycosis.
- Given orally in fungal infections of the gut.
- Topically in candidiasis.
- In kala azar and mucocutaneous leishmaniasis, amphotericin is used as an alternative.

Nystatin has actions similar to amphotericin B. But as it is too toxic for systemic use, it is used topically for local candidial infections, like oral thrush and vaginal candidiasis. **Hamycin** is similar to nystatin.

Griseofulvin is a fungi static. It is effective in superficial dermatophytosis.

It binds to microtubular protein in the nucleus, disrupts the mitotic spindle and inhibits mitosis in the fungus. It also causes abnormal metaphase configuration. It gets deposited in the newly forming skin, binds to keratin and protects the skin from getting newly infected.

Griseofulvin is poorly water soluble with poor bioavailability. Absorption can be enhanced by using microfined drug particles and by giving it with fatty food. Griseofulvin is used orally in superficial dermatophytosis.

Adverse effects include allergic reactions, hepatitis and neurotoxicity. Griseofulvin is a microsomal enzyme inducer.

Drug Interactions

Phenobarbitone reduces the absorption of griseofulvin. Griseofulvin enhances warfarin metabolism by inducing microsomal enzymes. Alcohol should be avoided because griseofulvin can cause intolerance to alcohol.

Anti-Metabolites

Flucytosine is a fluorinated pyrimidine effective against Cryptococcus neoformans and some strains of Candida. It is taken up by the fungal cells and converted to 5 fluorouracil which inhibits DNA synthesis. Bone marrow depression and gastrointestinal disturbances are the most common adverse effects.

Imidazoles and Triazoles

Azoles are newer synthetic anti-fungal drugs that are effective orally and are less toxic. They have a broad spectrum anti-fungal activity. They inhibit dermatophytes, candida, Cryptococcus neoformans, H. capsulatum and other deep mycoses.

Azoles inhibit the synthesis of ergosterol, an important component of the fungal cell membrane. They bind to the fungal cytochrome P450 enzyme dependent 14-alpha demethylase which catalyses the conversion of lanosterol to ergosterol which results in damaged leaky fungal cell membrane. They have low affinity for host cells. They also interfere with the function of some fungal enzymes and inhibit the growth of the fungi. They inhibit fungal respiration under aerobic conditions.

Ketoconazole (KTZ) is the first oral azole to be available. It is well absorbed from the gut. Food and low gastric pH enhance absorption. In large doses KTZ inhibits the biosynthesis of adrenal and gonadal steroids in humans resulting in gynaecomastia, infertility, decreased libido, oligozoospermia, menstrual irregularities and hypertension. It is useful in both mucocutaneous candidiasis and dermatophytosis. It is also used in Cushing's syndrome.

Clotimazole and miconazole are used topically in dermatophytic infections (ringworm) and mucocutaneous candidiasis.

Fluconazole is water soluble, well absorbed orally and attains good CSF concentration. Hence it is useful even in fungal meningitis.

Itraconazole is the most potent azole. Its effect on hepatic microsomal enzyme inhibition is less; does not affect steroid synthesis. Thus it is preferred over ketoconazole. Itraconazole is the drug of choice in most systemic mycoses, aspergillosis, chromomycosis candidiasis and dermatophytosis histoplasmosis but it is expensive.

Terbinafine is a synthetic anti-fungal that is effective against dermatophytes and Candida. It is orally effective and is fungicidal. It gets concentrated in the keratin used in tinea pedis/corporis/cruris. It is particularly preferred in onychomycosis, where it is superior to azoles and griseofulvin.

Econazole, terconazole, tibconazole, butaconazole, oxiconazole and sulconazole are available for topical use as creams and lotions.

ANTI-VIRAL DRUGS AND DRUGS USED IN THE TREATMENT OF HIV INFECTION

Anti-Viral Drugs

Viruses are intracellular parasites not only depend on the host cells for their food, growth and multiplication, but also direct its metabolic machinery to synthesize new particles. There are two types of viruses DNA and RNA viruses and there are minor differences in their replicative cycles. The DNA virus depends on host cell enzymes (mRNA polymerase) to synthesize mRNA while RNA viruses use their own enzymes for mRNA synthesis.

Retroviruses are type of RNA viruses which are known to cause AIDS. In retroviruses a viral enzyme reverse transcriptase is involved in replication.

Classification of Anti-Viral Drugs

1. **Anti-herpes virus agents:** Acyclovir, Ganciclovir, Famciclovir, Penciclovir, Valaciclovir, Idoxuridine* Trifluridine,* Vidarabine,* Foscarnet, Cidofovir (*very toxic, not used).
2. **Anti-influenza virus agent:** Amantadine, Rimantadine, Oseltamivir, Zanamivir (used as inhaler).
3. **Others:** Ribavirin, Interferons, Lamivudine.
4. **Anti-retroviral agents:**
   a. *Nucleoside Reverse Transcriptase Inhibitors (NRTI):* Zidovudine, Didanosine, Stavudine, Zalcitabine, Lamivudine, Abacavir.
   b. *Non Nucleaside Reverse Transcriptase Inhibitors (NNRTI):* Nevirapine, Efavirenz, Delavirdine.
   c. *Protease Inhibitors (PI):* Saquinavir, Indinavir, Ritonavir, Nelfinavir, Amprenavir, Lopinavir.
   d. *Fusion inhibitor:* Enfuvirtide.

Anti-Herpes Virus Agents

Acyclovir is synthetic purine nucleoside analogue and is effective against Herpes simplex virus (HSV) type 1 and type 2, Varicella zoster virus (VZV) and Epstein Barr virus (EBV).

Mechanism of Action

Acyclovir is taken up by the virus infected cell, converted to acyclovir tri-phosphate and this inhibits viral DNA synthesis by inhibiting viral DNA polymerases and causing DNA chain termination. Oral absorption of acyclovir is poor; it is well distributed, poor protein bound, attains good concentration in the CSF and aqueous humor.

Adverse effects include nausea, diarrhea and headache. Rashes may occur occasionally. Topical acyclovir can cause burning and irritation. Given IV, it may cause dose dependent renal and neurotoxicity. It is teratogenic.

Uses

1. It is effective in: Primary and recurrent genital and labial herpes.
2. HSV encephalitis and keratoconjunctivitis.
3. Herpes zoster and chickenpox.
4. Mucocutaneous HSV.

Valacyclovir is a prodrug of acyclovir and have greater bioavailability.
Famciclovir is a prodrug of pennciclovir, used in HSV and VZV infection.

Ganciclovir is éffective against herpes viruses especially Cytomegalovirus (CMV) and is more toxic.

Trifluride and Idoxuridine is effective in DNA viruses. It acts by inhibiting viral DNA synthesis is used topically in HSV keratitis (no systemic use).

Foscarnet is given intravenously to treat CMV retinitis as an alternative to ganciclovir. It is effective in resistant cases of herpes simplex; CMV infection (in AIDS patients). It causes nephrotoxicity.

Anti-Influenza Virus Agents

Oseltamivir and zanamivir inhibit viral replication. They act by inhibiting the neuraminidase enzyme activity which is essential for the release of daughter virions. Oseltamivir is given orally; zanamivir is given by inhalation which can occasionally cause respiratory distress.

Oseltamivir and zanamivir are indicated in the prevention and treatment of influenza, *e.g.*, A, B, H_5N_1 and H_1N_1 (swine flu).

Amantadine

Inhibits replication/uncoating of influenza A virus, and acts on M_2 proteins. It is well absorbed, well tolerated, cause anorexia, vomiting, insomnia, and ankle edema. It is used in influenza A infection and parkinsonism.

Contraindication: Epilepsy, gastric ulcer, pregnancy.

Interferons are cytokines produced by host cells in response to viral infections by recombinant DNA. There are three types alpha, beta and gamma interferons in man. They also have immune-modulating and anti-proliferative properties. They inhibit viral penetration, uncoating, synthesis of mRNA and the multiplication of many DNA and RNA viruses.

Adverse effects include myelosuppression, hypotension, arrhythmias, alopecia, headache and arthralgia, neurotoxicity and thyroid dysfunction.

Uses

1. Chronic hepatitis B and C.
2. Kaposi's sarcoma in AIDS patients.
3. Genital warts caused by papilloma virus–interferons are injected into the lesion.
4. Hairy cell leukemia.
5. HSV, herpes zoster and CMV infections in immune compromised patients.
6. Rhinovirus cold interferon is given intranasal for prophylaxis.

Anti-Retroviral Drugs

They are effective against acquired immunodeficiency syndrome results from infection with human immunodeficiency virus (HIV).

HIV has a high mutation rate and therefore easily develops resistance to the drugs. Multi-drug resistant strains have emerged and they further complicate treatment. Different drugs used in the treatment of HIV infection are:

(A) Nucleoside Reverse Transcriptase Inhibitors (NRTI)

Mechanism of Action

NRTI are converted to their corresponding triphosphate derivatives from cellular kinase, which have a high affinity for reverse transcriptase, an enzyme specific to HIV and required for DNA synthesis. The NRT inhibitors are nucleoside analogs. They competitively inhibit reverse transcriptase and terminate DNA chain elongation.

Zidovudine (AZT) is the first drug to be used in the treatment of HIV infection. Others including didanosine, stavudine, zalcitabine, lamivudine and abacavir were developed later.

Pharmacokinetics: NRT inhibitors are well absorbed when given orally. All NRT inhibitors (except abacavir) are excreted in the urine. They crosses placenta and are teratogenic. Bone marrow suppression is the most prominent adverse effect of zidovudine. Paracetamol increases its concentration by competing for glucuronide conjugations and increases toxicity.

AZT is the drug of choice in AIDS. It prolonged survival, decreased opportunistic infections (*e.g.*, CMV, Kaposi sarcoma), and weight gain and in early cases it delays disease progression. Given during pregnancy and continued in newborn for 6 weeks, AZT reduces the risk of transmission of infection to the baby. But it has no prophylactic value in those who are accidentally exposed to HIV infection.

Lamivudine is well tolerated with no significant adverse effects in therapeutic doses other than headache and nausea. **Abacavir** can cause a hypersensitivity syndrome with fever, rash and bronchitis which can be fatal. Hence abacavir should be withdrawn at the onset of such symptoms. Alcohol consumption should be avoided. Peripheral neuropathy, pancreatitis, rash, fever and headache can occur with didanosine, stavudine and zalcitabine.

(B) Non-Nucleoside Reverse Transcriptase Inhibitors (NNRTIs)

Mechanism of Action

The NNRT inhibitors bind to reverse transcriptase (are not converted to triphosphate derivatives) and bring about a change in the enzyme thereby inactivating the enzyme. NNRT inhibitors are effective only against HIV-1. Resistance develops due to mutation.

Adverse Effects

Allergic reactions ranging from skin rashes, pruritus to Stevens-Johnson syndrome and toxic epidermal necrolysis can occur. **Efavirenz** has teratogenic effects in monkeys and is contraindicated in pregnant women. Nevirapine can occasionally cause fulminant hepatitis. Enzyme inducer and enzyme inhibitors must be avoided with these drugs.

NNRTIs are used in the treatment of HIV infections in combination with other drugs. Nevirapine can be tried in pregnant women during labour and in newborn.

(C) Protease Inhibitors (PI)

Mechanism of Action

HIV protease activity is essential for the activation of viral enzymes and HIV replication. The protease inhibitors bind competitively to HIV protease and block viral maturation before they released from infected cells. This makes the daughter viral particles immature and non-infectious. They are effective in both newly and chronically infected cells.

Saquinavir has poor oral bioavailability while others are well absorbed. All PIs are extensively bound to plasma proteins. They are all metabolised by hepatic microsomal enzymes and are also microsomal enzyme inhibitors. Protease inhibitors are well tolerated. Gastrointestinal symptoms like nausea, vomiting and diarrhea can occur. Protease inhibitors are used in combination with other antiretroviral drugs in the treatment of HIV infections.

(D) Fusion Inhibitors

Enfuvirtide blocks the entry of HIV into the cells by preventing the fusion of virus with cellular membrane. It improves CD4 count and decreases viral titre when used with other ART drugs.

Maraviroc (Chemokine receptor-5 antagonist), Raltegravir (integrase inhibitor), Bevirimat (maturation inhibitors), Elvucitabine (new NRTI) and vicriviroc are newer drugs. They are used in combination with other drugs in resistant cases.

Drug Interactions of Anti-Retroviral Drugs

- Since AZT causes myelosuppression, it should not be combined with other myelosuppressants.
- Plasma levels of abacavir are increased by alcohol.
- Nevirapine and efavirenz are microsomal enzyme inducers concurrent administration of rifampicin and ketoconazole should be avoided. Failure of oral contraceptives can occur, hence alternative methods of contraception should be followed.
- Delavirdine is a microsomal enzyme inhibitor.

Objective of Therapy

1. To suppress HIV replication and improve immune system.
2. To prevent emergence of drug resistance.
3. To treat or prevent opportunistic infection.

A combination of drugs is used in AIDS to improve prognosis known as Highly Active Antiretroviral Therapy (HAART) which includes two NRT inhibitors with either NNRT or protease inhibitors. A HAART regimen suppresses HIV replication; plasma HIV-RNA levels are greatly reduced and prolong patient survival. HAART also has some disadvantages of being difficult to follow and is associated with adverse effects from drugs and has high relapse rate.

ANTI-MALARIAL DRUGS

Malaria is a parasitic disease caused by the protozoan of the genus Plasmodium. Four species of the genus Plasmodium cause human malaria: (i) Plasmodium falciparum, causes malignant tertian (MT) malaria; (ii) Plasmodium vivax, causes benign tertian (BT) malaria, and relapses are common. The term tertian indicates that the attacks of chills and fever typically tend to recur every third day; (iii) Plasmodium malariae, causes quartan (Q) malaria. The term quartan indicates that the spikes of fever come every fourth day; and (iv) Plasmodium ovale, causes a rare form of relapsing malaria. It is tertian in nature. Infections caused by P vivax, P malariae and P ovale are classified as 'relapsing malarias' because they have a secondary exoerythrocytic stage of development. In contrast, P falciparum has no exoerythrocytic stage in its life cycle.

Anti-Malarial Drug Act by Following Ways

1. **Causal prophylaxis:** A casual prophylactic agent prevents infection by its lethal effect on the plasmodia during their pre-erythrocytic stages, *e.g.*, primaquine for all species of malaria (but not for mass programme due to its toxicity).
2. **Suppressive treatment:** A suppressive drug causes inhibition of the erythrocytic stage of development of the parasite, *e.g.*, chloroquine, mefloquine, doxycycline (as an alternative) for travelers.
3. **Clinical cure:** Drugs in this category interrupt erythrocytic schizogony of the plasmodia and terminate the clinical attack, *e.g.*, chloroquine, amodiaquine, mefloquine, artimisinin etc. be used singly.
4. **Radical cure:** This refers to the eradication of both exoerythrocytic and erythrocytic phases of the infection, *e.g.*, primaquine.
5. **Suppressive cure:** This refers to the complete elimination of the malaria parasite from the body by continued suppressive therapy, *e.g.*, pyrimethamine for 10 weeks.
6. **Gametocidal therapy:** This category of drugs destroys the sexual forms of the malarial parasites in human blood, *e.g.*, primaquine.

Classification

A. *4 Aminoquinolines:* Chloroquine, Hydroxychloroquine, Amodiaquine, Piperaquine.
B. *Cinchona alkaloid:* Quinine.
C. *4 Quinoline methanol:* Mefloquine.
D. *Diaminopyrimidines:* Pyrimethamine.
E. *8 Aminoquinolines:* Primaquine, Bulaquine, Etaquine.
F. *Sesquiterpine lactone:* Artesunate, Artemether, Arteether.
G. *Sulfonamides and Sulfones, e.g.*, Sulfadoxine and Sulfamethoxazole.
H. *Antibiotics:* Doxycyclines, Tetracyclines, Clindamycin.
I. *Amino alcohols:* Halofantrine, Lumefantrine.
J. *Miscellaneous:* Pyronaridine, Atovaquone, Proguanil.

Aims of using anti-malarial drugs are:

1. To prevent and treat clinical attack of malaria.
2. To eradicate the parasite from the body of the patient completely.
3. To reduce the reservoir of infection.

A. Aminoquinolines

a. Chloroquine

Chloroquine was primarily developed as an anti-malarial, but in addition it is active against extra intestinal amoebiasis.

Chloroquine and its congeners block the enzymatic synthesis of DNA and RNA. It causes stabilization of lysosomes and have some anti-inflammatory and anti-histaminic activity.

Mechanism of action is not clear. Chloroquine is a base. Higher concentration is found in RBC. It concentrates in acidic food vacuoles (acidic) of the parasite and raises the vesicular pH. Malarial parasites digest the host hemoglobin and transport it into their acidic food vacuoles In this process a toxic product 'haeme' is formed. This haeme is converted to nontoxic 'haemazoin' a malarial pigment, by the enzyme haeme polymerase. Chloroquine, quinine and mefloquine inhibit the enzyme haeme polymerase resulting in accumulation of haeme which causes lysis of the parasite membrane and thereby death of the parasite. Chloroquine also prevents the digestion of haemoglobin by the parasite thereby depriving the parasite's amino acid supply.

Pharmacokinetics: Chloroquine is rapidly and well absorbed from the gut. It has high affinity for melanin rich tissues and nuclear chromatin. It is metabolized by hepatic microsomal enzymes and is largely excreted in the urine. Its selective accumulation in retina is responsible for the ocular toxicity.

Toxicity: Toxicity is low but side effects are frequent and include vomiting, vertigo, malaise, diarrhea, blurring of vision and urticaria. After high doses maculopapular eruptions, exfoliative lesions of the skin, alopecia and graying of the hair may develop. Hallucinations, agitation and peripheral neuropathies may occur. Parenteral administration can cause hypotension, cardiac depression and arrhythmia. Convulsions may occur in children.

Ocular Toxicity: Corneal deposits and retinopathy may occur.

Precautions and Contraindication of Chloroquine

- Chloroquine should be avoided or used carefully in patients with myopathy, porphyria, psoriasis and hepatic, gastrointestinal or neurological disorders.
- Avoided in patients with retinal diseases. When chloroquine is given in high doses for a long time, regular neurological and eye examination should be done.
- Concurrent use of gold or d penicillamine with chloroquine can cause more severe dermatitis.
- Chloroquine, quinine and mefloquine should not be given concurrently because they compete for accumulation in the parasite and may result in therapeutic failure. Also increased risk of seizures.
- Chloroquine + halofantrine increases risk of arrhythmias. Chloroquine is safe during pregnancy.

Therapeutic Uses

1. Acute malarial attacks.
2. Suppression of malaria.
3. Hepatic amoebiasis.
4. Rheumatoid arthritis, discoid lupus erythematosus, acute disseminated lupus erythematosus, photogenic reaction, lepra reaction and infectious mono nucleosis (IMN).

b. Amodiaquine

It is identical to chloroquine but faster acting than chloroquine. It is not recommended for prophylaxis as it causes agranulocytosis. It is now used in ACT regimen in chloroquine resistant P. falciparum malaria.

B. Cinchona Alkaloid

Quinine

Anti-Malarial Action: Quinine is an erythrocytic schizontocide for all species of plasmodia. It is less effective and more toxic to chloroquine.

Mode of Action: It has no effect on pre-erythrocytic stage. It is a weak base, get concentrated in the acidic vacuoles and cause pigment changes, inhibit polymerization of haeme to hemozoin and damage parasite membrane.

Pharmacokinetics: On oral administration, quinine is rapidly and effectively absorbed, mainly from the upper small intestine. Peak levels occur within 1–3 hours, and about 70–80% is protein bound. It is degraded in the liver by CYP3A4 and only 5 percent of the active drug is recoverable in the urine. It is non-cumulative.

Adverse Effect of Quinine includes:

(i) Cinchonism – ringing of ear, nausea, headache, vertigo, visual and hearing defects.
(ii) Local irritation.
(iii) Bone marrow depression.
(iv) Black water fever and kidney damage.
(v) Hypersensitivity reaction.
(vi) Cardiac toxicity: Hypotension, arrhythmia.
(vii) Hypoglycemia can be quite profound to result in coma. Quinine stimulates the insulin release.

Uses

1. Quinine is used in the treatment of resistant falciparum malaria and cerebral malaria.
2. Nocturnal muscle cramps.

C. Mefloquine

Mefloquine in a single dose is highly effective against erythrocytic forms of the malaria parasite including the multi-drug resistant (MDR) strains of P. falciparum. Mefloquine gets concentrated in the acidic vacuoles of the parasite. Mechanism of action is not exactly known but it is thought to act like quinine by inhibiting haeme polymerase in the parasite.

It is well absorbed orally and has a long $t_{1/2}$ of nearly 20–30 days as it undergoes extensive enterohepatic circulation. Nausea, vomiting, dizziness, confusion, abdominal pain and bradycardia are common. CNS effects like ataxia, disorientation, seizures, and encephalopathy and psychotic manifestations are rare and reversible.

Uses: Mefloquine is used in the prophylaxis and treatment of chloroquine resistant and multi-drug resistant falciparum malaria. Because of its potential toxicity, cost and long $t_{1/2}$ its use is being restricted to areas where resistant strains are prevalent. It should be avoided during pregnancy. It is not given parenterally because of pain and local irritation at the site of injection.

D. Pyrimethamine

Mode of Action: It is dihydrofolate reductase inhibitors, exert a plasmodicidal action by causing a deficiency of tetrahydrofolate which results in the inhibition of cell division and schizogony. It has poor action on bacterial DHFRase.

Pyrimethamine is effective as a prophylactic and suppressive agent, and has proved useful if given once weekly. But it does not eliminate the pre-erythrocytic cycle of P. falciparum.

Pyrimethamine in combination with sulfadoxine (Fansidar) is available for use in the treatment of multi-resistant infections. It is used in:

(a) *Acute attacks:* Pyrimethamine + sulfadoxine combination (S/P) is used as an alternative in uncomplicated, chloroquine resistant falciparum malaria. It is also used as an adjunct to quinine in acute attacks of malaria.
Prophylaxis 1–2 tablets once weekly for prophylaxis against MDR falciparum malaria is used.

(b) *Toxoplasmosis:* S/P combination is used.

E. Primaquine

Primaquine is the most effective and least toxic of the 8-aminoquinoline. Primaquine is a tissue schizonticide. It destroys the parasite in the liver cells and prevents the invasion of erythrocytes causal prophylactic. But it is generally not used for this purpose. Primaquine destroys the hypnozoites (exoerythrocytic form) in the liver and thereby prevents relapse of P. vivax and P. ovale malaria.

It is also effective against the gametocytes of all four species of the malaria parasite. It has weak and insignificant activity against the erythrocytic forms. It is used to induce radical cures of relapsing malarias. It is more effective against the pre-erythrocytic stage of P. falciparum than P. vivex. It is readily absorbed orally.

Side Effects include nausea, headache and disturbances of visual accommodation, pruritus and abdominal cramps. Severe reactions with high dose therapy include leucopenia and methaemoglobinaemia.

It may cause haemolysis in patients with G6PD deficiency.

Uses: Used for radical cure of malaria.

F. Artemisinin Derivatives

Artemisinin is an herbal product traditionally used in China for the treatment of malaria. The two commonly used derivatives are artemether and artesunate.

Mechanism of Action

The endoperoxide bridge in the molecule of artimisinin interacts with heme resulting in the generation of free radicals that bind to the membrane protein and damages ER, inhibits protein synthesis and lysis the parasite.

Artemether: It is a potent and rapidly acting blood schizonticide, and is highly efficacious in treating chloroquine resistant falciparum malaria, and complicated falciparum malaria including cerebral malaria. It is lipid soluble and given orally and IM (not IV).

Adverse reactions include nausea, vomiting, abdominal pain, bradycardia, first degree heart block, and transient increase in transaminases. Concurrent use of terfenadine, TCADs, increases the risk of cardiac toxicity.

Artesunate: It also is a potent blood schizonticide and is available for oral use in cases of chloroquine resistant falciparum malaria. It is given by oral, IM and IV routes.

Uses

- Uncomplicated/Severe and complicated chloroquine resistant malaria/ falciparum malaria.

  It is not used for prophylaxis due to its shorter duration of action.

G. Sulphonamides

Sulphonamides are active against the asexual blood forms of human malarial parasites. Sulfadoxine and sulfones have been used for suppression of infection caused by sensitive strains of P. falciparum.

H. Antibiotics

Antibiotics are weak erythrocytic scizontical also inhibits pre-erythrocytic stage of P. falciparum. They are not used alone but used with quinine or S/P combination.

I. Halofantrine

Halofantrine is schizontocidal but not used in India.

Lumefantrine is orally active, highly effective, long acting erythrocytic schizontocide, related with mefloquine. It is used only in combination with artemether and is available as fixed dose ACT combination.

J. Atovaquone

It is a naphthaquinone, effective against the erythrocytic forms of plasmodia. When combined with proguanil, the activity is synergistic and development of resistance is less common. Atovaquone inhibits the mitochondrial electron transport and collapses the mitochondrial membrane in the malaria parasite. It is not used in India.

Treatment regimen including ACT is shown in Table 6.2.

Table 6.2: Treatment regimen for malaria (as per NVBDCP)

A. Treatment of uncomplicated malaria

Chloroquine sensitive

- Chloroquine
  + Primaquine single dose in case of P. falciparum

Chloroquine resistant

- Artesunate (4 mg/kg/day orally for three days) + Sulfadoxine (1500 mg) - Pyrimethamine (75 mg) combination (single dose)
  Or Artesunate (as above) + Mefloquine (750 mg on 2nd day and 500 mg on 3rd day)
  Or Artesunate (as above) + Lumefantrine (480 mg twice daily for three days)
  Or Quinine (600 mg TDS for 7 days) + Doxycycline (100 mg/day for 7 days)

B. Treatment of severe and complicated falciparum malaria

- Artesunate (IV/IM) 2.4 mg/kg at 0,12, 24 hours, followed by 2.4 mg/kg/day for 7 days + Switch over to ACT orally for 3 days as mentioned above whenever patient is able to take oral therapy.

Or Artemether (IM) 3.2 mg/kg first day followed by 1.6 mg/kg/day for seven days. Switch over to ACT orally for 3 days as mentioned above whenever patient is able to take oral therapy.

Or Quinine 20 mg/kg diluted with 5% dextrose (10 ml/kg) infusion over 4 hours followed by 10 mg/kg over 4 hours 8 hourly.
Switch over to oral quinine 10 mg/kg TDS for 7 days.

CHEMOTHERAPY OF AMOEBIASIS (ANTI-AMOEBIC DRUGS)

Amoebiasis is an infection caused by entamoeba histolytica. It is an invasion of the gastrointestinal mucosa, liver and other tissues by the vegetative trophozoite forms of the protozoan.

Amoebiasis in man may presents as (i) asymptomatic intestinal infection, (ii) mild to moderate intestinal infection; (iii) severe intestinal infection (dysentery); (iv) amoebic liver abscess; and (v) amoeboma or extraintestinal infection.

Classification

The ameobicidal drugs may be classified according to their site of action:

1. **Tissue amoebicides:**
   a. For both intestinal and extraintestinal amoebiasis. Nitroimidazoles (Metronidazole, Tinidazole), Emetine Hydrochloride.
   b. For extra intestinal amoebiasis Chloroquine (mainly active in the liver).
2. **Luminal amoebicides:**
   a. *Halogenated hydroxyquinolines:* Iodoquinol, Clioquinol, Quindochlor.
   b. *Amides:* Diloxanide furoate, Teclozan, Etofamide, Nitazoxanide.
   c. *Antibiotics:* Tetracyclines, Paromomycin.

Ipecacuanha is obtained from the dried rhizomes or roots of cephaelis ipecacuanha. Its amoebicidal activity is due to its alkaloid content, mainly emetine. Emetine is seldom used today.

Metronidazole

Metronidazole is powerful amoebicidal at both intestinal and extra intestinal sites, and is currently the preferred drug for all amoebic infection. It is a nitroimidazole derivative.

Mechanism of Action

Metronidazole is a prodrug. Susceptible microorganisms reduce the nitro group of metronidazole by a nitro reductase and convert it to a cytotoxic derivative which binds to DNA and inhibits protein synthesis. It acts through ferredoxin-oxireductase (pyruvate FOR) enzyme. Aerobic bacteria lack this nitroreductase and are therefore not susceptible to metronidazole as they attenuate cytotoxicity of metronidazole by inhibiting its reductive activation. It also inhibits cell mediated immunity.

Metronidazole is well-absorbed and reaches adequate concentrations in the CSF, and its plasma $t_{½}$ is 8 hours. It is metabolized in the liver by oxidation and glucuronide conjugation and excreted in urine.

Toxicity: Frequent adverse effects are nausea and diarrhea. Other side effects include unpleasant taste, furry tongue, glossitis, stomatitis, anorexia, abdominal cramps and dark colour urine. It may cause peripheral neuropathy and CNS effects. Seizures may occur with large doses.

When taken with alcoholic beverages, metronidazole may produce a disulfiram type reaction caused by accumulation of acetaldehyde in the body.

Uses

1. Anaerobic bacterial infections.
2. Amoebiasis.
3. Trichomonas vaginitis.
4. Giardiasis.
5. H. pylori infection.
6. Pseudomembranous colitis.
7. Dracunculosis.
8. Topical preparations: like gel and ointment are used in skin infections and acne.

Tinidazole is longer acting and is better tolerated than metronidazole.

Secnidazole is long acting and can be given as a single 2 g dose.

Satranidazole: More potent and long acting than metronidazole. It is claimed to be better tolerated particularly because it does not cause nausea or metallic taste and disulfiram like reaction with alcohol.

Diloxanide Furoate

Diloxanide furoate is a highly effective luminal amoebicidal. Flatulence, nausea and occasionally abdominal cramps and rashes can occur. It is used alone in asymptomatic cyst passers, mild intestinal amoebiasis and along with metronidazole or tinidazole in amoebiasis.

Nitazoxanide is congener of niclosamide. It is prodrug and inhibitor of PFOR. It is used in giardiasis etc.

Guidelines for Amoebicidal Therapy

1. **Acute amoebic dysentery:** The drug of choice is metronidazole with or without an antibiotic.
2. **Chronic amoebic colitis:** It is best treated with a 3-week course of diloxanide plus chloroquine.
3. **Asymptomatic carrier state:** The asymptomatic carrier (cyst passer) is best treated with diloxanide furoate.

4. **Extraintestinal amoebiasis:** Chloroquine and emetine are the drugs of choice for either acute or chronic extra intestinal infection. Metronidazole is also recommended.

CHEMOTHERAPY OF HELMINTHIASIS (ANTHELMINTIC DRUGS)

Anthelmintics are drugs used to eradicate parasitic worms (known as helminths) from the human body.

Choice of Drugs for Helminthiasis

Sl	Worm	First choice drug	Second choice drug
1	Round worm (Ascariasis)	Mebendazole (M) Albendazole (A)	Piperazine, Levamisol
2	Hook worm A. duodenale N.americans	Pyrantel Pamoate (P), Mebendazole Albendazole (A)	Levamisol Pyrantel Pamoate
3	Thread worm E. (oxyuris) vermicularis	P, M & A	Piperazine
4	Strongyloides Stercoralis	Ivermectin (I)	A
5	Whip Worm (T.trichiura)	M	A
6	T. spiralis	A	M
7	Filaria W. brancrofti	I Diethyl Carbamazine (DEC)	A
8	Guinea worm Dracunculus medinensis	M	
9	Tapeworms		A
	T. saginata, Solium	Praziquantel, Niclosomid (N)	A
	H. Nana		N
	Neurocysticercosis	A	N
10	Hydatid disease	A	M

Albendazole

Albendazole is a broad spectrum oral anthelmintic. Albendazole blocks glucose uptake by larval and adult stages of susceptible parasites, depleting their glycogen stores. This results in immobilization of the parasite and its death. It inhibits microtubule polymerization by binding to beta-tubulin.

Therapeutic Uses

1. **Ascariasis, trichuriasis, hookworm and pin-worm infections:** A single dose of 400 mg orally is administered with a meal.
2. **Strongyloidosis:** A dose of 400 mg twice daily for 3–7 days.
3. **Hydatid disease:** A dose of 800 mg /day for 30 days is given.
4. **Neurocysticercosis:** The treatment schedule is 15 mg/kg/day for 30 days.

Adverse Reactions: Headache, diarrhea, epigastric distress, dizziness and insomnia have been reported. It may cause alopecia, liver damage and bone marrow depression.

Mebendazole

It is the primary drug of choice for enterobiasis and trichuriasis. It is particularly useful in the treatment of mixed infections with whipworms, roundworms, hookworms, and pinworms. No pretreatment or post treatment purging is required.

Diethylcarbamazine Citrate

Diethylcarbamazine is the drug of choice for the treatment of filariasis. It causes rapid disappearance of microfilariae of Wuchereria bancrofti, W. malayi and Loa loa from the blood of man. For filariasis combination of a single dose of DEC with albendazole or ivermectin is synergistic.

In the treatment of tropical eosinophilia, it causes a rapid disappearance of symptoms in a dose of 2 mg/kg tid for 7 days. For treatment of W bancrofti and W. malayi infections the usual dose is 2 mg/kg three times daily after meals for 7 days.

Ivermectin

It is the drug of choice for onchocerciasis. It acts by increasing the release and binding of gamma amino butyric acid (GABA), thereby producing paralysis. It is used in onchocerciasis, lymphatic filariasis, intestinal nematode infection scabies and head lice infestation.

Niclosamide

Niclosamide is the drug of choice for treating tapeworm infestations. It acts by inhibiting anaerobic phosphorylation of ADP by the mitochondria. This agent is administered orally and the concomitant use of a laxative is required, except for T. solium. Niclosamide may destroy T. solium segments (vermicidal), thereby releasing viable eggs. The laxative administered 1 to 2 hours after the anthelmintic avoids the possibility of cysticercosis. No serious side effects have been reported.

Piperazine

Currently piperazine is an alternative drug for the treatment of ascariasis. The main effect of piperazine on ascaris is to cause flaccid paralysis of the worm, which is expelled by peristalsis. A laxative is needed to expel the worms from the intestine.

Adverse reactions include nausea, vomiting, diarrhea and allergic reactions. With larger doses muscular incoordination, vertigo, speech difficulty confusion and myoclonic contractions have been reported. It can be given during pregnancy.

Pyrantel Pamoate

It is highly effective for the treatment of enterobius, ascariasis and strongyloides orientalis infestations. It has a depolarizing neuromuscular blocking action and causes spastic paralysis.

For round worms and pin worms, pyrantel is administered orally as a single dose. For hookworms this dose is given for 3 consecutive days. Fasting before treatment is not necessary.

Adverse reactions include anorexia, nausea, headache, drowsiness, rashes and elevated SGOT levels. It can be given during pregnancy.

Praziquantel

Praziquantel is effective against schistosome infestations of all species, and most other trematode and cestode infestations.

It is the drug of choice for treating schistosomiasis. Both S. mansoni and S. haematobiurm respond well to a single oral dose of 40 mg/kg.

OTHER PROTOZOAL INFECTIONS

Drugs Used in the Treatment of Pneumocystosis

Pneumocystis carinii is a microorganism having features of both protozoa and fungi though now considered to be a fungal infection caused by Pneumocystis firoveci while P. carinii causes pneumocystosis in animals.

It is treated by cotrimoxazole with high oral dose of trimethoprim (20 mg/kg) + sulfamethoxazole (100 mg/kg) daily.

Pentamidine 4 mg/kg daily for 14 days parenterally.

Atovaquone as an alternative to cotrimoxazole.

Leishmaniasis is caused by protozoa of the genus leishmania. Kala azar or visceral leishmaniasis is caused by Leishmania donovani; oriental sore by L. tropica and mucocutaneous leishmaniasis by L. braziliensis.

Drugs used in leishmaniasis include:

A. *Antimony compounds:* Sodium stibogluconate, Meglumine antimonite.
B. *Diamidines:* Pentamidine.
C. *Other drugs:* Amphotericin B, Ketoconazole, Allopurinol, Paramomycin, Miltefosin.

Sodium stibogluconate: It is also effective in mucocutaneous and cutaneous leishmaniasis. It is given as a 4% solution in the dose of 10–20 mg/kg IM (gluteal region) or IV for 20 days. Mechanism of action is unknown.

Adverse effects include a metallic taste in the mouth, nausea, vomiting, diarrhea, headache, myalgia, arthralgia, pain at the injection site, bradycardia, skin rashes, haematuria, pancreatitis, liver and kidney damage and jaundice. Some cases of sudden death due to shock have occurred. ECG should be done regularly as arrhythmias can occur during the later days of therapy.

Meglumine antimonate and **ethyl stibamine** can also be used in all forms of leishmaniasis.

Pentamidine is an aromatic diamidine effective against Leishmania donovani, Trypanosomes, Pneumocystis jiroveci and some fungi. It inhibits topoisomerase II.

Pentamidine liberates histamine which is responsible for vomiting, diarrhea, flushing, pruritis, rashes, tachycardia and hypotension apart from pain at the injection site. Other adverse effects include hepatotoxicity, renal impairment, ECG changes and in some patients diabetes mellitus may be precipitated.

Uses

1. Leishmaniasis.
2. Trypanosomiasis.
3. Pneumocystosis.

Trypanosomiasis is caused by protozoa of the genus Trypanosoma. African trypanosondasis or sleeping sickness is caused by T. gambiense and T. rhodesiense while South American trypanosomiasis is caused by

T. Cruzi. Drugs used in trypanosomiasis are suramin, pentamidine, melarsoprol, eflornithine, nifurtimox and benznidazole. **Suramin sodium** is the drug of choice for early stage of trypanosomiasis but it does not cross the BBB and therefore cannot be used in later stages of the disease. Suramin is also effective in eradicating adult forms of Onchocerca volvulus.

Toxicity of suramin is high; vomiting, shock and loss of consciousness may occur following IV injections. Rash, neuropathies, haemolytic anaemia and agranulocytosis may also occur.

Melarsoprol is the preferred drug in later stages of trypanosomiasis which is associated with encephalitis and meningitis.

Eflornithine is used as an alternative in CNS trypanosomiasis. Nifurtimox and benznidazole are useful in Chaga's disease (American trypanosomiasis).

CANCER CHEMOTHERAPY (ANTI-CANCER DRUGS)

The treatment of cancers is still unsatisfactory due to certain characteristics of the cancer cells like capacity for uncontrolled proliferation, invasiveness and metastasis. Moreover the cancer cells are our own cells unlike microbes, which means that drugs which destroy these cells also can affect normal cells. The host defense mechanisms which help us in infections is not doing so in cancers as these cancer cells are also host cells. Moreover, the cancer cells can be in a resting phase during which they are not sensitive to anti-cancer drugs but can start multiplying later resulting in recurrence. These features have made cancer chemotherapy more difficult.

Common Adverse Effects to Anti-Cancer Drugs

1. Bone marrow depression resulting in leucopenia, anaemia, thrombocytopenia and in higher doses aplastic anaemia. In such patients, infections and bleeding are common.
2. **Other proliferating cells:**
   a. Stomatitis and glossitis can occur. Good oral hygiene should be maintained. Antiseptic mouth washes may be given till the bone marrow recovers.
   b. GIT: Esophagitis and proctitis.
   c. Reduced spermetogenesis in men and amenorrhea in women (infertility).
   d. Alopecia.

3. **Immediate adverse effects:** Nausea and vomiting are very common with most cytotoxic drugs. They result from the stimulation of the vomiting centre situated in CTZ.
4. **Teratogenicity:** All cytotoxic drugs are teratogenic and are therefore contraindicated in pregnancy.
5. **Carcinogenicity:** Cytotoxic drugs themselves may cause secondary cancers.
6. Renal toxicity, hepatic and cardiac toxicity (precipitation of CCF), Pulmonary toxicity (Pulmonary fibrosis).

Classification of Anti-Cancer Drugs

1. **Alkylating agents:**
   a. *Nitrogen mustards:* Mechlorethamine, Cyclophosphamide, Ifosfamide, Chlorambucil, Melphalan.
   b. *Ethylenimines:* ThioTEPA.
   c. *Alkyl sulfonate:* Busulfan.
   d. *Nitrosoureas:* Carmustine, Streptazocin, Lomustine.
   e. *Triazine:* Dacarbazine.
2. **Antimetabolites:**
   a. *Folate antagonist:* Methotrexate.
   b. *Purine antagonist:* 6 Mercaptopurine Thioguanine, Azathioprine Pentostatin Fludarabin, Cladribin.
   c. *Pyrimidine antagonist:* 5 Fluorouracil, Floxuridine, Cytarabine (cytosine arabinoside), Gemcitabine.
3. **Antibiotics:** Actinomycin D (Dactinomycin), Daunorubicin, Doxorubicin Bleomycin, Mitomycin C, Mithramycin.
4. **Epipodophyllotoxins:** Etoposide, Teniposide.
5. **Camptothecins:** Topotecan, Irinotecan.
6. **Taxanes:** Paclitaxel, Docetaxel.
7. **Vinca alkaloids:** Vincristine, Vinblastine, Vinorelbine
8. **Miscellaneous:** Procarbazine, Mitotane, L-Asparaginase, Cisplatin, Interferon alpha, Imatinib.
9. **Hormones and their antagonists:** Glucocorticoids, Androgens, (anti-androgens), Estrogens (anti-estrogens), Progestins, Aromatase inhibitors.

Alkylating Agents

Alkylating agents exert cytotoxic, immunosuppressant and radiomimetic effects. These drugs form highly reactive derivatives which transfer alkyl groups to various cellular constituents which form highly reactive carbonium ion and bind them with covalent bonds. Thus such constituents are not available for normal metabolic reactions. Moreover, alkylation of DNA results in damage of the DNA strand which leads to cytotoxicity. They are cell cycle specific but not phase specific.

Mechlorethamine used in **Hodgkin's** (MOPP regime) and other lymphomas.

Cyclophosphamide causes haemorrhagic cystitis due to its metabolites. This can be prevented by giving IV Mesna, irrigating the bladder with acetylcysteine, and by taking in large amounts of fluids and increase urinary output.

Cyclophosphamide is used in **Hodgkin's lymphoma**, leukemia in children and as an immunosuppressive agent, neuroblastomia, Wilm's tumor multiple myeloma, ovarian, cervical and testicular carcinomas.

Chlorambucil is very effective against lymphoid series. It is the drug of choice in **chronic lymphocytic leukemia**. It is slow acting, less toxic.

Melphalan is given in **multiple myeloma**.

Busulfan is drug of choice in **chronic myeloid leukemia**.

Nitrosoureas Carmustine is effective in **meningeal leukemia and brain tumors** because it crosses the blood brain barrier.

Streptozocin is an antibiotic. It is used in **pancreatic islet cell tumors**.

Dacarbazine is useful in **malignant melanoma**.

Alkylating agents kill a fixed percentage of cells at a given dose. Tumor resistance develops due to capacity to repair damaged nucleic acid of the cells and to inactivate the drugs by conjugation with GSH.

Antimetabolites

Folate Antagonist

Methotrexate is a folic acid antagonist. It binds to dihydrofolate reductase (DHFR) and prevents the formation of tetrahydrofolate. THF is a coenzyme essential in several reactions in protein synthesis. The deficiency results in inhibition of protein synthesis. Thus rapidly multiplying cells are the most affected. It also has immunosuppressant and some anti-inflammatory properties. It causes neurotoxicity.

Methotrexate is curative in **choriocarcinoma** and is useful in **acute leukemias, breast cancer and soft tissue sarcomas**. It is also used in

rheumatoid arthritis and psoriasis. Toxicity of methotrexate can be minimized by giving folinic acid.

Purine Antagonists

6-Mercaptopurine, Thioguanine, Azathioprine, Fludarabine, Pentostatin and Cladribine are purine antagonists.

Purine antagonists enter the cells and get converted to active metabolites which are incorporated into DNA. They cause breakages in DNA strands and inhibit protein synthesis; purine ring biosynthesis and nucleotide inter conversion.

6 Mercaptopurine (6-MP) and Azothioprine are metabolized by xanthine oxidase. Allopurinol inhibits xanthine oxidase and thus prolongs the action of 6 MP.

6 MP is used in **acute leukemia in children**, choriocarcinoma and some solid tumors. Azothioprine is used in organ transplantation and in rheumatoid arthritis (RA).

Thioguanine is effective orally and is used in acute leukemias particularly **acute granulocytic leukemia.**

Fludarabine is used in the treatment of **chronic lymphocytic leukemia** (CLL) and **Hodgkin's lymphomas.**

Pentostatin can cause nausea, vomiting, diarrhea, skin rashes and bone marrow suppression.

Pentostatin is used intravenously in the treatment of **hairy cell leukemia** and other **chronic leukemia** and **non-Hodgkin's lymphomas**.

Cladribine is the drug of choice in **hairy cell leukemia**. It is also useful in CLL, AML and some lymphomas. Cladribine causes mild bone marrow suppression, nausea, vomiting, weakness and skin rashes.

Pyrimidine Antagonists

Pyrimidine antagonists are converted to active metabolites which resemble natural nucleotides. They compete with natural nucleotides, and incorporated into DNA in place of natural nucleotides and inhibit DNA synthesis.

5 Fluorouracil is inhibits the enzyme thymidylate synthetase due to which it inhibits the synthesis of thymine and thereby inhibits DNA synthesis. It is used in **carcinoma of the stomach, colon, rectum, breast and ovaries.**

Cytosine Arabinoside

In patients with renal dysfunction, it develops CNS toxicity. It is useful in **acute leukemia** particularly **myeloid leukemia** and in relapsed cases of acute lymphocytic leukemia, meningeal involvement with tumor.

Genicitabine, analog of cytarabine used in pancreatic, lung, cervical, ovarian and breast cancers.

Anti-Cancer Antibiotics

They are cell cycle non specific (CCNS), have direct action on DNA and interfere cell division. **Actinomycin D** acts by inhibiting DNA dependent RNA synthesis. It is used in Wilms' tumor, rhabdo myosarcoma, choriocarcinoma and some soft tissue sarcomas.

Daunorubicin and Doxorubicin causes cardio toxicity with hypotension, arrhythmias and CCF, is unique to both these drugs. They are used in **acute leukemia** while doxorubicin is useful in solid tumors and in acute leukemia.

Epirubicin and mitoxantrone are analogs of doxorubicin which are less cardio toxic.

Mitomycin C: It is used in cancers of the **stomach, lungs and cervix**.

Bleomycin: It binds with iron and forms free radicals and causes breakage in DNA strand. It has the advantage of the unique mechanism of action and is less toxic to the bone marrow this is advantageous in combination regimens.

Bleomycin is used in solid tumors **testicular tumors, squamous cell carcinoma of the head, neck and esophagus**.

Its most serious toxicity includes pulmonary fibrosis and cutaneous toxicity but does not cause significant bone marrow depression.

Mithramycin (Plicamycin) is highly toxic, used in disseminated testicular tumours and in severe hypercalcaemia due to bone metastasis cancers. It reduces plasma calcium levels by its action on the osteoclasts.

Epipodophyllotoxins

Etoposide and teniposide are plant extracts obtained from the mandrake plant. They bind to topoisomerase II as well as DNA resulting in DNA strand breakages. They are used in testicular and lung cancers (in combination with other drugs). They act on SG_2 phase of cell cycle.

Taxanes

Paclitaxel: It binds to beta tubulin of microtubules and arrests mitosis. It is metabolised by the liver microsomal enzymes.

Adverse effects include myelosuppression, myalgia and peripheral neuropathy.

Docetaxel is more potent and orally effective. It should be given before cisplatin in combination regimen.

Taxanes are useful in **breast cancers and ovarian cancers**. They are also found to be effective in the cancers of the head and neck, oesophagus and lungs.

Camptothecins

Topotecan and irinotecan are less toxic and useful. They inhibit topoisomerase I resulting in DNA strand breakages leading to cell death. They act on the S phase of the cell cycle. Topotecan is used in metastatic carcinoma of ovary and small cell lung cancer, after primary chemotherapy has failed.

Irinotecan inhibits the enzyme acetylcholinesterase resulting in accumulation of acetylcholine causing excessive salivation, abdominal cramps, miosis, bradycardia and sweating which respond to treatment with atropine. It is used in metastatic/advanced colorectal carcinoma, cancer lung/cervix/ovary etc.

Vinca Alkaloids

Vincristine and vinblastine: They bind to beta microtubules in the mitotic apparatus and arrest cell division in metaphase.

Vincristine is neurotoxic while bone marrow depression is less. It is used in leukemia, Hodgkin's lymphoma, Wilms' tumor and brain tumor.

Vinblastine causes bone marrow depression, alopecia and vomiting. It is used with bleomycin and cisplatin in testicular tumours, Hodgkin's lymphoma.

Vinorelbine is used intravenously in lung cancers.

Miscellaneous

Procarbazine is effective orally in Hodgkin's lymphoma (MOPP regime component).

Cisplatin gets converted to its active form and forms highly reactive platinum complexes in the cell, inhibits DNA synthesis and cell proliferation. It causes cytotoxicity, ototoxicity, nephrotoxicity, peripheral neuropathy, nausea and vomiting, anaemia and electrolyte imbalance. Anaphylactoid reactions also occur. It is relatively less toxic to bone marrow. Cisplatin is used in ovarian and testicular tumors and cancers of the head and neck. It is mutagenic, teratogenic and carcinogenic.

Carboplatin is a less toxic derivative of cisplatin but it causes myelosuppression.

Oxaliplatin is effective in **advanced colorectal cancer** and in other cancers like ovarian and cervical cancers.

L-Asparaginase: The amino acid asparagine is synthesized by normal cells but malignant cells are unable to synthesize asparagine and depend on the host for the supply. Asparaginase is an enzyme that converts asparagine to aspartic acid and deprives the malignant cells of asparagine supplies resulting in inhibition of protein synthesis. It is used in acute leukemia. It causes hypersensitivity, reaction, hemorrhage, hyperglycemia, headache and hallucination.

Imatinib is a recent introduction in cancer chemotherapy. It acts by inhibiting some selective tyrosine kinase which are considered to be involved in the pathogenesis of chronic myeloid leukemia. It also inhibits receptor tyrosine kinase for platelet derived growth factor receptor.

Hormones in Cancer Chemotherapy

Hormonal Agonist

Glucocorticoids: Due to their lympholytic action, glucocorticoids are used in acute leukemias and lymphomas.

Glucocorticoids are also of value in the following:

1. With radiation therapy to reduce radiation edema.
2. In intracranial tumors to reduce cerebral edema.
3. For symptomatic relief in critically ill patients.

Estrogens are useful in (i) prostatic carcinoma as it is an androgen dependent tumor, (ii) breast cancer in males and in postmenopausal women. They are used in advanced cases where surgery or radiotherapy cannot be employed.

Progestins are useful in the palliative management of **endometrial carcinoma.**

Androgens (methyl testosterone, fluoxymesterone) are used in the palliative treatment of breast cancer in postmenopausal women along with oophorectomy and stimulation of erythropoiesis.

Hormone Antagonists

Aromatase inhibitors: The enzyme aromatase catalyzes the conversion of androgens to estrogens. Inhibitors of aromatase have been found to be effective in breast cancers. Formestane, exemestane, anastrozole, vorozole and letrozole are the aromatase inhibitors used.

Aminoglutethemide and trilastane inhibit the conversion of cholesterol to pregnenolone and thereby inhibit the synthesis of adrenocorticoids. Aminoglutethemide is useful in advanced breast cancers when cancer cells contain oestrogen receptors.

Antiestrogen (Tamoxifen, Toremifen, Fulvestrant).

Antiestrogens tamoxifen is an estrogen receptor antagonist used in estrogen receptor containing breast cancer.

Anti-androgen (Bicalutamide, Flutamide, Nilutamide, Finasteride) used in prostatic carcinoma, reduces testicular androgen. They block the conversion of testosterone to dihydrotestosterone by inhibiting 5-alpha reductase.

GnRH analogs: Long term administration of leuprolide, goserelin and buserelin causes rise in FSH and LH and useful in **prostatic and breast cancers.** They may be combined with tamoxifen in breast cancers.

Radioactive Isotopes

Radio phosphorus ^{32}P is used in polycythemia vera.

Strontium chloride emits beta rays and has a longer $t_{½}$ in the bony metastases. It is used to alleviate pain in painful bony metastases. Radioactive iodine ^{131}I is used in the treatment of thyroid cancers.

Other Agents

Several agents are used to beneficially influence the patients' response to treatment and to overcome some adverse effects. These have also been termed **biological response modifiers**. They are as follows:

1. Haematopoietic growth factors like erythropoietin and myeloid growth factors like GMCSF, GCSF, MCSF and thrombopoietin are used to treat bone marrow suppression.

2. Interferons like interferon alpha are used in hairy cell leukemia, Kaposi's sarcoma and condylomata acuminata.
3. Monoclonal antibodies are immunoglobulins that react specifically with antigens present on the cancer cells. Trastuzumab also enhances host immune responses and is useful in breast cancers. Rituximab attaches to antigens on the B cells causing lysis of these cells. It is used in B cell lymphomas. Bevacizumab used in colorectal carcinoma.

General Principles in the Treatment of Cancers

1. Chemotherapy in cancers is generally palliative and suppressive. Chemotherapy is just one of the modes in the treatment of cancer. Other modes like radiotherapy and surgery are also employed.
2. Combination of drugs is preferred for synergistic effect to reduce adverse effects and to prevent rapid development of resistance.
3. Drugs which do not depress bone marrow are useful in combination regimens to avoid overlapping of adverse effects. With appropriate treatment, cure can now be achieved in a few, cancers. Maintenance of good nutrition, treatment of anaemia, protection against infections, adequate relief of pain and anxiety and good emotional support all go a long way in the appropriate management of this dreaded disease.

MULTIPLE CHOICE QUESTIONS

Q. 1 Bone marrow aplasia is seen with all *except:*

(A) Methicillin
(B) Chloramphenicol
(C) Flucytosine
(D) Zidovudin

Q. 2 All of the following anti-bacterial agents act by inhibiting cell well synthesis *except:*

(A) Carbapenems
(B) Monobactams
(C) Vancomycin
(D) Nitrofurantoin

Q. 3 All of the following are therapeutic uses of penicillin G *except:*

(A) Bacterial meningitis
(B) Syphilis
(C) Anthrax
(D) Rickettsial infection

Q. 4 Which of the following drugs is an anti-pseudomonal beta-lactam?

(A) Cephalaxin (B) Cloxacillin
(C) Piperacillin (D) Dicloxacillin

Q. 5 All of the following drugs are used in an epileptic patient developing cellulitis due to MRSA *except:*

(A) Vanomycin (B) Imipenem
(C) Teicoplanin (D) Linezolid

Q. 6 Which antibiotic acts by inhibiting cell wall synthesis?

(A) Cefepime (B) Lomefloxacin
(C) Erythromycin (D) Tetracyclines

Q. 7 Which one is penicillinase resistant antibiotic?

(A) Amoxicillin (B) Cloxacillin
(C) Penicillin G (D) Piperacillin

---

1 (A) 2 (D) 3 (D) 4 (C) 5 (B) 6 (A) 7 (B)

Q. 8 Which group of antibiotic possess additional anti-inflammatory and immune-modulatory action?

(A) Tetracyclines
(B) Polypeptide antibiotic
(C) Fluroquinolones
(D) Macrolide

Q. 9 All of the following are topically used sulfonamides *except:*

(A) Sulfacetamide
(B) Sulfadoxine
(C) Silver sulfadiazine
(D) Mafenide

Q. 10 Tetracycline inhibits protein synthesis by:

(A) Inhibiting initiation and causing misreading of mRNA
(B) Binding to 30S subunit and inhibits binding of aminoacyl tRNA
(C) Inhibiting peptidyl transferase activity
(D) Inhibiting translocation

Q. 11 Which of the following fluoroquinolone does not require dose adjustment in patient with renal dysfunction?

(A) Ciprofloxacin (B) Trovafloxacin
(C) Lomefloxacin (D) Sparfloxacin

Q. 12 Which of the following is a fourth generation cephalosporin?

(A) Cefrixone (B) Cefaclor
(C) Cefepime (D) Cefuroxime

Q. 13 Which of the following statement is not true regarding sulfonamides?

(A) Sulfasalazine is absorbed well from GIT
(B) Crystalluria can occur with sulfonamide administration
(C) Sulfonamides may cause kernicterus in newborn
(D) Sulfonamides are effective in Nocardia infection

Q. 14 Which of the following drug cause pseudotumor cerebri?

(A) Sparfloxacin (B) Tetracycline
(C) Gentamicin (D) Clofazimine

---

8 (D) 9 (B) 10 (B) 11 (B) 12 (C) 13 (A) 14 (B)

Q. 15 Thalidomide can be used in all *except:*

(A) Multiple myeloma
(B) Erythema nodosum leprosum
(C) Melanoma
(D) Chronic myeloid leukemia

Q. 16 Antimicrobial agent preferred in a patient with Pneumocystis carinii infection:

(A) Vancomycin (B) Gentamicin
(C) Co-trimoxazole (D) Ceftriaxone

Q. 17 All of the following cephalosporins have good activity against P. aeruginosa *except:*

(A) Cephadroxil (B) Cefpime
(C) Cefoperazone (D) Ceftazidime

Q. 18 Risk of renal toxicity with aminoglycosides increases in all *except:*

(A) Elderly persons
(B) Patients on loop diuretics
(C) Simultaneous use of penicillin
(D) Aminoglycoside given in recent past

Q. 19 All of the following statements are true about fluoroquinolone *except:*

(A) Suspected of having teratogenic potential
(B) Arthropathy of limb in children may occur
(C) Increases theophylline toxicity
(D) Increases neuromuscular blocking action

Q. 20 Clindamycin acts by inhibiting:

(A) Protein synthesis (B) DNA gyrase
(C) Cell wall synthesis (D) Lysosomal enzyme

Q. 21 Drug induced interstitial nephritis is caused by:

(A) Methicillin (B) Cloxacillin
(C) Azlocillin (D) Piperacillin

---

15 (D) 16 (C) 17 (A) 18 (C) 19 (D) 20 (A) 21 (A)

Q. 22 Photosensitivity is seen maximum with which fluoroquinolone?

(A) Ciprofloxacin
(B) Sparfloxacin
(C) Ofloxacin
(D) Norfloxacin

Q. 23 All of the following is true about co-trimoxazole *except:*

(A) Resistance is delayed due to drug combination
(B) Ratio of trimethoprim and sulfamethoxazole is 1:5
(C) Similar pharmacokinetics for both components
(D) Trimethoprim increases absorption of sulfamethoxazole

Q. 24 Which of the following drug is not effective against anaerobes?

(A) Penicillin (B) Chloramphenicol
(C) Gentamicin (D) Clindamycin

Q. 25 Duration of action of penicillin is increased by combining with any of the following *except:*

(A) Probenecid (B) Procaine
(C) Benzathine (D) Clavulanic acid

Q. 26 Rational use of drug combination in microbial infection includes all of the following *except:*

(A) Mixed bacterial infections
(B) Life threatening infections (reports of sensitivity awaited)
(C) Supra-additive effects
(D) Reduction in individual doses and thus toxicity

Q. 27 Which of the following cephalosporin is not very useful in meningitis?

(A) Cefuroxime (B) Cefoxitin
(C) Ceftriaxone (D) Cefotaxime

Q. 28 Drug of choice for acute gonorrhea in a patient allergic to penicillin is:

(A) Cephalosporin (B) Amoxicillin
(C) Ampicillin (D) Spectinomycin

---

22 (B) 23 (D) 24 (C) 25 (D) 26 (D) 27 (B) 28 (D)

Q. 29 Bacterial resistance to penicillin is due to all of the following effects *except:*

(A) Failure to activate autolysins
(B) Beta-lactamase inactivation
(C) Inability to reach inside cell wall
(D) Failure to bind to penicillin binding proteins

Q. 30 All are true about methenamine *except:*

(A) It act by releasing formaldehyde
(B) Resistance is not a problem clinically
(C) It antagonizes sulfonamide action
(D) It is very useful for acute urinary tract infection

Q. 31 Rifampicin chemoprophylaxis is indicated in all infections *except:*

(A) H. influenzae (B) Staph. aureus
(C) N. meningitides (D) Tuberculosis

Q. 32 A bactericidal antibiotic has the following features:

(A) It has pronounced post antibiotic effect
(B) It has efficacy in the absence of host defense
(C) Useful when carrier state is possible
(D) All of the above

Q. 33 Which of the following condition is mostly treated with combination of anti-microbial agents?

(A) Lobar pneumonia (B) Syphilis
(C) Peritonitis (D) Typhoid

Q. 34 In which condition trimethoprim alone is as effective as of co-trimoxazole?

(A) Respiratory tract infection (B) Prostatitis
(C) Typhoid fever (D) Bacillary dysentery

Q. 35 All of the following are the advantages of fluoroquinolone over quinolones *except:*

(A) They have extended anti-microbial spectrum
(B) They have longer plasma half life
(C) Development of resistance is slow and infrequent
(D) They have higher antimicrobial potency

---

29 (A) 30 (D) 31 (D) 32 (D) 33 (C) 34 (B) 35 (B)

Q. 36 Which fluoroquinolone is most effective against gram positive bacteria and anaerobes?

(A) Pefloxacin (B) Ciprofloxacin
(C) Norfloxacin (D) Sparfloxacin

Q. 37 Combination of clavulanic acid with amoxicillin have following advantage:

(A) It kills bacteria that are not killed by amoxicillin
(B) It inhibits beta lactamase enzyme that destroy amoxicillin
(C) It reduces renal clearance of amoxicillin
(D) It minimize the adverse effects of amoxicillin

Q. 38 Tetracyclines are still the first choice drug in following:

(A) Granuloma inguinale
(B) Chancroid
(C) Syphilis
(D) Gonorrhea in patients allergic to penicillin

Q. 39 Most important reason which restrict the use of chloramphenicol clinically is:

(A) Its narrow spectrum of activity
(B) Its potential to cause super infection
(C) Its potential to cause bone marrow depression
(D) Emergence to develop resistance

Q. 40 Which anti-tubercular drug impart orange color to urine?

(A) Rifampicin (B) Isoniazid
(C) Ethambutol (D) Pyrazinamide

Q. 41 Transient memory loss is caused by which anti-tubercular drug?

(A) Isoniazid (B) Rifampicin
(C) Pyrazinamide (D) Ethambutol

Q. 42 Patient showing resistant tuberculosis (MDR) can be treated with all of the following *except:*

(A) Ciprofloxacin (B) Amikacin
(C) Tobramycin (D) Clarithromycin

---

36 (D) 37 (B) 38 (A) 39 (C) 40 (A) 41 (A) 42 (C)

Q. 43 Which anti-tubercular drug should not be used during pregnancy?

(A) Streptomycin
(B) Isoniazid
(C) Rifampicin
(D) Ethambutol

Q. 44 Clinically significant interaction with pyridoxine occur with all of the following *except:*

(A) Cyclosporine
(B) Levodopa
(C) Hydralazine
(D) Isoniazid

Q. 45 All of the following are true about anti-tubercular drug therapy *except:*

(A) Flu like syndrome is seen with rifampicin
(B) Hyper uricemia is recognized effect of pyrazinamide
(C) Isonizid may cause seizures
(D) Ethambutol causes impairment/discrimination of yellow colour

Q. 46 Dose adjustment is not required in which of the anti-tubercular drug in a patient with renal failure?

(A) Rifampicin (B) Ethambutol
(C) Isoniazid (D) Pyrazinamide

Q. 47 Neuropsychiatric symptoms can occur with which of the following drug?

(A) Ethionamide (B) Cycloserine
(C) Rifampicin (D) Cephalosporin

Q. 48 All are the features of ethambutol toxicity *except:*

(A) Retrobulbar neuritis (B) Hyperuricemia
(C) Hypercalcemia (D) Colour vision defect

Q. 49 Effect of oral contraceptive is inhibited by:

(A) Rifampicin (B) Ethambutol
(C) Streptomycin (D) Pyrazinamide

---

43 (A) 44 (D) 45 (D) 46 (A) 47 (B) 48 (C) 49 (A)

Q. 50 The primary reason to use multi-drug combination in the treatment of tuberculosis is:

(A) Enhance activity against metabolically inactive mycobacteria
(B) Delay or prevent the emergence of resistance
(C) Reduce the incidence of adverse effects
(D) Ensure patients compliance with the drug regimen

Q. 51 Which of the following agent is not effective on intracellular tubercular bacilli?

(A) Streptomycin (B) Pyrazinamide
(C) Isoniazid (D) Ethinonamide

Q. 52 Corticosteroids are indicated in tuberculosis in all patients *except* with:

(A) Miliary dissemination (B) Meningitis
(C) Haemetemesis (D) Endobronchial lesion

Q. 53 Isoniazid is indicated in all *except:*

(A) Active apical lobe disease
(B) Recently positive Mantoux test
(C) Residual fibrotic lesion in untreated elderly
(D) Tuberculin anergy

Q. 54 The mechanism of high level INH resistance of M. tuberculosis is:

(A) Change in the pathway of mycolic acid synthesis
(B) Decreased intracellular accumulation of INH
(C) Reduced expression of the Kat G gene
(D) Mutation in the inh A gene

Q. 55 Dapsone is used in the treatment of all *except:*

(A) Rhinosporidiosis (B) Malaria
(C) Dermatitis herpetiformis (D) Leprosy

Q. 56 Ichthyosis and hyperpigmentation is common with which anti-leprotic drug?

(A) Clofazimine (B) Dapsone
(C) Ethambutol (D) Rifampicin

---

50 (B) 51 (A) 52 (C) 53 (D) 54 (D) 55 (A) 56 (A)

Q. 57 The most effective drug against M. leprae is:

(A) Clofazimine (B) Protionamide
(C) Dapsone (D) Rifampicin

Q. 58 The most common dose dependent toxicity of dapsone is:

(A) Methemoglobinemia (B) Haemolysis
(C) Hepatitis (D) Dermatitis

Q. 59 The tetracycline with highest anti-leprotic activity is:

(A) Minocycline (B) Doxycycline
(C) Methacycline (D) Oxytetracycline

Q. 60 The multi-drug therapy (MDT) of leprosy is superior to monotherapy because:

(A) It prevents development of dapsone resistance
(B) It shorten the total duration of the drug therapy
(C) It is also effective in case of primary dapsone resistance
(D) All of the above

Q. 61 Which of the following is common adverse effect with amphotericin B?

(A) Hypokalemia (B) Hyperkalemia
(C) Hyponatraemia (D) Hypermagnesaemia

Q. 62 All of the following anti-fungal drugs act on cell membrane *except:*

(A) Nystatin (B) Griseofulvin
(C) Amophotericin B (D) Polymyxin B

Q. 63 The drug of choice in the treatment of cryptococcal meningitis is:

(A) Fluconazole (B) Itraconazole
(C) Flucytosine (D) Amphotericin B

Q. 64 Which statement about fluconazole is accurate?

(A) It is a potent enzyme inducer
(B) It does not penetrate BBB
(C) It is highly effective in the treatment of aspergillosis
(D) It inhibits demethylation of lanosterol

---

57 (D) 58 (B) 59 (A) 60 (D) 61 (A) 62 (B) 63 (D) 64 (D)

Q. 65 Which drug is least likely to be effective in the treatment of esophageal candidiasis used by oral route?

(A) Amphotericin B (B) Griseofulvin
(C) Fluconazole (D) Ketoconazole

Q. 66 Ketoconazole is useful in:

(A) Blastomycosis (B) Aspergillosis
(C) Sporotrichosis (D) Cryptococcal meningitis

Q. 67 The drug of choice for monilial diarrhea is:

(A) Flucytosine (B) Nystatin
(C) Natamycin (D) Ketoconazole

Q. 68 The distinctive feature of terbenafine is:

(A) It is highly effective in histoplasmosis
(B) It can be used topically as well as orally for dermatophytosis
(C) It inhibits mucor and aspergillosis as well
(D) When applied intravaginally, it cures both candidal as well as trichomonas vaginitis

Q. 69 Which of the following is not the topical anti-fungal drug?

(A) Ciclopiroxolamine (B) Tolnaftate
(C) Crotamiton (D) Terbinafine

Q. 70 Which statement about the mechanism of action of anti-viral drugs is accurate?

(A) Activation by phosphorylation is not required for the action of cidofovir
(B) Ganciclovir inhibits viral DNA polymerase but does not cause chain termination
(C) Increased activity of host cell ribonucleases that degrade viral mRNA is one of the antiviral actions of interferon alpha
(D) The initial step in activation of foscarnet in HSV-infected cell is its phosphorylation by viral thymidine kinase

Q. 71 The drug most likely to suppress herpetic infection and provide prophylaxis against CMV retinitis in immunocompromised patient is:

(A) Ganciclovir (B) Indinavir
(C) Acyclovir (D) Rifabutin

---

65 (B) 66 (A) 67 (B) 68 (B) 69 (C) 70 (C) 71 (A)

Q. 72 Regarding interferon alpha which statement is false?

(A) At the start of treatment most patients experience flu like symptoms
(B) Indications includes treatment of genital warts, hepatic B&C
(C) Toxicity includes bone marrow suppression
(D) Lamivudin interfere with the activity against hepatitis B

Q. 73 Which statement is true about stavudine is accurate?

(A) Bone marrow depression is dose limiting
(B) It cause marked neurotoxicity
(C) It inhibits HIV protease
(D) Resistance occurs via mutations in the gene that code for thymidine kinase

Q. 74 Nevirapine belongs to the following group:

(A) Non-nucleoside reverse transcriptase inhibitor (NNRTI)
(B) Protease inhibitor
(C) Fusion inhibitor
(D) Nucleoside reverse transcriptase inhibitor (NRTI)

Q. 75 All of the following drugs are protease inhibitors *except:*

(A) Nelfinavir (B) Abacavir
(C) Saquinavir (D) Ritonavir

Q. 76 Resistance to zidovudine develops due to:

(A) Mutations at reverse transcriptase
(B) Increased efflux of the drug from inside the cell
(C) Increased metabolism of the drug
(D) Decrease zidovudine 5 triphosphate formations

Q. 77 Which anti-retroviral drug does not cause peripheral neuritis:

(A) Lamivudine (B) Zalcitabine
(C) Stavudine (D) Didanosine

Q. 78 A patient with AIDS and a CD_4 cell count of 100/μL develops M. avium infection. The management of this patient is:

(A) Selection of antibiotic regimen based on susceptibility of the cultured organism
(B) Treat with rifabutin
(C) Treat with clarithromycin, ethambutol and rifabutin
(D) Start treatment with INH and pyrazinamide

---

72 (D) 73 (B) 74 (A) 75 (B) 76 (A) 77 (A) 78 (C)

Q. 79 Zidovidin treatment affords the following benefits in HIV infection *except:*

(A) It increases CD_4 leucocyte count
(B) It reduces the incidence of opportunistic infection in AIDS patients
(C) It increases survival time in AIDS patients
(D) It protects exposed subjects from contracting HIV infections

Q. 80 Mefloquine is contraindicated in combination with which of the following drug?

(A) Quinine (B) Atenolol
(C) Verapamil (D) Enalapril

Q. 81 Which of the following anti-malarial drug is a slow schizonticide?

(A) Artemether (B) Mefloquine
(C) Pyrimethamine (D) Quinine

Q. 82 Plasmodial resistance to chloroquine is due to:

(A) Change in receptor structure
(B) Decreased accumulation of the drug in the vacuole
(C) Increase in the activity of DNA repair mechanism
(D) Increased synthesis of dihydrofolate reductase

Q. 83 The drug of choice for a traveler's move to a geographical area where chloroquine resistant P. falciparum is endemic (for prophylaxis) is:

(A) Mefloquine (B) Primaquine
(C) Quinine (D) Atovaquine

Q. 84 The drug which is a causal prophylactic for both falciparum and vivax malaria but is not used on mass scale due to risk of severe reaction is:

(A) Mefloquine (B) Amodiaquine
(C) Primaquine (D) Pyrimethamine

Q. 85 Chemoprophylaxis of malaria is recommended for the following category of subjects:

(A) Residents of non-endemic areas
(B) Residents of endemic areas
(C) Travelers from non-endemic to endemic area
(D) Travelers from endemic to non-endemic area

---

79 (D) 80 (A) 81 (C) 82 (B) 83 (A) 84 (C) 85 (C)

Q. 86 Chloroquine is indicated in the following disorders *except:*

(A) Rheumatic fever
(B) Lepra reaction
(C) Discoid lupus erythematosus
(D) Photogenic skin reaction

Q. 87 The drug of choice for cerebral malaria due to P. falciparum is:

(A) Mefloquine
(B) Chloroquine
(C) Pyrimethamine + sulfadoxine
(D) Quinine

Q. 88 Intravenous injection of quinine produces:

(A) Rise in blood pressure
(B) Neuromuscular block
(C) Hyperglycemia
(D) Hypoglycaemia

Q. 89 Drug of choice for malaria during pregnancy is:

(A) Chloroquine (B) Quinine
(C) Primaquine (D) Mepacrine

Q. 90 All of the following anti-amoebic drugs produce disulfiram like reaction with alcohol *except:*

(A) Metronidazole (B) Tinidazole
(C) Secnidazole (D) Satranidazole

Q. 91 Tinidazole differs from metronidazole in the following way:

(A) It is not active against anaerobic bacteria
(B) It has a broad spectrum of activity
(C) It has a longer half life
(D) It has better oral absorption

Q. 92 The following drug is effective in hepatic amoebiasis but not in intestinal amoebiasis:

(A) Emetin (B) Chloroquine
(C) Tetracycline (D) Diloxanide furoate

---

86 (A) 87 (D) 88 (D) 89 (A) 90 (D) 91 (C) 92 (B)

Q. 93 All of the following drugs can be used in kala azar *except:*

(A) Pentamidine (B) Amphotericin B
(C) Ketoconazole (D) Sodium stibogluconate

Q. 94 Albendazole may be used for the treatment of all of the following conditions *except:*

(A) Enterobius (B) Ascariasis
(C) Ankylostoma (D) Schistosomiasis

Q. 95 The following anthelmintic has been found to be safe during pregnancy:

(A) Thiabendazole (B) Piperazine
(C) Albendazole (D) Praziquantel

Q. 96 The following is not true of levamisole:

(A) A single dose cures over 90% cases of round worm infestation
(B) It is more effective against Necator amaricanus than against Ancylostoma duodenale
(C) It has immunomodulating action
(D) Its prolonged use causes severe reaction

Q. 97 The following anti-cancer drug has high emetogenic potential:

(A) Vincristine (B) Chlorambucil
(C) Cisplatin (D) 6-mercaptopurine

Q. 98 Practically all neoplastic drugs can produce the following toxic effects *except:*

(A) Depression of leukocyte count
(B) Mucositis
(C) Cardiomyopathy
(D) Oligozoospermia

Q. 99 The following is not true about use of prednisolone in malignant diseases:

(A) It is curative in acute childhood leukemia
(B) It is used in Hodgkin's disease
(C) It controls hypercalcaemia in patients with bony metastasis
(D) It affords symptomatic relief in most cancer patients

---

93 (C) 94 (D) 95 (B) 96 (B) 97 (C) 98 (C) 99 (A)

Q. 100 Which of the following does not apply to cancer chemotherapy?

(A) Each treatment with cytotoxic drug kills a constant number of malignant cell
(B) Drugs are used at maximum tolerated doses
(C) The same regimen which is palliative for a large solid tumor may be curative after surgical removal of the tumor
(D) Combination regimens using several drugs in succession are superior to single drugs used continuously

Q. 101 All drugs can be used for long-term in prostatic carcinoma *except:*

(A) Flutamide (B) Goserelin
(C) Diethyl stilbestrol (D) Finasteride

Q. 102 All of the following statements are true regarding methotrexate *except:*

(A) Folinic acid enhances its action (toxicity)
(B) It inhibits dihydrofolate reductase
(C) It has resistance against non-proliferative cells
(D) It is used in the treatment of psoriasis

Q. 103 Drug therapy in the treatment of chronic myelocytic leukemia (CML) in adult is:

(A) Anastrozole (B) Rituximab
(C) Imatinib (D) Amifostine

Q. 104 All of the following anti-cancer agents can be used in leukemia *except:*

(A) Chlorambucil (B) Daunorubicin
(C) Doxorubicin (D) Flutamide

---

100 (C) 101 (D) 102 (A) 103 (C) 104 (D)

ANSWERS

Ans. 1 (A) Methicillin is a beta lactamse resistant, AMA having narrow spectrum. It causes nephrotoxicity, but not bone marrow depression, so no more use in the treatment of S. aureus strains and is replaced by cloxacillin flucloxacin and dicloxacin. All other three causes bone marrow depression.

Ans. 2 (D) Beta lactam antibiotics, vancomycin, Teicoplanin, monobactams, carbapenems and some antitubercular drugs act by inhibiting cell wall synthesis. Nitrfurantoin, a nitrofuran, used exclusively as a urinary antiseptic in the treatment of UTI. Nitrofurans (Nitrofurantoin, Furazolidine, Nifuroxime, Nitrofurazone) undergoes enzymatic reduction, resulting into a formation of highly reactive intermediate which cause damage to DNA. They also have mutagenic as well as radiomimetic activity.

Ans. 3 (D) The various preparations of penicillin can be used in the treatment of meningococcal meningitis, anthrax, diphtheria, tetanus, gas gangrene gonorrhea, syphilis and actinomycosis, listeriasis and rat bite fever. It is not effective against rickettsial infection. Tetracyclines are very effective in murine, epidemic and scrub typus, Q fever and Rocky mountain spotted fever. Tetracyclines (Doxycline) are also effective in Chlamydia infection, in cholera and in plague.

Ans. 4 (C) Carbenicillin, Ticarcilin, Piperacillin, Mezlocillin and Aziocilin are penicillin having extended spectrum. These are acid labile so given parenterally. These are effective against pseudomonas and indole positive proteus which are not inhibited by penicillin G or amino penicillin. These drugs are mainly used in the treatment of severe burn, septicemia caused by Pseudomonas, Proteus and Klebsiella. Cloxacillin and Dicloxacillin are anti-staphylococcal penicillins. Cephalaxin, a first generation cephalosporin is effective against Proteus and Klebsiella but not against Pseudomonas infection. Cefaperazone, ceftazidine and cefotaxim (third generation cephalosporins) are effective against pseudomonas.

Ans. 5 (B) Vancomycin and teicoplanin (glycopeptide beta lactam, cell wall inhibitor) and Linezolid (oxazolidinones) acting by inhibiting proteins synthesis by binding to 50S sub-units of ribosome. They are effective against MRSA infection. Imipenem (a carebapenem) is not a preferred drug as it may cause seizures. It is hydrolysed by renal dehydropeptidase so administered with cilastatin which inhibits this enzyme.

Ans. 6 (A) Cefepime, a fourth generation cephalosporin act by inhibiting cell wall synthesis. Lomefloxacin a fluoroquinolone act by inhibiting DNA gyrase enzyme. Erythromycin is a macrolide act by inhibiting protein synthesis by binding with 50S subunit of ribosome. Tetracyclines inhibit protein synthesis by binding with 30S sub-unit.

Ans. 7 (B) Cloxacillin is a beta lactamase resistant AMA and thus effective against penicillinase producing organism (See Ans. 1 also).

Ans. 8 (D) Macrolides, *e.g.*, erythromycin possesses anti-inflammatory effect and act by decreasing proinflammatory cytokines release from phagocytes, so useful in the treatment of rheumatoid arthritis, cystic fibrosis, chronic sinusitis and asthma.

Ans. 9 (B) Sulfacetamide (as eye drops), silver sulfadiazine (in burns) and mafenide (in burns, pseudomonas and clostridia infection) are topically used sulfonamides. Sulfadoxine with pyrimethamine is used to treat chloroquine resistant falciparum malaria.

Ans. 10 (B) Tetracycline inhibits the bacterial protein synthesis by binding to their 30S subunit of ribosome and thus blocking the attachment of the mRNA ribosome complex. So the formation of peptide chain does not form. They are bacteriostatic.

Ans. 11 (B) Trovafloxacin is eliminated by bile, while all other eliminated in urine. So dose adjustment is not required in patients with renal dysfunction.

Ans. 12 (C) Cefepime, cefpirone and cefozopran are fourth generation cephalosporins.

Ans. 13 (A) Sulfonamides are effective against gram positive bacilli, indole positive Proteus, Neisseria, and Actinomycetes (Nocardia, Rickettsia). The main adverse effects of sulfonamides are crystalluria and renal toxicity, hypersensitivity reaction, hemolytic anaemia (in G-6PD deficiency) and kernicterus in neonates. Sulfasalazine is used widely in the treatment of ulcerative colitis, and rheumatoid arthritis. It is poorly absorbed through GIT.

Ans. 14 (B) Tetracyclines, nowadays is less commonly used due to its adverse effects, *e.g.*, hepatotoxicity, staining of teeth, fanconi syndrome and pulmonary eosinophilia syndrome. Pseudomotor cerebri and bulging fontanelles in adult is another complication of chronic use of tetracycline which resolves by stopping the therapy.

Ans. 15 (D) Thalidomide is used in the erythema nodosa (type II), melanoma and in multiple myeloma but not used in CML. It is contraindicated during pregnancy due to its teratogenic effect. It also have potent anti-inflammatory action.

Ans. 16 (C) Intravenous co-trimoxazole in 5% dextrose is preferred to treat moderate to severe P. carinii pneumonia.

Ans. 17 (A) Cephadroxil, a first generation cephalosporin, is not effective against pseudomonas infection (See Ans. 4).

Ans. 18 (C) Aminoglycosides, *e.g.*, Streptomycin, Gentamicin etc are nephrotoxic due to NH_2 group. The chances of toxicity are more when they are used for prolonged period in elderly in presence of renal insufficiency, biliary obstruction or hepatitis. Concurrent use of loop diuretics, vancomycin, amphotericin B cisplatin, and cyclosporine potentiate the nephrotoxicity. Combination of streptomycin and penicillin act synergistically particularly in SABE.

Ans. 19 (D) Neuromuscular blockade occur by aminoglycosides not by fluoroquinolone, due to displacement of Ca^{2+} from NMJ, by blocking post synaptic Nm receptors and by inhibiting Ca^{2+} mediated release acetylcholine.

Ans. 20 (A) Clindamycin is a lincosamide act like macrolides and inhibit bacterial protein synthesis by binding with 50S ribosomal subunit.

Ans. 21 (A) Methicillin causes severe nephrotoxicity and no more in use.

Ans. 22 (B) Photosensitivity occurs commonly with sparfloxacin (5%) lomefloxacin (2%) and pefloxacin (1%). Ciprofloxacin causes ligament damage. Hypo and hyperglycemia with gatifloxacin, change in QT interval (prolongation) with gatifloxacin, levofloxacin and moxifloxacin, hepatotoxicity with travafloxacin are common adverse effects with fluoroquinolone.

Ans. 23 (D) Co-trimoxazole is combination of trimethoprim and sulfamethoxazole in fixed dose (1:5 ratio). They are having similar plasma half life. The combination is bactericidal due to blockade of folic acid synthesis at two sites in sequence (dihydrofolate reductase with trimethoprim and sulfamethoxazole compete for PABA for the synthesis of folic acid).

Ans. 24 (C) Gentamicin inactivated by purulent exudates of wound, hence it is not useful in presence of pus.

Ans. 25 (D) Benzyl penicillin have short duration of action due to its rapid urinary elimination and necessitates its parenteral administration at 4-hourly interval. So repository preparations are prepared, though they are not useful for treating severe infections where an immediate high concentration of benzyl penicillin is desirable. These are prepared by adding procaine (procaine penicillin) benzathine penicillin (a dibenzyl ethylenediamine salt). Probenecid is a uricosuric drug which competes with penicillin for tubular transport and delays its excretion. Clavulinic acid is used with amoxicillin to widen its anti-bacterial spectrum.

Ans. 26 (D) More than one anti-microbial agents are frequently used for the specific purpose, *e.g.*, to achieve synergism (sulfonamide + trimethoprim), to reduce severity of adverse effects (streptomycin + penicillin for SABE), to prevent emergence of resistance (for chronic infections like tuberculosis) and to broaden the spectrum of anti-microbial action (to treat mixed infections) for empirical treatment. But disadvantages of such combination are increased incidence of adverse effects, increased chance of super-infection and increase in cost of therapy.

Ans. 27 (B) Cefoxitin is a second generation cephalosporin (not effective in meningitis as they do not cross BBB). Only cefuroxime (a second generation), among this group crosses BBB. Ceftriaxone, cefixime cefotaxim, cefodoxime etc., are third generation crosses BBB and achieve adequate levels in CSF.

Ans. 28 (D) Spectinomycin, is not a true aminoglycoside, used as a single dose as an alternative treatment for gonorrhea in patients who are allergic to penicillin.

Ans. 29 (A) The micro-organism may develop resistance to penicillin due to structural difference in the PBPs and failure to bind (due to decrease affinity), due to formation of beta lactamase enzyme which open the beta lactam ring and inactivate penicillin. Also failure to reach inside as with gram-negative bacteria where the outer membrane function as an impenetrable barriers (except few which penetrates through porin channels) is responsible for development of resistance.

Ans. 30 (D) This is a salt of mandelic acid and methenamine. At an acidic pH of less than 5.5, it liberates formaldehyde which is active against many gram negative organisms and C. albicans. This is not effective in acute upper UTI as it is washed down too rapidly. It should not be used along with sulfonamides as it forms an insoluble precipitate. Bacteria donot develop resistance with it.

Ans. 31 (D) Rifampicin is used for prophylaxis of meningococcal and H. influenzae meningitis and carrier state in MRSA, diphtheroid (2nd or 3rd choice) and in brucellosis (with doxycycline). For prophylaxis of tuberculosis, standard drug is INH (effective in HIV patients). Rifampicin can be used in those patients who are resistant to INH.

Ans. 32 (D) Several acute infections resolve faster with a bactericidal drug. They also exert prolonged post antibiotic effect so that maintenance of drug level continuously above the MIC is not essential. They are also superior to bacteriostatic drug, in impaired host defense, life threatening infections at less accessible sites (SABE) or when carrier state is possible.

Ans. 33 (C) Combination of AMA is used to broaden the spectrum of anti-microbial action, to treat mixed infections, *e.g.*, bronchiectasis, peritonitis, certain UTI, brain abscess, diabetic foot infections (both to cover anaerobic and aerobic organism). Clindamycin or metronidazole may be added to cover anaerobic infection (See also Ans. 26).

Ans. 34 (B) Trimethoprim alone may be as effective as in combination of sulfonamides in UTI and prostatitis.

Ans. 35 (B) Fluoroquinones (ciprofloxacin, norfloxacin etc.) has a broader antimicrobial activity with fewer side effects and comparatively slower rate for microbial resistance, but difference in plasma $t_{½}$ is not very much.

Ans. 36 (D) Sparfloxacin, a second generation F.Q. has enhanced activity against gram positive bacteria, bacteroids fragilis, anaerobes and mycobacteria which are not affected by first generation F.Q. (ciprofloxacin,. norfloxacin etc).

Ans. 37 (B) Clavulinic acid does not possess any antibacterial activity of its own. It improves anti-bacterial spectrum of amoxicillin by inhibiting beta lactamase enzyme which destroys amoxicillin. It is a progressive and suicidal as it gets inactivated after binding to the enzyme. It inhibits beta lactamase produced by various gram positive and gram negative organism but not cephalosporinase.

Ans. 38 (A) Tetracyclines are first drug of choice in various venereal diseases (Chlamydial urethritis, lymphogranuloma venerum, granuloma inguinale), mycoplasma pneumonia, cholera, plague, and rickettsial infections (for gonorrhea, ampicillin, for syphilis penicillin and for chancroid ceftriaxone or macrolides, *e.g.*, azithromycin are first drug of choice).

Ans. 39 (C) Chloramphenicol is broad spectrum antibiotic. Super-infection is less common with this drug. It has higher potential to cause bone marrow depression which restricts its use. Other adverse effects are hypersensitivity reactions and grey baby syndrome (when high doses are used in premature neonates).

Ans. 40 (A) Rifampicin, a first line bactericidal anti-tubercular drug, acts against both intra and extracellular organism. It is the only drug act on persister. It imparts harmless orange color to urine, saliva, sputum, tears, sweat, faeces and even to contact lenses.

Ans. 41 (A) Isoniazid is a bactericidal, potent anti-tubercular drug. It act on the bacilli in the walls of the cavities as well as those inside the macrophage, but not effective against persisters. The main toxicities includes peripheral neuropathy (in slow acetylator), hepatotoxicity (in rapid acetylator). CNS toxicities include psychosis, euphoria, transient loss of memory and personalities changes. Large dose may cause ataxia, muscle twitching and toxic encephalopathy.

Ans. 42 (C) MDR is defined as resistance to INH and rifampicin along with / without resistance to other drugs. F.Q. (ciprofloxacin) macrolides (clarithromycin, azithromycin) and some reserved (second line drugs, *e.g.*, amikacin, cycloserine, ethionamide, PAS etc) can be used. Tobramycin is not used. Linezolid is another drug found effective against M.Tb. (both drug susceptible as well as drug resistance), but its adverse effects on prolonged use may limits its usefulness.

Ans. 43 (A) Rifampicin, isoniazid, pyrazenamide and ethambutol (in last trimester not earlier), can be used during pregnancy and breast feeding. Streptomycin is contraindicated during pregnancy.

Ans. 44 (D) Pyridoxine is rather added in the anti-tubercular regimen to prevent peripheral neuropathy because isoniazid inhibits pyridoxine kinase which converts pyridoxine to its active metabolitic pyridoxyl phosphate and promotes (causes) its excretion leads to deficiency and neuropathy.

Ans. 45 (D) Ethambutol causes impairment of visual acuity and red green color discrimination.

Ans. 46 (A) Rifampicin penetrates all tissue including CSF. It is mainly excreted through liver into bile and undergoes enterohepatic circulation. So dose adjustment is not required in renal dysfunction.

Ans. 47 (B) Cycloserine, a second line anti-tubercular drug, act by inhibiting bacterial cell wall synthesis. It is bacteriostatic and is mainly excreted unchanged in urine. So, it is very useful in the treatment of renal tuberculosis. It is also effective against bacilli resistant to INH or streptomycin. But its use is limited due to its neurological adverse effects, *e.g.*, peripheral neuropathy, ataxia, slurred speech and seizures. Psychic effects includes nervousness insomnia, delusion hallucination etc. Pyridoxine may help to reduce neurotoxicity.

Ans. 48 (C) The main adverse effects of ethambutol are retrobulbar optic neuritis, color vision defects and anorexia. It also decreases renal excretion of uric acid and precipitate gouty arthritis. Pyrazenamide also causes hyperuricaemia. Hypercalcaemia is not an adverse effect of anti-tubercular drugs.

Ans. 49 (A) Rifampicin is an enzyme inducer, so may decrease plasma concentration of oral contraceptives, anti-coagulants and protease inhibitors used in HIV patients (*e.g.*, zidovudin lamivudin and indinavir but not ritonavir) and cause treatment failure. Rifabutin which is a weak enzyme inducer can be added instead of rifampicin.

Ans. 50 (B) The goal of anti-tubercular chemotherapy is to kill dividing bacilli, kill persisting bacilli and to prevent emergence of resistance. Though combination of drugs act synergistically but main reason is to prevent the development of resistance.

Ans. 51 (A) Streptomycin is effective only on extracellular bacilli (because of poor penetration into cells). Thus host defense mechanisms are needed to eradicate the disease. Rifampicin, isoniazid pyrazinamide, ethionamide are effective on both extra and intracellular bacilli. Pyrazinamide is more lethal to intracellular bacilli, so it reduces the risk of relapse.

Ans. 52 (C) Corticosteroids are not routinely used in tuberculosis. It is used in special circumstances, *e.g.*, in seriously ill patients (miliary tuberculosis), when hypersensitive reaction occur with anti-tubercular drugs, in meningeal or renal tuberculosis, in pleural effusion and in patients with AIDS. Corticosteroids are contraindicated in intestinal tuberculosis, in which silent perforation can occur which may leads to haemetemesis.

Ans. 53 (D) Isoniazid is a primary anti-tubercular drug and used in all types of tuberculosis (category I to IV). Isoniazid is also used for chemoprophylaxis (contact of open case in children with positive TB patient in family, neonates of tubercular mother, patient of leukemia, diabetes silicosis or those who are HIV positive but are not tubercular anergie and in patients with old inactive disease with inadequate therapy).

Ans. 54 (D) The mechanism of INH resistance is by mutation of the catalase peroxidase gene, so that the bacilli do not generate active metabolite of INH. It also involve the mutation in the target inh A gene.

Ans. 55 (A) Dapsone is chemically related with sulfonamides. It is leprostatic in low doses and have cidal effect in higher doses. It is commonly used in the treatment of both multi and paucibacillary leprosy (common constituent of MDT). It is also used in dermatitis herpetiformis (characterized by itching papule), in penumocystitis jiroveci infection and with pyrimethamine used in MDR falciparum malaria. It should not be used in patients with severe anaemia (Hb <7gm%), G-6PD deficiency and in those showing hypersensitivity reaction.

Ans. 56 (A) The major adverse effect of clofazimine is reddish-black discoloration of skin specially on exposed parts. It also gets deposited in the intestine and causes segmental thickening which leads to cramps and diarrhea. It acts by inhibition of mycobacterial DNA synthesis.

Ans. 57 (D) Rifampicin is most effective drug against M. leprae and up to 99.99% of mycobacteria are killed in 3-7 days. It is added in MDT as once in a month dose which is relatively non-toxic and does not induce metabolism of other drugs. It should not be given in patients with hepato renal dysfunction.

Ans. 58 (B) Dose dependent hemolytic anaemia is very common with dapsone. Patients with G-6PD deficiency are more prone. Methemoglobenemia hepatitis, drug fever, cutaneous lesions are other effect (which are not dose related).

Ans. 59 (A) Minocycline is used due to its high lipophilicity. Other antibiotics, *e.g.*, ofloxacin, pefloxacin, gatifloxacin clarithromycin and sparfloxacin are also highly active. Combination of clarithromycin and minocycline give beneficial effects.

Ans. 60 (D) MDT in leprosy is superior to monotherapy. It is effective in both multi and paucibacillary leprosy and relapse rate is reduced. It also improves efficacy, safety and acceptability with MDT, with less drug toxicity. Resistance does not develop with rifampicin in MDT regimen. In patients with HIV same regimen can be used.

Ans. 61 (A) Amphotericin B, an anti-fungal drug (polyenes) have high affinity for ergosterol present in fungal cell membrane. It is effective against a wide range of yeast and fungi. It can be given orally, and topically for oral, vaginal and cutaneous candidiasis and otomycosis. It is very toxic drug. Its adverse effect includes acute reaction (due to release of IL and TNF alpha), nephrotoxicity (azotemia, reduced GFR, hypokalemia) anaemia (due to bone marrow depression) and CNS toxicity (headache, nerve palsies). It does not cause hyperkalemia or alteration of other electrolytes.

Ans. 62 (B) Grisiofulvin act by disruption of mitotic spindle and inhibition of fungal mitosis. All other act on cell membrane (by binding with ergosterol). 5-flucytosin act by inhibiting nucleic acid synthesis.

Ans. 63 (D) Amphotericin B use is decline because of its toxicity and due to advent of azole group of drugs (*e.g.*, fluconazole) but still it is used (first choice drug) in invasive aspergillosis, mucormycosis, histoplasmosis, cryptococal meningitis, (non-AIDS) blastomycosis, meningeal coccidomycosis.

Ans. 64 (D) Fluconazole and other imidazole and triazoles (ketoconazole, clotrimazole (topical), itraconazole, voriconazole etc.) inhibits the fungal cytochrome P-450 enzyme (lanosterol-14 demethylase) and thus impair ergosterol synthesis leading to formation of damaged leaky fungal cell membrane. Its penetration to brain (CSF) is good but has less activity against aspergillosis.

Ans. 65 (B) Grisiofulvin is not used orally for candidiasis due to its systemic toxic effects. It is used orally only for dermatophytosis.

Ans. 66 (A) Ketoconazole is ineffective in the treatment of sporotrichosis, cryptococcal infection, aspergillosis. It is useful in silent non CNS blastomycosis and in silent coccidiodomycosis, oropharyngeal candidiasis.

Ans. 67 (B) Nystatin, being a toxic drug used only locally in superficial candidiasis. When given orally it is not absorbed, so can be used for monilial diarrhea.

Ans. 68 (B) Terbinafine is a fungicidal, act as a non-competitive inhibitor of squalene epoxidase (an early step of ergosterol synthesis), accumulation of which is responsible for its fungicidal effect. It is used topically and orally against dermatophytes and candida (tinea pedis /corporis/ cruris/ capitis) and pityriasis versicolor.

Ans. 69 (C) Topical anti-fungal drugs includes tolnaftate, ciclopirox olamine, butenafine, undecylenic acid, benzoic acid, quiniodochlor, sodium thiosulphate, topical azole (clotrimazole etc). Crotamiton is an effective scabicide, pediculoside and anti-pruritic.

Ans. 70 (C) Cidofovir is activated by host cell kinases. Ganciclovir, like acyclovir inhibits viral DNA polymerase and cause chain termination. Foscarnet inhibits viral polymerase without requiring bio-activation. Interferon alpha act through host cell surface receptor and increase the activity of kinase.

Ans. 71 (A) Ganciclovir is the most commonly used drug for prevention and treatment of CMV infection. It act by inhibiting DNA polymerase of virus and cause chain termination cidofovir is also effective (specially in those who are resistant to acyclovir).

Ans. 72 (D) Interferon alpha is rather used in chronic HBV as an individual agent or in combination with lamivudine. Other use includes treatment of Kaposi sarcoma, papillomatosis and genital warts (topical). Toxicity includes flu like syndrome, neutropenia, fatigue, myalgia, thyroid dysfunction, depression etc.

Ans. 73 (B) Stavudine is a nucleoside reverse transcriptase inhibitor (NRTI). The drug is markedly neurotoxic and cause peripheral neuropathy. Resistance caused by mutation in the pol gene which encode for several proteins.

Ans. 74 (A) Nevirapine, Delavirdine, Efavirenz are NNRTI.

Ans. 75 (B) Abacavir, Didanosine, Lamivudine, Zidovudine, Stavudine etc are NRTI while Amprenavir, Atazanavir, Indianvir, Ritonavir, Nelfinavir, Saquinavir are protease inhibitors.

Ans. 76 (A) Zidovudine is a NRTI, resistance develops due to mutation at reverse transcriptase.

Ans. 77 (A) Pancreatitis and peripheral neuropathy are rare with lamivudine.

Ans. 78 (C) M. avium infection in patients with AIDS is treated by clarithromycin (or azithromycin), ethambutol, rifabutin + one F.Q./Clofazimine/ethionamide given for 2–6 months.

Ans. 79 (D) Zidovudine along with one or two drug is the standard choice for post exposure prophylaxis of HIV, as well as for mother to offspring transmission. But it does not protect exposed subjects from contracting HIV infections.

Ans. 80 (A) Chances of arrhythmia or bradycardia were more when mefloquine is given to patients on CCBs, beta-blockers, digitalis and anti-depressants, but nowadays, they are no more contraindicated. It is the quinine/quinidine, which when given with mefloquine cause QTc lengthening and causes cardiac arrest.

Ans. 81 (C) Pyrimethamine is inhibitor of DHFRase and due to which schizogony of malarial parasites are gradually stops. It is potent and slow acting schizontocide. It is used in combination with sulfonamide, as resistance develop rapidly by mutation when used alone.

Ans. 82 (B) Chloroquine resistance among P. falciparum is mostly of low grade and is associated with a decrease ability of the parasite to accumulate chloroquine. As higher concentration is found in infected RBS by accumulating in the acidic vacuoles.

Ans. 83 (A) Mefloquine is an effective drug for multi-resistant P.falciparum but because of its cost, toxicity and development of resistance it is recommended to use with artisunate (ACT) for uncomplicated as well as complicated chloroquine resistance malaria. It can be given for prophylaxis of malaria among travelers (not recommended for resident of the endemic area for prophylaxis).

Ans. 84 (C) Primaquine is a causal prophylactic for all species of malaria but not used due to its toxicity. Particularly with G-6PD deficiency. So used only in those subjects who cannot take other drugs (if used, chloroquine is combined and given once a week for 8–10 weeks).

Ans. 85 (C) When resident of non-endemic area move to an endemic area, anti-malarial (chemoprophylaxis) drugs are recommended and chloroquine is drug of choice (mefloquine in resistant cases can be used).

Ans. 86 (A) The therapeutic uses of chloroquine are malaria, hepatic amoebiasis, giardiasis, Chinese liver fluke (Clonorchis sinensis), rheumatoid arthritis (not rheumatic fever), DLE, lepra reaction, IMN and photogenic reaction.

Ans. 87 (D) Quinine has been used as the drug of choice for cerebral malaria. But nowadays parenteral artimisinins are considered more effective, faster acting, better tolerated and more convenient for cerebral or complicated malaria (see text also).

Ans. 88 (D) Severe and even fatal hypoglycemia has been reported when quinine is given IV in patients with cerebral malaria.

Ans. 89 (A) Chloroquine is not contraindicated in acute malarial attack during pregnancy. For chloroquine resistant malaria; chloroquine + clindamycin combination is safe.

Ans. 90 (D) Satranidazole is the only anti-amoebic drug which does not produce disulfiram like reaction with alcohol.

Ans. 91 (C) Tinidazole is a analogue of metronidazoel and has longer half life and better tolerated.

Ans. 92 (B) Chloroquine is effective in hepatic amoebiasis and has minimal effect in intestinal amoebiasis in which metronidazole is very effective (another effective drug is emetin, which is very toxic).

Ans. 93 (C) Sodium stibogluconate, meglumine, amphotericin B, pentamidine are some drugs used in leishmaniasis (kala azar). Ketoconazole is not effective.

Ans. 94 (D) Albendazole/ mebendazole are drug of choice in all types of worm infestation except in nematodes (Ivermectin is effective) and cestodes *e.g.*, Teniasis and schistosomias in which praziquantel is drug of choice (see text also).

Ans. 95 (B) Piperazine, pyrantal pamoate are safe to be used during pregnancy.

Ans. 96 (B) Levamisol is more effective against ascariasis as single dose.

Ans. 97 (C) Cisplatin has high emetogenic potential.

Ans. 98 (C) Cardiomyopathy is very unusual toxic effect with anti-cancer drugs.

Ans. 99 (A) Prednisolon (glucocorticoids) are primarily used in acute childhood leukemia and lymphomas. They induce remission rapidly due to its marked lympholytic action but relapse occur after variable interval and the response is loss gradually. They also control complication like hypercalcaemia, hemolysis, bleeding and potentiate the antiemetic effect of ondansetron/metoclopramide.

Ans. 100(C) The same therapy cannot be effective.

Ans. 101(D) Flutamide, Bicalutamide, Nilutamide are androgen receptor blockers and inhibit testosterone binding to ARs. Goserelin is GnRH agonist which inhibits gonadotropin release and suppresses gonadal function. DES is estrogen which suppress pituitary LH and thus inhibit testosterone. Finasteride is alpha blocker and is used for BPH but long term use of this increases risk of prostatic carcinoma.

Ans. 102(A) Folinic acid reduces the risk of toxicity and rescue normal cells from toxicity.

Ans. 103(C) Imatinib is an orally active small molecule inhibitor of tyrosine kinase (the oncogenic bcr-abl kinase) produced as a result of the Philadelphia chromosome used to treat CML. It also inhibits the c-Kit receptor and can be used in GI stromal tumors (GISTs).

Ans. 104(D) Flutamide is a non-steroidal anti-androgen compound and is used in the treatment of prostatic cancer while all other three are myelosuppressive and used in cases of leukemias.

7

CENTRAL NERVOUS SYSTEM (CNS)

GENERAL CONSIDERATION

CNS Neurotransmitters

Neurotransmitters are released into the synaptic cleft to stimulate or inhibit the post-synaptic neuron. Criteria for a substance to be a neurotransmitters are:

1. It must be synthesized and released in the pre-synaptic nerve terminals and stores in synaptic vesicles.
2. Released on nerve stimulation and should be rapidly inactivated after its action is over.
3. Exogenous application of this substance should produce the same effect as does its endogenous release.
4. Its action should be blocked by known antagonist.

Neuromodulators

Their action is less defined. These have a latent action of longer duration and arise from the neurons as well as from non neuronal cells. They are neither store nor released like neurotransmitters, but may increase or decrease their efficacy without participating directly as neurotransmitter, *e.g.*, prostaglandins, adenosine.

Neuromediators are second messengers like cAMP, cGMP and inositol phosphate, which play an important role to elicit response (excitatory/ inhibitory) produced by various neurotransmitters.

A large number of CNS neurotransmitters have been (either tentatively or positively) identified.

1. **Acetylcholine** (ACh) is mainly excitatory neurotransmitter in the brain. Cholinergic neurons are particularly abundant in the basal ganglia, and are involved in cortical arousal responses and in memory. Hence, atropine-like drugs can impair memory.

2. Biogenic Amines

The catecholamines generally have inhibitory effects when applied locally onto central neurons. They are:

a. *Dopamine* is the most important neurotransmitter in the CNS, while norepinephrine and epinephrine are important amine neurotransmitters in the peripheral sympathetic system. Dopamine pathways project from the substantia nigra in the midbrain to the basal ganglia. It is inhibitory neurotransmitter and its deficiency causes extra pyramidal disturbances.

b. *Norepinephrine* containing cell bodies are located in the brainstem. Fibers from these nuclei innervate a large number of cortical and sub-cortical areas. Functions ascribed to noradrenergic neurons include learning and memory, sleep-wake cycle and a role in affective disorders. **Epinephrine** is found only in very low concentration in the mammalian CNS. It is of minor importance in the brain.

c. *Serotonin (5 Hydroxytryptamine)* 90% of the total serotonin in the body is found in enterochromaffin cells in the GIT and the remaining 10% is in platelets and the brains. It is localized in the raphe nuclei, and considerable amounts are also present in the hypothalamus, limbic system, brainstem and pituitary gland. Serotonin is involved in the regulation of several aspects of behavior, sleep-wake cycle, temperature control, pain perception, depression, sexual activity, aggressiveness and hypothalamic control of the release of pituitary hormones.

d. *Histamine* present in the brain, particularly in certain hypothalamic neurons, and evidences strongly suggests that histamine is a neurotransmitter. Histaminergic neurons play a major role in arousal in coupling neuronal activity, with cerebral metabolism and in neuroendocrine regulation.

3. Amino Acids

a. *Gamma amino butyric acid (GABA)* is present in all areas of the CNS; mainly in local inhibitory inter neurons. They are linked with Cl^- ion channels. They cause hyperpolarization and reduce the membrane excitability.

Drugs which are thought to act by modifying GABAnergic synaptic transmission include benzodiazepines, barbiturates, alcohols, valproate and general anesthetics.

b. *Glycine* is another inhibitory CNS neurotransmitter. Whereas, GABA is primarily located in the brain, glycine is found predominantly in medulla, spinal inter neurons. Glycine is antagonized by *strychnine,* and its release is prevented by *tetanus toxin,* thereby both substances cause convulsions.

c. *Glutamate* and *aspartate* are excitatory neurotransmitter.

4. **Neuropeptides:** They form a big group of possible central transmitters. They depend on transcription, translation and post translational processing in the body.
5. **Nitric oxide.**
6. **Miscellaneous:** Endocannabinoids, Purine (adenosine).

GENERAL ANAESTHETIC AGENTS

General anaesthetics are agents that bring about loss of all the modalities of sensation specially pain with reversible loss of consciousness. They also cause varying degree of amnesia, muscle relaxation and loss of reflexes (both somatic and autonomic).

Stages of General Anaesthesia

1. **Stage of analgesia** is from the beginning of inhalation of the anaesthetic to loss of consciousness. Reflexes and respiration remain normal. Some minor operation can be carried out during this stage.
2. **Stage of delirium:** This stage is from loss of consciousness to beginning of surgical anaesthesia. It may be associated with excitement–shouting, crying and violent behavior. There is irregular rise in BP and respiratory rate and pupil is dilated. With new anaesthetic agent this stage is not very evident.
3. **Stage of surgical anaesthesia:** As anaesthesia passes to deeper planes, respiratory depression is seen. There is gradual loss of reflexes and relaxation of skeletal muscles, fall in BP, HR increases and respiration decreases in depth. This has 4 planes:

   Plane 1: Presence of roving eyeball.

   Plane 2: It is characterized by progressive loss of corneal, light and laryngeal reflexes. Respiration is slow and regular, surgical process performed in this stage.

   Plane 3: Marked muscle relaxation, eyeball movement is absent and all reflexes absent.

Plane 4: Complete muscle relaxation, intercostals muscle paralysis, respiration is abdominal.

4. **Stage of medullary paralysis:** This is seen only with overdose. It is the stage of medullary depression. This leads to cessation of breathing, circulatory failure and death may follow. With pre-anaesthetic medication and newer anaesthetic agent, these stages are not very characteristic.

Mechanism of Action of General Anaesthetics

The most accepted mechanisms of action are as follows:

1. Inhaled and some intravenous anaesthetics bind to specific sites on GABA receptor chloride channels and activate these receptors. By this the increase Cl^- flux and inhibit neurotransmission and depress the CNS.
2. Inhalational anaesthetics (barbiturates, propofol) also enhance the sensitivity of glycine gated chloride channels to glycine. These glycine receptors bring about inhibitory neurotransmission in the brainstem. They also decrease duration of opening of nicotine receptor activated Na^+ channels.
3. Some anaesthetics like ketamine and nitrous oxide bind to and inhibit the N-methyl D aspartate (NMDA) receptors.

Classification of General Anaesthetic Agents

1. **Inhalational:**
   a. *Gases:* Nitrous oxide, Cyclopropane.
   b. *Liquids:* Ether, Halothane, Enflurane, Isoflurane, Methoxyflurane, Desflurane, Sevoflurane.
2. **Intravenous:**
   a. *Inducing agents:*
      (i) ***Barbiturates*** – Thiopentone sodium, Methohexitone.
      (ii) *Non-barbiturates* – Propofol, Etomidate.
   b. *Dissociative anaesthesia:* Ketamine.
   c. *Neuroleptanalgesia:* Fentanyl + Droperidol.
   d. *Benzodiazepines:* Diazepam, Lorazepam, Midazolam.

Inhalational anaesthetics are either gases or volatile liquids. Given by inhalation they are absorbed by the pulmonary circulation. On attaining adequate concentration in the brain, they produce general anaesthesia.

Since the brain is a highly perfuse organ, steady state can be achieved quickly. When the steady state is reached, the partial pressure of the anaesthetic in the lung and the brain are equal and this makes it possible to monitor the anaesthesia. But, for anaesthetics with high solubility in blood and tissues, rise in alveolar partial pressure (and thereby induction) is slower. Such anaesthetics need to be administered at higher pressures. Factors affecting the partial pressure (PP) of anaesthetic agents attained in the brain are:

1. PP of anaesthetic in inspired gas.
2. Pulmonary ventilation.
3. Alveolar exchange.
4. Solubility of anaesthetic in blood.
5. Solubility of anaesthetic in tissues.
6. Cerebral blood flow.

Inhaled anaesthetics are largely eliminated unchanged by the lungs.

The potency of inhaled anaesthetic is measured by minimum alveolar concentration (MAC). It is the concentration that immobilizes 50% of subjects in response to a surgical skin incision. Potent anaesthetic agent shows small MAC.

Inhalational Anaesthetic Agent

Nitrous oxide is a gas with a slightly sweetish odour. It produces light anaesthesia without significant depression of respiration or vasomotor centre.

Advantages

1. Strong analgesic, non-irritating and non-inflammable.
2. Induction is rapid and smooth. Recovery is rapid.
3. Post-operative nausea is not significant.
4. Has little effect on respiration and cardiovascular functions, hence ideal for combination. It reduces the requirement of other volatile anaesthetic agent.
5. It is nontoxic to liver, kidney and brain and is quickly removed from lungs.

Disadvantages

1. It is less potent, poor muscle relaxant and should be used with other agents.
2. N_2O displaces nitrogen from the airfilled cavities and while doing so, it enters the cavities faster, *i.e.*, even before nitrogen escapes.

This results in expansion of such cavities like in patients with pneumothorax. Hence N_2O should be avoided in such patients (have second gas effect and cause diffuse hypoxia).

3. It is used along with oxygen (30%).

Ether is color less volatile liquid. It is highly inflammable; vapours are irritating.

Advantages

1. Potent and reliable anaesthetic with good analgesic activity.
2. Effect on cardiovascular and respiratory functions is not significant in therapeutic doses; reflexes are well-maintained.
3. It is a bronchodilator. Provides full muscle relaxation in deep anaesthesia.
4. Does not sensitize the heart to epinephrine.
5. Easy to administer as complicated equipment is not necessary.
6. Inexpensive.

Disadvantages

1. It is inflammable hence diathermy is contraindicated.
2. Highly soluble in body tissues, induction is slow and unpleasant.
3. It is irritating and therefore enhances respiratory secretions. Laryngeal spasm may occur during induction. Recovery is slow.
4. Postoperative nausea and vomiting are frequent.
5. Not used commonly nowadays.

Halothane is a colorless volatile liquid with a sweet odour. It is non-irritant and non-inflammable.

Advantages

1. Potent, non-inflammable anaesthetic. Non-irritant.
2. Induction is smooth and rapid. Recovery is rapid.
3. Postoperative nausea and vomiting are of low incidence.
4. It is bronchodilator, so preferred in asthma.

Disadvantages

1. Neither a good analgesic nor a muscle relaxant.
2. Halothane is a direct myocardial depressant, causes respiratory depression and severe hepatitis.
3. Malignant hyperthermia occurs in genetically predisposed cases. Succinylcholine accentuates this effect of halothane.
4. Relatively expensive.

Enflurane is similar to halothane except that:

1. It is metabolized to a lesser extent than halothane.
2. Does not sensitize the heart to epinephrine.
3. Enflurane may precipitate seizures in epileptics and should be avoided in these patients.

Isoflurane is similar to halothane. It differs as follows:

1. More potent than halothane.
2. Does not sensitize the heart to adrenaline. It does not provoke seizures.
3. Metabolism is negligible, therefore organ toxicity are rare.
4. It is expensive.
5. Low concentration does not increase cerebral blood flow.
6. Though coronary circulation is maintained, so safer in patients with myocardial ischemia. But it may cause coronary steal phenomenon and precipitate regional myocardial ischemia.
7. It can cause hypotension and reflex tachycardia.

Desflurane and **sevoflurane** are newer agents which allow very rapid induction and recovery because of low solubility in blood. Desflurane may induce coughing and sometimes laryngospasm. Recovery is more rapid to any other anaesthetic. Sevoflurane get degraded to a compound that is nephrotoxic. Acceptance is better, even in children. It may trigger malignant hyperthermia.

Intravenous Anaesthetics

Intravenous anaesthetics allow an extremely rapid induction because the blood concentration can be raised rapidly, due to their rapid diffusion in the brain; there is no channel for quick elimination like the lungs. Moreover, elimination of inhaled anaesthetics can be hastened by inducing hyperventilation. Hence IV anaesthetics are used for induction.

Thiopentone sodium is an ultra-short acting barbiturate which when administered IV, rapidly induces hypnosis and anaesthesia without analgesia. It is redistributed to body fats and other tissues and results in termination of its action. Extravasations of the solution produce intense pain, necrosis and gangrene.

It produces unconsciousness in 20–30 sec. Duration of action is 4–7 minutes. It is highly lipid soluble and gets rapidly redistributed in the body tissues. It reduces cerebral metabolic rate of O_2 consumption.

Advantages

Quick onset of action; induction is smooth, rapid and pleasant.

Disadvantages

1. Not a good analgesic and not a muscle relaxant.
2. It cannot be used alone as the dose required results in delayed recovery, respiratory and circulatory depression.
3. A short period of apnea occurs. Overdosage results in profound respiratory depression. Artificial ventilation has to be given.
4. Severe hypotension, hiccoughs may occur.
5. May precipitate acute intermittent porphyria.

Methohexitone is similar to thiopentone but is more potent. It is not preferred due to toxicity.

Propofol is an oily liquid. Quick induction (30 sec) and recovery (4 minutes) is possible from a single dose. It is used for induction and maintenance for short procedures of upto 1 hour duration. The effect of a single dose is terminated by distribution. It can be used for IV anaesthesia as continuous infusion or intermittent injection. It is antiemetic, non-irritant, causes dose dependent cortical depression and marked fall in systemic BP.

Etomidate is similar to thiopental but it differs in that:

1. It is rapidly metabolized, so recovery is fast.
2. Less cardiovascular and respiratory depression.

But it may cause:

1. Involuntary movements and excitatory effects during induction.
3. Pain at the injection site.
4. Adrenocortical suppression on longterm use.

Etomidate is preferred for induction in patients with cardiovascular problems, as it causes less hypotension.

Benzodiazepines: They are now also used for induction, maintaining and supplement anaesthesia. They are preferred for minor procedures. Diazepam, lorazepam and midazolam are used as anaesthetic agents.

Ketamine: In anaesthetic doses ketamine produces a translike state known as dissociative anaesthesia, characterized by intense analgesia, immobility, amnesia and a feeling of dissociation from ones own body and surroundings with or without actual loss of consciousness. Ketamine acts by blocking the NMDA receptor which is an excitatory amino acid receptor.

Ketamine is highly lipid soluble and gets rapidly distributed into highly perfuse organs and then redistributed to less vascular structures. Amnesia lasts for 1–2 hours. Premedication with atropine is needed. Return to consciousness is gradual. Delirium with vivid dreams may be accompanied. If diazepam is administered, preoperatively and postoperatively, delirium can be avoided. Heart rate, cardiac output and BP are increased due to sympathetic stimulation. Pulse and BP should be closely monitored during recovery, patients must be undisturbed and under observation. Respiration is not depressed.

It has less chance to induce vomiting. Pharyngeal and laryngeal reflexes are only slightly affected. It is of particular value in children and poor risk patients and also in asthmatic patients since it does not induce bronchospasm.

Contraindications: Hypertension, CCF, cerebral hemorrhage, increased intracranial tension, psychiatric disorders and pregnancy before term.

Pre-Anaesthetic Medication

Prior to anaesthesia, certain drugs are administered in order to make anaesthesia safer and more pleasant. This is known as pre-anaesthetic medication.

The drugs used are:

1. *Sedative hypnotics*: Benzodiazepines are used to relieve anxiety and for sedation.
2. *Anti-histamines* have sedative, antiemetic and anti-cholinergic properties, *e.g.*, promethazine.
3. *Anti-emetics*: Metoclopramide, domperidone or ondansetron may be used.
4. *Anti-cholinergic drugs*: Atropine, scopolamine or glycopyrrolate can be used. They reduce the secretions, prevent bradycardia due to vagal stimulation, laryngospasm which is due to excessive secretion. **Glycopyrrolate** is nowadays preferred, as it is long acting, is a better anti-sialogogue and is less likely to cause significant tachycardia.
5. *Drugs that reduce acidity*: H_2 blockers like ranitidine decrease gastric acid secretion and are given on the night before surgery.
6. *Opioid like morphine and pethidine* reduced anxiety and apprehension, provide analgesia and reduce the dose of the anaesthetic but not used due to toxicity.

Balanced Anaesthesia

Since it is not possible to achieve ideal anaesthesia with a single drug, multiple drugs are used. To attain this, pre-anaesthetic medication, IV anaesthesia for induction, inhalational agents for maintenance, oxygen, skeletal muscle relaxants and analgesics are given. This is termed as balanced anaesthesia.

LOCAL ANAESTHETIC AGENTS

Local anaesthetics are drugs that which upon topical application causes reversible loss of sensory perception, specially pain in the particular area without affecting the level of consciousness. They block nerve conduction when applied locally to nerve tissue in appropriate concentrations. They act on axons, cell body, dendrites, synapses and other excitable membranes that utilize sodium channels as the primary means of action potential generation. They are used to perform minor surgeries.

Classification

- **i. Injectable**
  - a. *Short acting:* Procaine, Chloroprocaine.
  - b. *Intermediate acting:* Lignocaine, Prilocaine.
  - c. *Long acting*: Tetracaine (amethocaine), Bupivacaine, Dibucaine, Ropivacaine, Etidocaine.
- **ii. Surface anaesthetics:** Lignocaine, Cocaine, Tetracaine, Benzocaine, Oxethazaine, Butamben (Butyl amino benzoate).

Mechanism of Action

Local anaesthetic must possess high lipid as well as water solubility for better action (penetration). Local anaesthetics prevent the generation and the conduction of nerve impulses. The primary mechanism of action is blockade of voltage gated sodium channels.

Local anaesthetics diffuse through the cell membrane and bind to the voltage sensitive sodium channels from the inner side of the cell membrane. They decrease the entry of Na^+ during upstroke. With increasing concentration, impulse conduction slows, rate of rise of action potential (AP) declines, AP amplitude decreases and finally the ability to generate an AP is abolished. These result from binding of LA to more and more sodium channels and finally local depolarization fails to reach the threshold potential. Thus they prevent the generation of an AP and its conduction.

They have membrane stabilizing effect.

Resting nerve fibers are resistant to blockade. Degree of blockade depends on the pKa value of LA.

Small nerve fibers are more susceptible as they present a greater surface area per unit volume and are blocked first. The autonomic fibers are blocked first followed by sensory fibers conducting pain, temperature, then touch, pressure and vibration sensations in the same order. Non-myelinated fibers are blocked more readily than the myelinated. The recovery occurs in reverse order.

Systemic Actions

i. **CNS:** LA (Cocaine) depresses the cortical inhibitory pathway thereby allowing unopposed activity of excitatory components. This loss of inhibition is manifested as restlessness, tremors and may proceed to convulsions. This central stimulation is followed by generalized CNS depression and death may result from respiratory failure.

ii. **CVS:** Lignocaine decreases excitability, conduction rate and force of contraction (quinidine like effects). Procainamide is used as an anti-arrhythmic. They cause hypotension, primarily due to blockade of sympathetic activity followed by relaxation of arteriolar smooth muscle.

iii. **Smooth muscle:** LAs depress contractions in the intact bowel. They also relax vascular and bronchial smooth muscles.

Pharmacokinetics

Local anaesthetics are rapidly absorbed from the mucous membranes. Rate of absorption is dependent on the vascularity of the area. Toxicity depends on the balance between absorption and metabolism. Ester linked LAs are rapidly hydrolyzed by plasma pseudo cholinesterase and in the liver and have short duration of action. Amides linked LAs are metabolized by the liver microsomes by dealkylation and hydrolysis. They have longer duration of action and are not effective orally. They undergo extensive first pass metabolism. So not used orally.

Addition of a vasoconstrictor like adrenaline (1:1,00,000 to 1: 2,00,000) or phenylephrine (1:20,000) prolongs the duration of action of LAs by slowing the rate of absorption from the site of administration and reduces systemic toxicity of LAs since the absorption rate is reduced and as it gets absorbed, it is metabolized.

Adverse Effects

1. Hypersensitivity reactions include skin rashes, dermatitis, asthma or rarely anaphylaxis (with ester type LA, *e.g.*, procaine).
2. **CNS:** Dizziness, auditory and visual disturbances, mental confusion, disorientation, anxiety, muscle tremors, convulsions and respiratory failure (more common with cocaine).
3. **CVS:** Hypotension, bradycardia and arrhythmias may be encountered. Rarely cardiac arrest can occur (with bupivacaine and etidocaine).
4. Local irritation can be seen with bupivacaine. Wound healing may be delayed.
5. Large doses may cause neuromuscular blockage.
6. Large doses of prilocaine may cause methaemoglobinemia.

Individual Drugs

Injectable

1. **Lignocaine** is the most widely used LA. It is fast and long acting. It is useful for all types of blocks. Though it is good corneal anaesthetic, it is not generally preferred because it causes irritation.
2. **Bupivacine:** Potent long acting, used for all types of block, causes adequate analgesia with motor block when epidural injection is given. So preferred in obstetric practice. It can cause more cardio toxicity than levobupivacine.
3. **Ropivacaine:** Its analgesic action lasts longer, it is used for epidural and all types of infiltration and regional anaesthesia (relief of labour pain).
4. **Mepivacaine:** It have more rapid onset of action and more prolonged action than lignocaine.
5. **Cocaine** produces euphoria and is a drug of dependence and abuse, used rarely. It also damages corneal surface.
6. **Procaine** was widely used once. But is now replaced by other agents.
7. **Tetracaine** is a PABA derivative and is 10 times more toxic and more active than procaine, used topically only (as surface anaesthesia).

8. **Benoxinate** produces corneal anaesthesia, enough to perform tonometry without mydriasis.
9. **Oxethazaine** remains unionized in acidic pH, so when swallowed with antacids, give symptomatic relief in gastritis, peptic ulcer and GERD.

Uses of Local Anaesthetics

Surface Anaesthesia

Anaesthesia of mucous membrane of the eye, nose, mouth, tracheobronchial tree, oesophagus and genitourinary tract can be produced by direct application of the anaesthetic solution and is useful in:

1. On the eye (a) for tonometry, surgery (b) to remove foreign bodies from the cornea and conjunctiva (c) for preoperative preparation
2. Others: Nasal lesions, stomatitis, sore throat, tonsillectomy, endoscopies, intubation, gastric ulcer, bums and proctoscopy.

Infiltration Anaesthesia

Injection of a local anaesthetic solution directly into the tissue can be (i) superficial–only into the skin, or (ii) into deeper structures including intra-abdominal organs. It is used for minor procedures like incisions, drainage of an abscess, excision, etc.

Field Block

Subcutaneous injection of a LA solution proximal to the site to be anaesthetized interrupts nerve transmission in the region distal to the injection. Thus lesser dose can be used to provide a greater area of anaesthesia.

Nerve Block

LA is injected around anatomically localized nerve trunk. They last longer than field block/infiltration anaesthesia.

Nerve block anaesthesia is useful for:

1. Blocks of brachial plexus for procedures on the arm.
2. Intercostal nerve blocks to anaesthetize anterior abdominal wall.
3. Cervical plexus block for surgery of the neck.
4. Sciatic and femoral nerve blocks for surgeries distal to the knee.
5. Blocks of nerves at wrist and ankle.

6. Radial and ulnar nerve block at the elbow.
7. Sensory cranial nerves block.
8. Facial and lingual nerves block.
9. Inferior alveolar nerve block for extraction of lower jaw teeth.

Spinal Anaesthesia (SA)

Local anaesthetic solution is injected into the subarachnoid space between L_2–L_3 or L_3–L_4, below the lower end of the spinal cord. The drug acts on nerve roots. Lower abdomen and lower limbs are anaesthetized and paralyzed. The level of anaesthesia can be altered by the volume of injection and specific gravity of the solution. Generally a hyperbaric solution is injected. Isobaric and hypobaric (rarely) solutions can also be given. Level of sympathetic block produced is two segments higher and motor paralysis is two segments lower than sensory or cutaneous anaesthesia. Lignocaine, tetracaine, bupivacaine and ropivacaine are used for spinal anaesthesia.

Advantages

Safer, affords good analgesia and muscle relaxation and there is no loss of consciousness. In cardiac, pulmonary and renal diseases, SA may be preferred over general anaesthesia whenever possible.

Complications of SA

1. Hypotension – due to sympathetic blockade, decrease venous return, decrease C.O.P. (treated with IV fluids and by raising foot and by mephenteramine).
2. Respiratory paralysis.
3. Headache – due to leakage of CSF from site of injection.
4. Cauda equina syndrome – due to traumatic damage to nerve roots.
5. Sepsis.
6. Nausea and vomiting.

Epidural Anaesthesia

LA is injected into the epidural space with semi-liquid fat. It acts on nerve roots while small amounts diffuse into subarachnoid space. It may be thoracic, lumbar or caudal depending on the site of injection.

Advantages

1. Sensory blockade is 4–5 segments higher than motor blockade.

Useful for obstetric analgesia, as the mother has painless labour and can still cooperate in the process of labour and is conscious throughout.

2. There are no chances of infection; headache and neurological complication are less.

Intravenous Regional Anaesthesia

This type of anaesthesia is useful for rapid, anaesthetization of an extremity (upper limb). A rubber bandage is used to force the blood out of the limb (veins) and a tourniquet is applied to prevent the reentry of the blood. A dilute solution of the local anaesthetic is then injected intravenously. It is commonly used on the upper limbs, though it can also be used on the legs and the thighs.

SEDATIVE HYPNOTICS

Sedative is a drug that produces a calming effect and reduces excitement. Hypnotic is a drug that induces sleep ideally resembling with the natural sleep. Tranquillizers are those drugs which quiet an agitated person without causing sedation and hypnosis. Sleep can be classified into two types:

1. Non-rapid eye movement (NREM) sleep.
2. Rapid eye movement (REM) sleep.

Throughout the night, NREM and REM sleep cycles repeat alternately for brief periods.

Classification

1. **Benzodiazepines**
   a. *Long acting*: Diazepam, Chlordiazepoxide, Clonazepam, Flurazepam, Chlorazepat, Clobazam.
   b. *Short acting*: Temazepam, Lorazepam, Oxazepam, Nitrazepam, Alprazolam, Halazepam.
   c. *Ultra short acting*: Triazolam, Midazolam.
2. **Newer agents:** Zolpidem, Zopiclone, Zaleplon, Eszopiclone.
3. **Barbiturates:** Phenobarbitone, Mephobarbitone, Secobarbitone, Pentobarbiton, Thiopentone, Hexobarbitone.
4. **Atypical anxiolytic:** Buspirone, Ispapirone, Gepirone.
5. **Non-sedative anxiolytic:** Propranolol.
6. **Miscellaneous:** Paraldehyde, Chloral hydrate, Glutethimide, Meprobamate.

Benzodiazepines (BZD)

Pharmacological actions of BZD:

1. **Sedation and hypnosis:** BZDs hasten the onset of sleep and increase the duration of sleep. The quality of sleep resembles natural sleep more closely when compared to other hypnotics.
2. **Anxiolytic or anti-anxiety effects:** BZDs reduce anxiety and aggression and thus produce a calming effect.
3. **Muscle relaxant:** BZDs reduce muscle tone by a central action.
4. **Anticonvulsant effects:** BZDs increase the seizure threshold and act as anticonvulsants. BZDs like clonazepam is used in the treatment of absence seizures and myoclonic seizures in children.
5. **Amnesia:** BZDs produce loss of memory for the events happening after the administration of BZDs. This property is an advantage when BZDs are used in surgical procedures as the patient does not remember the unpleasant events.
6. **Other actions:** In higher doses BZDs decrease BP and increase heart rate. Diazepam decreases nocturnal gastric acid secretion.

Mechanism of Action

Benzodiazepines bind to the $GABA_A$ receptor (BZD receptor) at a site which is different from the GABAbinding site of barbiturates. They increase the frequency (not duration) of chloride channel opening. This in turn leads to increased flow of chloride ions into the neurons, resulting in hyper polarization.

Advantages of BZDs

1. BZDs induce sleep which closely resembles with natural sleep and has less hangover, they do not cause hyperalgesia, no affect on respiration or cardiovascular functions and have a higher safety margin.
2. In case of BZD over dosage, a specific BZD antagonist flumazenil can be used.
3. BZDs do not cause microsomal enzyme induction.
4. BZDs have lower abuse liability, no drug automatism.

Pharmacokinetics

BZDs are completely absorbed on oral administration. Intramuscular absorption is slow hence oral route is preferred. They are extensively bound to plasma proteins. No displacement reactions occur due to their marked volume of distribution. BZDs metabolized in the liver by glucuronide conjugation. Long acting BZDs are converted to active metabolites, thereby prolonging their effects.

Adverse Effects

BZDs are generally well tolerated. The common side effects include drowsiness, confusion, amnesia, lethargy, weakness, headache, blurred vision, ataxia, day time sedation and impaired motor coordination such as driving skills.

Tolerance and dependence liability are less with BZDs. The withdrawal symptoms are milder but they may be abrupt and more intensive with short acting agents. When given to a pregnant mother during labour, BZDs cause hypotonia and respiratory depression in the neonate.

Uses of BZDs

1. *Insomnia:* Lorazepam, oxazepam, temazepam, nitrazepam or triazolam may be used.
2. In anxiety states BZDs except the ultra short acting may be used.
3. As anti-convulsants and as muscle relaxant diazepam is the drug of choice.
4. As pre-anaesthetic medication.
5. During alcohol withdrawal.

Benzodiazepine Antagonist

Flumazenil is a BZD receptor antagonist which competes with BZDs. It may rarely induce seizure and used to reverse sedation/anaesthesia due to BZDs and in BZD overdose.

Newer Agents

Newer agents include zolpidem, zopiclone and zaleplon.

- They are not BZDs but produce their effects by binding to benzodiazepine site on the $GABA_A$ receptors and facilitate the inhibitory actions of GABA. They are all rapid and short acting agents and produce minimum hangover.
- Their actions are blocked by flumazenil.
- They are used when short acting hypnotics are needed.

- **Zolpidem** is a good hypnotic but has weak anticonvulsant and muscle relaxant effects. **Zaleplon** is rapidly absorbed from the gut. It has the advantages that no withdrawal symptoms are reported after stopping. **Zopiclone** is longer acting.

Barbiturates

Barbiturates were the largest group of hypnotics in clinical use until the 1960s. But, due to their toxicity and availability of better drugs they are not preferred as sedative hypnotics now-a-days.

Classification

- *Long acting*: Phenobarbitone, Mephobarbitone (used as anticonvulsant).
- *Short acting*: Pentobarbitone, Butobarbitone (used as sedative hypnotics).
- *Ultra-short acting*: Thiopentone, Hexobarbitone, Methohexitone (used as anesthetic).

Mechanism of Action

Barbiturates cause inhibition by binding to a specific site on the $GABA_A$ receptor Cl^- channel complex. They facilitate inhibitory neurotransmission by opening chloride ion channels and hyperpolarize the neural membrane. They increase the binding of BZD rather than displacing them from binding site.

Pharmacological Actions

1. **CNS:** Barbiturates cause dose dependent depression of CNS ranging from mild sedation to general anaesthesia.
   a. *Sedation and hypnosis:* In hypnotic doses, barbiturates induce sleep and prolong the duration of sleep. On waking up there is hangover with headache and residual sedation. Barbiturates reduce anxiety; impair short-term memory and judgment. They can produce euphoria and are drugs of addiction. Barbiturates produce hyperalgesia. Barbiturates decrease the duration of REM sleep.
   b. *General anaesthesia:* In higher doses barbiturates produce general anaesthesia.
   c. *Anticonvulsant actions*: Phenobarbitone and mephobarbitone have specific anticonvulsant activity in sub-hypnotic doses and are used in the treatment of epilepsy.

2. **Respiratory system:** Barbiturates depress the respiration. High doses bring about a direct paralysis of the medullary respiratory centre and can be fatal.
3. **Cardiovascular system:** It causes slight reduction in blood pressure and heart rate in therapeutic doses. Toxic doses of barbiturates produce a significant fall in BP due to direct decrease in myocardial contractility and vasomotor centre depression.
4. **Skeletal muscles:** Higher doses depress the excitability of the neuromuscular junction and potentiate the effect of tubocurarine and decamethonium.
5. It decreases tone and amplitude of GIT muscles.

Pharmacokinetics

Barbiturates are well absorbed and widely distributed in the body. The highly lipid soluble barbiturates like thiopentone have a fast onset of action and short duration of action due to redistribution into adipose tissues. They are hepatic microsomal enzyme inducers.

Adverse Reactions

Han gover due to residual depression of the CNS may be accompanied by nausea, vomiting, vertigo and diarrhoea. Distortions of mood, impaired judgement and fine motor skills may be evident.

Respiratory depression, hypersensitivity reactions like skin rashes, swelling of the eyelids and lips and rarely exfoliative dermatitis may be seen.

Barbiturates are contraindicated in porphyrias (because they increase porphyrin synthesis), in severe respiratory insufficiency and hepatorenal disease.

Dependence and Tolerance

On repeated administration, tolerance develops to the effects of barbiturates. Both psychological and physical dependence make them one of the drugs with abuse liability.

Treatment of Acute Barbiturate Poisoning

There is no specific antidote. The measures include:

1. Gastric lavage followed by administration of activated charcoal to prevent further absorption of barbiturates.
2. General supportive measures like maintenance of BP, patent airway, adequate ventilation and oxygen administration.

3. Forced alkaline diuresis with furosemide and alkalinization of urine by sodium bicarbonate.
4. Haemodialysis should be done especially if there is renal failure.

Uses

1. *Anaesthesia:* Thiopentone sodium is used IV for the induction of general anaesthesia.
2. *Antiepileptic:* Phenobarbitone is used as an antiepileptic.
3. *Neonatal jaundice:* Phenobarbitone is a microsomal enzyme inducer and thereby enhances the production of glucuronyl transferase, the enzyme required for metabolism and excretion of bilirubin. It therefore helps in the clearance of bile in the neonates.

Miscellaneous

Chloral hydrate: It produces hypnosis without affecting respiratory and cardiovascular functions.

Meprobamate has sedative and anti-anxiety properties but is now not recommended. It produces respiratory depression, ataxia and is a drug of abuse.

ETHYL ALCOHOL

Ethyl alcohol is a monohydroxy alcohol. It is a colorless, volatile, inflammable liquid. The ethanol content of various alcoholic beverages ranges from 4–55%.

Actions

1. **Local:** On topical application, it has a cooling effect. It is an astringent, precipitates surface protein and hardens the skin. 40–50% alcohol is rubefacient and counter irritant and 70% acts as antiseptic.
2. **CNS:** Alcohol is a CNS depressant. Small doses cause euphoria, relief of anxiety and loss of social inhibitions. Moderate doses impair muscular coordination and visual acuity making driving dangerous. Higher doses cause mental clouding, impaired judgment, drowsiness and loss of self-control. Toxic doses cause stupor and coma. Death is due to respiratory depression. Alcohol may precipitate convulsions in epileptics. Tolerance develops on long-term use.
3. **CVS:** The actions are dose dependent. Small doses cause cutaneous vasodilatation resulting in flushing and feeling of

warmth. Large doses cause hypotension due to depression of myocardium and vasomotor centre.

4. **GIT and liver:** Alcohol increases gastric secretion and feeling of warmth. It is an appetizer. Chronic alcoholism results in peptic ulcer. Chronic consumption of moderate amounts of alcohol results in accumulation of fat in the liver, enlargement of the liver, followed by fatty degeneration and cirrhosis.
5. **Other effects:** Though alcohol is called an aphrodisiac, this effect could be due to loss of inhibition. It increases HDL and lowers LDL cholesterol. It causes diuresis due to decrease in ADH secretion. It interferes with folate metabolism and may cause megaloblastic anaemia. Food value is 7 calories/gram.

Mechanism of Action

Ethanol acts by:

1. Inhibiting central neuronal nicotinic acetylcholine receptors.
2. Inhibiting excitatory NMDA (N-methyl D-asparate) receptors mediate excitatory responses in the CNS and cAMP dependent protein kinase activity.

Pharmacokinetics

Alcohol is rapidly absorbed from the stomach and is metabolized in the liver by alcohol and aldehyde dehydrogenase. Food and milk delays its absorption by slowing gastric emptying. It has wide volume of distribution, it cross BBB and placental barrier.

Metabolism follows zero order kinetics, *i.e.*, a constant amount is metabolized per unit time, *i.e.*, about 10 ml of absolute alcohol is metabolized per hour (80 mg/100 ml of ethanol in blood is equivalent to 35 μ / 100 ml of ethanol in expired air, which forms the basis of the breath analysis test).

Drug Interactions

1. Alcohol potentiates effect of other CNS depressants including hypnotics, opioids and antipsychotics.
2. Sulfonylurea, metronidazole and griseofulvin have disulfiram like effects on alcohol consumption.
3. Alcohol is an enzyme inducer.
4. It enhances hypoglycemic effect of insulin and sulfonylureas.

Uses

1. As antiseptic (in bedsores), in fever, as appetite stimulant.

2. In neuralgias.
3. In methanol poisoning.

Acute Alcohol Poisoning

Treatment measures include gastric lavage, airway maintenance, positive pressure ventilation and maintenance of fluid and electrolyte balance. Haemodialysis is needed in severe intoxication.

Chronic alcoholism causes dependence, Wernicke's encephalopathy, Korsakoff's psychosis, tremors, cirrhosis of liver hypertension and cardiomyopathy. Nutritional deficiencies such as polyneuritis, anaemia and pellagra can occur. Alcohol is teratogenic. It can produce 'fetal alcohol syndrome' with manifestations like mental retardation, microcephaly, growth retardation and facial anomalies in the foetus. Children are more susceptible to infection.

Treatment of Chronic Alcoholism

Disufiram inhibits the enzyme aldehyde dehydrogenase. If alcohol is consumed after taking disulfiram, acetaldehyde accumulates and within few minutes it can produce flushing, throbbing headache, nausea, vomiting, sweating, hypotension and confusion called the antabuse reaction.

Orally effective opioid antagonists **naltrexone** and **nalmefene** reduce the urge and craving to drink and are recommended as adjuvant to other measures. **Ondansetron**, a 5-HT_3 antagonist, antiemetic has been shown to reduce alcohol consumption and is being evaluated for use. **Benzodiazepines** reduce the symptoms like anxiety and insomnia. **Clonidine** an $alpha_2$ agonist also reduces symptoms of sympathetic overactivity like tremors and tachycardia. **Acamprosate** an antagonist of NMDA receptor is also found to prevent relapse of heavy drinking. Topiramate, decreases dopamine release and causes improvement.

Methyl Alcohol

Ingestion of methanol results in methanol poisoning. Methanol is converted to formaldehyde which is catalyzed by alcohol dehydrogenase; formaldehyde is converted to formic acid by the action of aldehyde dehydrogenase. Toxic effects are due to formic acid.

Manifestations of toxicity are vomiting, headache, vertigo, severe abdominal pain, hypotension, delirium, acidosis and coma. Formic acid has affinity for optic nerve and causes retinal damage resulting in blindness.

Treatment

1. Protect eyes.
2. Gastric lavage.
3. BP and ventilation should be maintained, correction of acidosis by sodium carbonate.
4. Ethyl alcohol should be given immediately. It competes with methanol for alcohol dehydrogenase. Thus slows the metabolism of methanol and prevents the formation of toxic metabolites.
5. Antidote: Formepizole specifically inhibits the enzyme alcohol dehydrogenase and thereby prevents the formation of toxic metabolites, *e.g.*, formaldehyde and formic acid.
6. Haemodialysis, folate therapy.

ANTI-EPILEPTIC DRUGS

Epilepsy is a common neurological abnormality that affects about 0.5–1% of the population. Epilepsy is a chronic disorder characterized by recurrent occasional, sudden rapid discharge of grey matter. Seizures often accompanied by episodes of unconsciousness and/or amnesia.

Seizure indicates paroxysmal, abnormal discharge at high frequency which cause transient alteration in behavior because of disordered firing of groups of brain neurons. **Convulsions** are involuntary violent, and spasmodic or prolonged contraction of skeletal muscles.

Seizures have been classified into:

(A) **Generalized seizures** which are further divided into:

a. Grandmal seizures (Tonic-clonic convulsion).
b. Petitmal seizures.
c. Myoclonic seizures.
d. Atonic seizures.
e. Clonic seizures.
f. Tonic seizures.

(B) **Partial seizures** account for about 60% of all epilepsies. Partial seizures are divided into:

a. Simple partial seizures (Jacksonian epilepsy).
b. Complex partial seizures.
c. Secondary generalized seizures.
d. Status epilepticus.

Etiology of Seizures and Epilepsy

The normal brain contains billions of neurons which fire asynchronously due to inhibitory mechanism. When this inhibitory mechanism is defective, a large number of cells in the given area of the brain fires at the same time and produce a self regenerating electrical impulse, which become an epileptic focus. Epilepsy can be due to imbalance or defect in:

a. Na^+ or Ca^+ ion conductance.
b. Inhibiting GABA neuronal circuit, *i.e.*, defect in GABA transmission.
c. Excitatory mechanism involving NMDA channels.

Mechanism of Action of Anti-Epileptic Drugs

Anti-epileptic drug may act by one or more of the following mechanisms:

- Blockade of Na^+ channels and prolongation of their inactive state, delaying their recovery, *e.g.*, phenytoin, carbamazepine, lamotrigine, valproate.
- Blockade of low threshold Ca^{++} current in the thalamic neurons, controls absence seizures, *e.g.*, ethosuccimide.
- Enhancing GABA mediated inhibition:
  - By acting on GABA receptors, *e.g.*, benzodiazepines.
  - By inhibiting GABA metabolism, *e.g.*, valproic acid, vigabatrin.
  - By blocking excitatory glutamate receptors, *e.g.*, topiramate.
  - Blockade of NMDA and AMPA receptors, *e.g.*, felbamate, phenobarbitone, valproate etc.

Classification

1. **Hydantoins:** Phenytoin, Mephenytoin, Fosphenytoin.
2. **Barbiturates:** Phenobarbitone, Mephobarbitone, Primadone.
3. **Iminostilbene:** Carbamazepine, Oxycarbazepine.
4. **Succinimide:** Ethosuccimide.
5. **GABA transaminase inhibitors:** Valproic acid, Vigabatrin.
6. **Benzodiazepines:** Diazepam, Clonazepam, Lorazepam, Clorazepate, Clobazam.

Newer Agents

1. **GABA analogues:** Gabapentin, Vigabatrin, Tiagabine, Pregabolin.
2. **Others:** Lamotrigine, Levetiracetam, Felbamate, Topiramate, Zonisamide.

Phenytoin

Pharmacological Actions

CNS: Phenytoin has good antiseizure activity and is one of the most effective drugs against generalised tonic-clonic seizures and partial seizures.

It causes blockade of the voltage dependent sodium channels and stabilizes the neuronal membrane. It inhibits the generation of repetitive action potentials.

Phenytoin blocks the Na^+ channels which are in an inactivated state and delay the recovery of these channels from inactivation. Phenytoin preferentially blocks high frequency firing state. At higher doses, it also reduces the influx of Ca^{2+}, and facilitates GABA action and inhibits glutamate activity.

Pharmacokinetics

Oral absorption is slow but complete. Phenytoin is 90% bound to plasma proteins. It is metabolized in the liver initially by first order and later by zero order kinetics as the dose increases. Therefore, monitoring of plasma concentration is useful.

Adverse Effects

1. GIT: Nausea, vomiting, epigastric pain, anorexia.
2. Nystagmus, diplopia, ataxia, blurred vision are common.
3. Gingival hyperplasia.
4. Peripheral neuropathy.
5. Endocrine: It causes hirsutism, acne, coarsening of facial features, hyperglycaemia decrease release of ADH, osteomalacia, hypocalcaemia (due to altered metabolism of vitamin D and inhibition of intestinal absorption of Ca^{2+}).
6. Hypersensitivity rashes, hepatic necrosis.
7. Megaloblastic anaemia because phenytoin decreases absorption and increase excretion of folate (folic acid).
8. Teratogenicity phenytoin produces foetal hydantoin syndrome characterized by hypoplastic phalanges, cleft palate, harelip and microcephaly in the offspring.
9. In toxic doses cerebellar and vestibular effects are prominent; followed by drowsiness, delirium, confusion, hallucinations, altered behavior and coma.

Uses

1. Generalized tonic-clonic seizures and partial seizures.
2. Status epilepticus.
3. Trigeminal neuralgia (an alternative to carbamazepine).
4. Cardiac arrhythmias.
5. To enhance wound healing.

Drug Interactions

1. Phenytoin is an enzyme inducer. Given with phenobarbitone and carbamazepine, they enhance each other's metabolism. It also increases the metabolism of corticosteroid, OCP, rifampicin, tetracycline etc.
2. Valproate displaces protein bound phenytoin and may result in phenytoin toxicity.
3. Cimetidine and chloramphenicol inhibit the metabolism of phenytoin resulting in toxicity.
4. Antacids decrease absorption of phenytoin.

Phenobarbitone

It remains one of the widely used drugs. Phenobarbitone has specific antiepileptic activity and raises the seizure threshold. Primidone which is rarely used now is metabolised to phenobarbitone. Phenobarbitone is effective in tonic-clonic seizures and is ineffective in absence seizures.

Mechanism of Action: Barbiturates:

1. Enhance the inhibitory neurotransmission in the CNS by enhancing the activation of $GABA_A$ receptors and thus facilitating the $GABA_A$ mediated opening of chloride ion channels.
2. Inhibit glutamate mediated excitatory effect through AMPA receptor blockade.
3. At higher doses they block L-type of Ca^{+2} channels.

Pharmacokinetics: Oral absorption of phenobarbitone is slow but complete. About 50% is bound to plasma proteins. It is enzyme inducer.

Sedation is the most common side effect. Tolerance develops to some extent, allergic reaction, confusion, irritability, megaloblastic anaemia may occur.

Carbamazepine

Carbamazepine is a tricyclic compound closely related to imipramine.

Carbamazepine has good antiseizure activity. Its mechanism of action and antiepileptic actions are similar to phenytoin, *i.e.*, it blocks sodium channels, modifies maximal electro shock (MES) seizures and raises threshold to PTZ and inhibits kindling.

Carbamazepine is also useful in the treatment of trigeminal neuralgia and beneficial in mood disorders. Carbamazepine has mild anti-diuretic effects.

Adverse Effects

Drowsiness, vertigo, ataxia, diplopia, blurring of vision, nausea, vomiting and dizziness are common. It also causes water retention due to anti-diuretic effects. Hematological toxicity includes leucopenia, thrombocytopenia and rarely agranulocytosis and aplastic anaemia. It is a teratogenic drug and cause finger nail hypoplasia, craniofacial defects and delayed development of fetus. It is also enzyme inducer.

Uses

1. Generalized tonic-clonic seizures (grandmal epilepsy). Simple and complex partial seizures.
2. Trigeminal neuralgia and glosso-pharyngeal neuralgia.
3. In chronic neuronathic pain, *e.g.*, diabetic pain, post herpetic pain.
4. Bipolar mood disorder.

Oxcarbazepine is similar to carbamazepine in action and uses. It has fewer hypersensitivity reactions, mild inducer of microsomal enzymes as compare to carbamazepine.

Ethosuccimide (Ethosuximide)

Ethosuccimide reduces the low threshold calcium currents in the thalamic neurons. These T currents are thought to be responsible for absence seizures. It raises seizure threshold.

Absorption is complete on administration of oral dosage forms. It is metabolized in the liver. The most common adverse effects are nausea, vomiting, epigastric pain, gastric irritation and anorexia. CNS effects like drowsiness, fatigue, lethargy, euphoria, dizziness, headache and hiccough are dose related adverse effects.

Ethosuccimide is the drug of choice for absence seizures. It can be used in myoclonic spasm and akinetic epilepsy.

Valproic Acid

Valproic acid is useful in many types of epilepsies including absence seizures, partial and generalized tonic-clonic seizures.

Mechanism of Action

It acts through several mechanisms:

1. It enhances the level of GABA by:
   - Increasing the synthesis of GABA.
   - By increased activity of GABA synthetase enzyme; and
   - Decreasing the metabolism of GABA by inhibiting GABA transaminase enzyme.
2. Like phenytoin, valproic acid blocks the sodium channels, causing prolonged recovery from inactivation.
3. Like ethosuccimide, valproate decreases low threshold Ca^{++} (T currents) current in the thalamus.
4. It activates glutamate decarboxylase.
5. Decrease the release of aspartate in the brain.

Adverse Effects

Gastrointestinal symptoms like nausea, vomiting, epigastric distress occur initially. Tremors, sedation, ataxia, rashes, alopecia, increase appetite and weight gain are rare. Fulminate hepatitis though rare can be fatal. Valproic acid is teratogenic; it can cause neural tube defects including spina bifida.

It is useful in partial and generalized seizures. Valproic acid is particularly useful in absence seizures. In patients with both absence seizures and generalized tonic-clonic attacks, valproate is the drug of choice. It is also used in cluster headache and tardive dyskinesia.

Valproate is also useful as a mood stabilizer in bipolar mood disorder when lithium is not effective. It can be used in trigeminal neuralgia (as an alternative to carbamazepine).

Benzodiazepine

Diazepam is the drug of choice in status epilepticus. Clonazepam is a potent anti-epileptic useful in absence and myoclonic seizures. Clobazam causes less sedation and is effective in most types of epilepsies and used as an adjuvant to other antiepileptic drugs.

Newer Anti-Epileptic

Gabapentin, vigabatrin, tiagabine, lamotrigine, levetiracetam, topiramate, felbamate, zonisamide, all are generally well tolerated newer drugs, except felbamate which can rarely cause aplastic anaemia and hepatitis. Presently they are recommended as add on drugs in refractory cases.

Gabapentin is a highly soluble analogue of GABA. It crosses BBB and increases the synthesis and release of GABA, thus increase its concentration in the brain. It is well tolerated. It does not influence the plasma concentrations of other anti-epileptics. It is neither metabolized nor bound to plasma proteins.

It is also used in migraine, neuropathic pain and in bipolar mood disorder.

Lamotrigine has a broad spectrum of antiepileptic activity. It inhibits the sodium channels and also inhibits the release of the excitatory amino acids like glutamate. It is used either alone or with other drugs in partial and generalized seizures, in myoclonic seizures.

Vigabatrin acts by irreversibly inhibiting the enzyme GABA transaminase thereby raising brain GABA levels. It should not be used in cases of absence seizure or myoclonic seizures and in patients with pre-existing visual field defects.

Levetiracetam: It can be used as an add on drug in refractory partial seizures.

Tiagabine, inhibits the reuptake of GABA into neurons and thereby enhances extracellular GABA levels, primarily used for partial complex seizures.

Topiramate a monosaccharide acts by multiple mechanisms. It blocks the sodium channels, enhances $GABA_A$ receptor currents and blocks AMPA receptors (glutamate receptor). It is effective in partial and generalized seizures.

Felbamate, an analogue of meprobamate is found to have good antiepileptic action. It blocks the NMDA receptors in addition to weak sodium channel blocking effect.

Zonisamide is a sulfonamide derivative, acts by inhibiting T type Ca^{++} currents and also by blocking Na^{+} channels. It is well tolerated and is indicated in refractory partial seizures. It has good bioavailability.

Therapeutic spectrum of various drugs

Type of seizures	First drug	Alternative therapy
(A) Generalized seizures		
a. Grand mal seizures	Carbamazepine, Phenobarbitone, Phenytoin, Valproic acid	Primadone
b. Petit mal seizures	Ethosuccemide, Lamotrigine	Clonazepam valproate
c. Atonic	Valproic acid, Lamotrigine	Clonazepam, Clobazem
d. Myoclonic	Valproic acid, Lamotrigine	Clonazepam, Levetiracetam
e. Clonic	Valproic acid, Lamotrigine	
f. Tonic	Valproic acid, Lamotrigine	
(B) Partial seizures		
a. Simple partial	Carbamazepine, Valproic acid, Phenytoin, Phenobarbitone	Levetiracetam, Gabapentin, Tiagabin
b. Complex partial	Carbamazepine, Valproic acid, Phenytoin, Phenobarbitone	Gabapentin, Lamotrigine
c. Secondary generalized	Valproic acid, Phenytoin, Phenobarbitone	Carbamazepine, Gabapentin
(C) Unclassified		
a. Infantile spasm	BZD, Vigabatrin	Glucocorticoids
b. Febrile seizure	Midazolam (rectal), Diazepam	Phenobarbitone (for prophylaxis)
(D) Epilepsy in pregnancy	Phenobarbitone	Magnesium sulphate in PET

Status Epilepticus (Treatment)

1. Lorazepam or clonazepam or diazepam IV. If not respond.
2. Phenytoin or phenobarbitone (IV/IM/IVslow infusion).
3. In refractory cases – General anaesthesia, *e.g.*, thiopental sodium or propofol.

Drugs used in Psychiatric Disorders

Psychiatric conditions are broadly divided into psychoses, neuroses and personality disorders. Psychoses are the more severe psychiatric disorders of the three and involve a marked impairment of behavior, inability to think coherently and to comprehend reality. Psychoses could be due to:

(i) An organic cause when there is a definable toxic, metabolic or pathological changes, following head injury.

(ii) Functional or idiopathic disorders like in schizophrenia, paranoia and affective disorders.

Schizophrenia: It has a strong hereditary tendency and is characterized by delusions, hallucinations, irrational conclusions, interpretations and withdrawal from social contacts. Negative symptoms include poor concentration, lack of initiative and energy. Overactivity of the neurotransmitters mainly dopamine and probably others including glutamate and 5-HT may be the cause.

Neuroses are the milder forms of psychiatric disorders and include anxiety, mood changes, panic disorders, obsessions, irrational fears and reactive depression. Personality disorders include paranoid, schizoid, histrionic, avoidant, antisocial and obsessive compulsive personality types.

ANTI-PSYCHOTIC DRUGS (NEUROLEPTICS)

Classification

1. **Classical/typical neuroleptics:**
   a. *Phenothiazines:* Chlorpromazine, Triflupromazine, Thioridazine, Mesoridazine, Trifluoperazine, Fluphenazine.
   b. *Butyrophenones:* Haloperidol, Droperidol, Trifluperidol, Penfluridol.
   c. *Thioxanthenes:* Thiothixene, Chlorprothixene, Flupenthixol, Zuclopenthixol.
2. **Atypical neuroleptics:** Clozapine, Olanzapine, Risperidone, Quetiapine, Ziprasidone, Amisulpride, Remoxipride, Aripiparazole.
3. **Miscellaneous:** Reserpine, Pimozide, Loxapine.

Chlorpromazine (CPZ)

It is a typical neuroleptics act by blocking the dopamine D_2 receptors in the CNS. Since dopaminergic overactivity, mainly in the limbic area, is thought to be responsible for schizophrenia, DA (D_2) receptor blockade helps. Phenothiazines also block D_1, D_3 and D_4 receptors.

Pharmacological Actions

1. **CNS:** In normal subjects CPZ reduces motor activity, produces drowsiness and indifference to surroundings. In psychotic agitated patients, it reduces aggression, initiative and motor

activity, relieves anxiety and brings about emotional quietening and drowsiness. It normalizes the sleep disturbances characteristic of psychoses. Other CNS actions are:

1. CPZ lowers seizure threshold and can precipitate convulsions in untreated epileptics.
2. CPZ decreases gonadotropin secretion and may result in amenorrhea in women. It increases the secretion of prolactin resulting in galactorrhoea and gynaecomastia in males.
3. CPZ acts as a dopamine antagonist and therefore results in extra pyramidal motor symptoms.
4. Vasomotor reflexes are depressed leading to a fall in BP.
5. Neuroleptics block the dopamine (DA) receptors in the CTZ and thereby act as anti-emetics.

2. Autonomic nervous system: Actions on the ANS are complex. Anti-cholinergic properties leads to side effects like dryness of mouth, blurred vision, reduced sweating decreased gastric motility, constipation and urinary retention.
It also produces orthostatic hypotension due to alpha blockade action and reflex tachycardia. CPZ also has a direct myocardial depressant effect like quinidine.

3. CPZ has local anaesthetic properties but is not used for the purpose since it is irritant.

4. Kidney: CPZ depresses ADH secretion and has weak diuretic effects.

Tolerance develops to the sedative and hypotensive actions while no tolerance is seen to the antipsychotic actions.

Pharmacokinetic: CPZ is incompletely absorbed following oral administration and also undergoes significant first pass metabolism. It is highly lipophilic, extensively protein bound and crosses BBB and placenta freely, have long plasma half life.

Adverse Reactions

Anti-psychotics have a high therapeutic index and are fairly safe drugs. Common adverse effects are:

1. Cardiovascular and autonomic effects include postural hypotension, palpitation, blurred vision, dry mouth, constipation, nasal stuffiness and urinary retention (due to blockade of alpha adrenergic and muscarinic receptors) and prolongation of Q.T. interval (dose dependent).

2. *CNS effects:* Drowsiness and mental confusion are common, extra pyramidal syndrome (EPS) is the most troublesome side effects and includes, Acute dystonia, Parkinsonism, Perioral tremors, Akathesia, Tardive dyskinesia and Malignant neuroleptic syndrome.
3. *Endocrine disturbances:* Gynaecomastia, amenorrhoea and galactorrhoea due to DA receptor blockade and increase in prolactin levels.
4. Hyperglycemia.
5. Ocular toxicity due to granular deposits in the cornea and lens.

Drug Interactions

Neuroleptics enhance the sedative effects of CNS depressants, alpha blockers and of anticholinergic drugs. Neuroleptics antagonize the actions of dopamine agonists and levodopa.

Uses

1. **Psychiatric conditions** psychoses including schizophrenia and organic brain syndromes like delirium and dementia all respond to anti-psychotics.
2. **Nausea, vomiting** CPZ is a good anti-emetic.
3. **Hiccough** CPZ can control intractable hiccough.
4. **Neuroleptics** are useful in the treatment of several syndromes with psychiatric features like psychoses associated with chronic alcoholism, Huntington's disease and Tourette's syndrome.

Atypical Antipsychotics

The newer atypical antipsychotics like clozapine and others are weak D_2 blocking and potent 5-HT_2 antagonist activity and have the following advantages:

1. Causing fewer side effects like less sedation by unique receptor affinity.
2. Effective in suppressing both positive and negative symptoms of schizophrenia.
3. Effective in resistant cases of psychoses.
4. Less liability to induce EPS.

Clozapine: It blocks the dopamine D_1 and D_4, receptors but has low affinity for D_2 receptors. It also blocks 5-HT_2, adrenergic and muscarinic receptors. Clozapine has the following advantages over of conventional antipsychotics.

1. Very low incidence of EPS.
2. Sedation is low.
3. No endocrine side effects (no galactorrhoea and gynaecomastia).
4. It is effective in patients not responding to conventional antipsychotics.

The most important disadvantage with clozapine is that it may cause agranulocytosis in some patients, which can be fatal.

Olanzapine is similar to clozapine except that, olanzapine does not cause agranulocytosis.

Risperidone blocks serotonin (5-HT_{2A}) and dopamine (D_2) receptors. It is effective against both positive and negative symptoms of schizophrenia. It causes no EPS and sedation.

ANTI-ANXIETY DRUGS

Anxiety is tension or apprehension which is a normal response to certain situations in life.

Classification of Anti-Anxiety Drugs

1. **Benzodiazepines:** Lorazepam, Alprazolam etc.
2. **5-HT agonist antagonists:** Buspirone, Gepirone, Ipsapirone.
3. **Beta blockers:** Propranolol.
4. **Others:** Meprobamate, Hydroxyzine.

Benzodiazepines are already discussed earlier.

Buspirone is an azapirone with good anxiolytic properties. It is a selective 5-HT_{1A} partial agonist. 5-HT_{1A}', receptors are inhibitory auto receptors and binding of buspirone inhibits the release of 5-HT. Buspirone is also a weak D_2 antagonist. It is useful in mild to moderate anxiety.

Unlike diazepam, it is not a muscle relaxant, not an anti-convulsant, does not produce significant sedation, tolerance or dependence, does not modify GABAergic transmission and is not useful in panic attacks.

Buspirone is particularly beneficial when sedation is to be avoided. ipsapirone and gepirone are similar to buspirone.

Beta blockers: In patients with prominent autonomic symptoms of anxiety like tremors, palpitation and hypertension propranolol may be useful.

ANTI-DEPRESSANT DRUGS

Affective disorders are a group of psychoses associated with changes of mood, *i.e.*, depression and mania.

Depression could be:

1. **Unipolar**
   a. Endogenous depression is major depression and results from a biochemical abnormality in the brain. Deficiency of monoamine (NA, 5-HT) activity in the CNS is thought to be responsible for endogenous depression.
   b. Reactive depression is due to stressful and distressing circumstances in life.
2. **Bipolar mood disorder or manic depressive illness.**

Classification of Antidepressant Drugs

1. **Tricyclic antidepressants (TCAs):** Imipramine, Desipramine, Clomipramine, Amitriptyline, Nortriptyline, Doxepin.
2. **Selective serotonin reuptake inhibitors (SSRI):** Fluoxetine, Fluvoxamine, Paroxetine, Citalopram, Sertraline, Escitalopram.
3. **Monoamine oxidase inhibitors (MAOI):** Phenelzine, Tranylcypromine, Isocarboxazid, Moclobemide, Clorgyline, Selegeline.
4. **Atypical antidepressants:** Trazodone, Nefazodone, Venlafaxine, Bupropion, Mianserine, Mirtazapine, Reboxetine.

Tricyclic Antidepressants (TCAs)

Pharmacological Actions

1. In normal subjects, TCA cause dizziness, drowsiness, confusion and difficulty in thinking. In depressed patients, patient shows more interest in the surroundings and the sleep pattern becomes normal.
2. *CVS:* Postural hypotension and tachycardia (due to blockade of alpha adrenergic and muscarinic receptors) can be severe in over-dosage.
3. *ANS:* TCAs have anticholinergic properties and cause dry mouth, blurred vision, constipation and urinary retention.

TCAs block the reuptake of amines (norepinephrine or 5-HT) into the pre synaptic terminal and thereby prolong their action on the receptors. Thus they potentiate amine neurotransmission in the CNS. On prolonged administration accumulation can cause cumulative toxicity.

Adverse Effects

Sedation, postural hypotension, tachycardia, sweating and anticholinergic side effects like dry mouth, constipation, blurred vision and urinary retention are relatively common. They lowered seizure threshold.

Acute toxicity is manifested as delirium; excitement, hypotension, convulsions, fever, arrhythmias, respiratory depression and coma (mimic symptoms of atropine poisoning). Physostigmine is given to overcome atropine like effects; sodium bicarbonate for acidosis, phenytoin for seizures and arrhythmias and diazepam to control convulsions.

TCAs should be gradually withdrawn, because withdrawal symptoms like headache, anxiety and chills can occur due to physical dependence.

Drug Interactions

1. Tricyclics potentiate sympathomimetics even small amounts of adrenaline used with local anaesthetics can cause serious hypertension.
2. Highly protein bound drugs like phenytoin, aspirin and phenylbutazone displace TCAs from binding sites resulting in toxicity.
3. TCAs potentiate the effects of alcohol and other CNS depressants.

Selective Serotonin Reuptake Inhibitors (SSRIs) (Fluoxetine, Fluvoxamine, Paroxetine Citalopram and Sertraline)

Mechanism of Action

SSRIs blocks the reuptake of serotonin into the serotonergic nerve endings. Hence they enhance serotonin levels in these synapses. SSRIs have the following advantages over TCAs:

- Low cardiovascular side effects.
- Anticholinergic side effects are negligible, preferred in elderly because of low anticholinergic effects.
- Less sedation.
- Safer in overdose.
- Due to low side effect profile, SSRIs are generally well tolerated and accepted by patients.

Adverse effects to SSRIs include nausea, vomiting, insomnia, anxiety and sexual dysfunction.

Among the SSRIs, fluoxetine is the most commonly used.

MAO Inhibitors

Monoamine oxidase (MAO) is an enzyme which metabolizes NA, 5-HT and DA. Drugs which inhibit this enzyme enhance the neuronal levels of NA, DA and 5-HT. MAO exists as two isoenzymes – MAO-A and MAO-B, MAO-A is selective for 5-HT. Reversible and selective MAO-A inhibitors like moclobemide are now developed. Nonselective and irreversible MAO inhibitors phenelzine and tranylcypromine are associated with several side effects and risk of many food-drug interactions, so not used nowadays.

Tranylcypromine and Phenelzine

- Irreversibly inhibit the enzyme MAO and enhance neuronal levels of norepinephrine, dopamine and 5-HT.
- Antidepressant actions develop slowly over weeks of treatment.
- Most of them are long acting and require 12 weeks for recovery of MAO activity after stopping the drug.
- Side effects are hypotension, weight gain, restlessness, insomnia (due to CNS stimulation), anticholinergic effects and rarely liver dysfunction.
- They interact with many drugs and food.
- Patients on MAO inhibitors taking tyramine containing foods like cheese, beer, wine, yeast, buttermilk and fish–develop severe hypertension and is known as 'cheese reaction'. Tyramine is normally metabolized by MAO in the gut wall. On inhibition of MAO by drugs, tyramine escapes metabolism and displaces NA from nerve endings leading to hypertension.

Moclobemide is a reversible, competitive, selective MAO- A inhibitor. It is short acting and MAO activity recovers within 1–2 days after stopping the drug and has the advantages that it is not a sedative, does not produce cardiovascular and anticholinergic side effects. No significant drug interactions are seen.

Moclobemide is used in mild to moderate depression as an alternative to TCA.

Atypical Antidepressants

Trazodone, Bupropion, Mianserin, Nefazodone and Mirtazapine.

Advantages

- Fewer side effects particularly sedation and anticholinergic effects.
- Safer in overdose.
- Effective in patients not responding to TCA.

Trazodone is a weak serotonin reuptake inhibitor and lacks anticholinergic activity. It blocks H_1 and $alpha_1$ adrenergic receptors. It causes desensitization of $alpha_2$ receptors. It can cause postural hypotension and priapism due to its blocking effects.

Nefazodone blocks serotonin reuptake and is an effective antidepressant. Nefazodone is used in the prophylaxis of recurrent depression.

Venlafaxine: It inhibits the uptake of norepinephrine in addition to 5-HT (serotonin and norepinephrine reuptake inhibitor SNRI). It is thought to be faster acting and may be useful in patients not responding to other antidepressants. It does not interact with cholinergic, adrenergic or histamine receptors, so no side effects.

Mirtazapine blocks $5\text{-}HT_2$, $5\text{-}HT_3$, and $alpha_2$ auto-receptors and enhances the release of NA and 5-HT. It is faster acting.

Bupropion is a weak DA reuptake inhibitor and has CNS stimulant effects. Bupropion is also used to help to stop smoking (along with nicotine patch).

Uses of Antidepressants

1. Endogenous depression.
2. Panic attacks.
3. Obsessive compulsive disorders.
4. Nocturnal enuresis.
5. Psychosomatic disorders.
6. **Other indications:** Attention deficit hyperactivity disorder, chronic pain and chronic alcoholism may result in depression so antidepressants are tried.

MOOD STABILIZERS

Mood stabilizers control the mood swings that are seen in bipolar mood disorders. These include:

Lithium, Sodium valproate, Carbamazepine, Lamotrigine, Gabapentin.

Lithium: Lithium is a monovalent cation and has been used for several decades but several anti epileptics like carbamazepine, valproic acid and gabapentin are now being tried.

Mechanism of action of lithium is complex. It is thought that lithium blocks the formation of inositol from IP_3 and thereby inhibits the regeneration of phosphotidyl inositol (PI). Depletion of membrane phosphotidyl inositol results in inhibition of receptor mediated effects through IP_3 and DAG.

Lithium is a small ion and mimics the role of sodium in excitable tissues. It partly replaces body Na^+ and equally distributed in all tissue. Thus, alter a variety of physiological processes linked to the functioning of Na^+/K^+ ATPase and inhibit Ca^{++} dependent biochemical phenomenon. It may also increase 5-HT release and post synaptic activity, neuronal uptake and storage of catecholamine.

Lithium is secreted in sweat, saliva and breast milk. Since safety margin is narrow, plasma lithium concentration needs to be monitored. 0.5–1m Eq/L is the therapeutic plasma concentration and >1.5 m Eq/lit can cause toxicity.

Nausea, vomiting, mild diarrhoea, thirst and polyuria occur initially in most patients. Weight gain can also occur. As the plasma concentration raises, hypothyroidism, CNS effects like coarse tremors, drowsiness, giddiness, confusion, ataxia, blurred vision and nystagmus are seen. In overdosage, delirium, muscle twitching, convulsions, arrhythmias and renal failure develop. Prolonged use causes diabetes insipidus.

(On prophylactic use in bipolar mood disorder, lithium acts as a mood stabilizer. It prevents swings of mood and thus reduces both the depressive and manic phases of the illness.)

Precautions

1. Minimum effective dose should be used.
2. Patients should always use the same formulation.
3. Patients should be made aware of the first symptom of toxicity.
4. Lithium is contraindicated in pregnancy.

Drug Interactions

1. Diuretics enhance sodium loss and lithium absorption from the kidney. This increases plasma lithium levels resulting in toxicity.
2. NSAIDs reduce lithium elimination and enhance toxicity.

Uses

1. Prophylaxis of bipolar mood disorder.
2. Acute mania.
3. Depression.
4. Cancer chemotherapy induced leucopenia and agranulocytosis.
5. Other uses: Lithium is tried in recurrent neuropsychiatric disorders, childhood mood disorders, hyperthyroidism and inappropriate ADH secretion syndrome.

Carbamezipine, sodium valproate, clonazepam, verapamil, clonidine can be used in manic disorders.

CNS STIMULANTS

Drugs that have a predominantly stimulant effect on the CNS may be broadly divided into:

1. **Respiratory stimulants:** Doxapram, Nikethamide.
2. **Psychomotor stimulants:** Amphetamine, Cocaine, Methylxanthines.
3. **Convulsants:** Leptazol, Strychnine, Picrotoxin, Bicuculline.

Respiratory stimulants are also called analeptics. These drugs stimulate respiration and are sometimes used to treat respiratory failure. They have a low safety margin and may produce convulsions.

Doxapram appears to act mainly on the brainstem and spinal cord and increase the activity of respiratory and vasomotor centers.

Uses

1. Doxapram is occasionally used IV as an analeptic in acute respiratory failure.
2. Apnoea in premature infants not responding to theophylline.

Psychomotor stimulants: Amphetamine and dextro amphetamine are sympathomimetic drugs.

Cocaine is a CNS stimulant, produces euphoria and is a drug of abuse.

Methylxanthines: Caffeine, theophylline and theobromine are the naturally occurring xanthine alkaloids. The beverages like coffee contain caffeine; tea contains theophylline and caffeine; cocoa has caffeine and theobromine.

Nootropics

Nootropics are drugs that improve memory and cognition. They are also called cognition enhancers or cerebral activators.

Piracetam described as a 'nootropic agent' is thought to protect cerebral cortex from hypoxia and improve learning and memory. In higher doses it also inhibits platelet aggregation. Adverse effects include insomnia, weight gain, nervousness, depression and gastrointestinal disturbances.

Piracetam has been tried in dementia, myoclonus, stroke and other cerebrovascular accidents; alcoholism, behavioral disorders and learning problems in children and in vertigo. The beneficial effects in all these are not proved.

ANALGESICS

Pain is an unpleasant sensation associated with actual or potential tissue damage. Analgesics are drugs which relieves pain without loss of consciousness. They only afford symptomatic relief from pain without affecting the cause.

Analgesics can be divided into two groups:

A. Opioid analgesics.

B. Non-steroidal anti-inflammatory drugs.

OPIOID ANALGESICS

Opioid is the term used for drugs with morphine like actions.

Classification

1. **Agonists:**
   a. *Natural opium alkaloids:* Morphine, Codeine, Levorphanol, Diomorphine.
   b. *Synthetic opioid derivatives:* Pethidine, Fentanyl, Diphenoxylate*, Loperamide*, Dextropropoxyphene, Methadone, Tramadol, Ethoheptazine, Dextromethorphane (*devoid of analgesic activity).
   c. *Semi-synthetic derivatives:* Heroin, Oxymorphone, Pholcodeine.
2. **Antagonists:** Naloxone, Naltrexone, Nalmefene.
3. **Mixed agonist antagonists:** Pentazocoine, Nalbuphine, Butorphanol, Buprenorphine, Nalorphie, Levollorphan, Cyclazocine.

Chemically the opium alkaloids can be grouped into:

1. **The Phenanthrene group:** Morphine, Codeine, Thebaine.
2. **The Benzyl isoquinoline group:** Papaverine, Noscapine, Narcine.

Endogenous Opioid Peptides

There are 3 families of endogenous opioid peptides released in the body in response to pain. They are enkephalins, endorphins and the dynorphins. These opioid peptides act on opioid receptors and relieve pain. Endorphins are endogenous ligands for μ receptors. Dynorphins are endogenous ligands for k receptors while enkephalins bind with delta receptors.

Recently two more endogenous peptides are found:

1. Endomorphine which are released during stress and in anticipation of pain. These have affinity for μ receptors.
2. Nociceptin: They are orphanin receptor and have action opposite to "μ" (mu) receptors.

Opioid Receptors

Morphine and other opioids produce their effects by acting on specific opioid receptors, which are weekly distributed in the CNS and other tissues. They are mu (μ), kappa (k) and delta receptors. Most of the pharmacological effects of opioids including analgesia, sedation, euphoria, respiratory depression, miosis and constipation are mediated through μ receptors.

Mechanism of Action

All opioid receptors are G protein coupled receptors. Stimulation of these receptors inhibits adenylyl cyclase resulting in decreased intracellular cAMP formation (mainly through mu and delta receptors). They also facilitate the opening of K^+ channels leading to hyper polarization and inhibit the entry of calcium into the cell. In addition to this, they inhibit the opening of calcium channels (through 'k' receptors). All these result in a decrease in the intracellular calcium which, in turn, decreases the release of neurotransmitters. Details of receptor action are mentioned in following table:

Table 7.1

μ (mu) receptors	k (kappa)	Delta receptors
Analgesia (supra spinal and spinal) (μ_1 and μ_2)	Analgesia (spinal) k_3	Analgesia (spinal + affective component of supra spinal)
Respiratory depression (μ_2)	Respiratory depression	Respiratory depression
Sedation, euphoria	Dysphoria	Affective behavior
Miosis	Miosis	
Reduced gut motility (μ_2)	Reduced gut motility	Reduced gut motility
Affinity for morphine and endorphine	Affinity for ketacyclozocine	Affinity for enkephalin

Opioids also directly inhibit the transmission in the dorsal horn ascending pathway. Opioid receptors are abundant in these areas including the periaqueductal grey (PAG) area, substantia gelatinosa and the spinal cord. They decrease the release of substance P and glutamate from nociceptive terminals.

Pharmacological Actions

Morphine is the most important alkaloid of opium.

(A) Central Nervous System

1. **Analgesia:** Morphine is a potent analgesic and relieves pain in doses that usually does not cause motor in coordination and loss of consciousness (as alcohol and GA do). Dull aching visceral pain is relieved better than sharp pricking pain. But in higher doses it relieves even the severe pain as that of biliary colic. Morphine alters both the perception and reaction to pain. It raises the pain threshold and thus increases the capacity to tolerate pain. It alters the emotional reaction to pain. Analgesic action is mediated through 'μ' receptors. Euphoria and sedation also contribute to its analgesic effects.
2. **Euphoria, sedation and hypnosis:** Morphine produces a feeling of well-being termed euphoria. Rapid intravenous injection of morphine produces a warm flushing of the skin and an immensely pleasurable sensation in the lower abdomen lasting for about 45 seconds which is known as 'high', 'rush' or 'kick'. It also produces drowsiness, a calming effect, inability to concentrate, feeling of detachment and indifference to surroundings. Sometimes it causes dysphoria, restlessness, malaise and anxiety. It increases mono and polysynaptic response, without ataxia (in contrast to alcohol which also causes ataxia).
3. **Respiration:** Morphine produces significant respiratory depression. It directly depresses the respiratory centre in the brainstem. It depresses all phases of respiratory activity–rate and tidal volume. It may also alter the rhythm to produce irregular and periodic breathing.
   Morphine suppresses neurogenic, chemical and hypoxic drive directly proportional to its analgesic effect. The respiratory centre is insensitive to increased plasma CO_2 concentration. With toxic doses, breathing is maintained by hypoxic drive. No effect on other function controlled by medullary centre.
4. **Cough centre:** It directly depresses the cough centre.
5. **Nausea and emesis:** Morphine directly stimulates the CTZ in the medulla causing nausea and vomiting. In higher doses it depresses the vomiting centre and hence there is no vomiting in poisoning.

6. **Miosis:** Morphine produces miosis resulting in a characteristic pinpoint pupil in high doses due to stimulation of E.W. nucleus of the third cranial nerve. Tolerance does not develop with this effect.
7. **Vagal centre:** Morphine stimulates vagal centre causing bradycardia.
8. **Heat regulation:** Opioids shift the equilibrium point of heat regulating centre in the hypothalamus, so that body temperature falls slightly and causes hypothermia.
9. **Excitatory effect:** In high doses, opioids produce convulsions. They may increase the excitability of the spinal cord.
10. **Vasomotor centers:** Morphine depresses VMC and causes fall in BP.

(B) Cardiovascular System

CVS actions are usually minor in analgesic doses. In higher doses it causes depression of the vasomotor centre, inhibition of adrenergic tone centrally and releases histamine which contributing to postural hypotension and bradycardia. Increase PCO_2 levels causes cerebral vasodilatation and an increase in intracranial pressure.

(C) GIT

Opioids decrease the motility of the gut.

Esophageal reflux may increase. Gastric acid secretion is reduced, increase the tone of the antrum and first part of the duodenum which contribute to delay emptying by almost 12 hours and this can retard the absorption of orally given drugs.

Intestines

Morphine diminishes all intestinal secretions, delays digestion of food in the small intestine; resting tone is increased. Tone of the sphincters is increased leading to spasm. The intestinal motility (propulsive) is markedly diminished. The resulting delay in the passage of the intestinal contents in the large intestine, together with reduced secretions and inattention to the sensory stimuli for defecation reflex produce marked constipation (mediated through μ and delta receptors in the gut).

(D) Other Smooth Muscles

Biliary tract: Morphine causes spasm of the sphincter of Oddi.

Urinary bladder and ureter: Tone and amplitude of ureter is increased; with increased tone of external sphincter and volume of the bladder. Thus it inhibit urinary voiding reflex. All these result in urinary retention especially in the elderly male with prostatic hypertrophy.

No significant effect, on uterus is observed.

Morphine causes release of histamine from the mast cells and causes bronchoconstriction.

(E) Neuroendocrine Effects

Morphine acts on the hypothalamus to inhibit the release of gonadotrophin releasing hormone and CRF, thus decreasing blood levels of FSH, LH, ACTH and beta endorphins and increase the release of prolactin.

(F) Immune System

Morphine suppresses various immune function and increase susceptibility to infection.

(G) Skin

Morphine causes dilation of cutaneous blood vessels and cause flushing. It also causes urticaria due to release to histamine.

Pharmacokinetics

Given orally, absorption of morphine is slow and incomplete. Morphine undergoes extensive first pass metabolism. Bioavailability is 20 to 40%. Highly lipid soluble opioids are available as transdermal preparation.

Given subcutaneously, onset of action is in 15–20 min, peak effect occur in 1 hour, duration of action is 3–5 hours. Morphine is metabolized in the liver by glucuronide conjugation. The active metabolite morphine 6 glucuronide is more potent than morphine and have high affinity for μ receptors. It is excreted through the kidneys. Morphine undergoes enterohepatic circulation.

Adverse Effects

Morphine can produce a wide range of adverse effects like nausea, vomiting, dizziness, mental clouding, respiratory depression, constipation, dysphoria, urinary retention postural hypotension and bronchospasm.

Allergic reactions including skin rashes, pruritus urticaria and wheal at the site of injection may occur. Rarely intravenous injection can cause anaphylaxis.

Tolerance

Repeated administration of morphine, results in the development of tolerance (cellular adaptive type) to some of its effects including respiratory depression, analgesia, sedation, euphoria and other CNS depressant effects. Tolerance does not develop to miosis and constipation. Tolerance may develop due to long term desensitization or down regulation of receptor or due to return of neurotransmitters to normal level.

Dependence

Its ability to produce euphoria makes it a drug of addiction. Opioids produce both psychological and physical dependence. Sudden cessation of opioids produces significant withdrawal symptoms. The person craves for the drug. Withdrawal symptoms are generally not life-threatening and include pain, hyperventilation, coughing, mydriasis, hypertension, diarrhea, dysphoria agitation and piloerection.

Withdrawal symptoms in the newborn appear in babies born to mothers who were addicts prior to delivery. These are irritability, excessive crying, tremors, frantic suckling of fists, diarrhea, sneezing, yawning, vomiting and fever.

Management of Addiction

Morphine is slowly withdrawn over several days and substituted by oral methadone. The dose is adjusted as per the degree of dependence (1 mg methadone for every 4 mg of morphine). Methadone is then gradually withdrawn.

Symptoms like insomnia, malaise, restlessness, irritability, fatigue and GI hyperactivity may last upto several months. Clonidine a central $alpha_2$ agonist can suppress some of the autonomic withdrawal symptoms like anxiety, nausea, vomiting and diarrhea.

Acute Morphine Poisoning

Signs and symptoms include respiratory depression with shallow breathing, pinpoint pupils, hypotension, shock, cyanosis, flaccidity, stupor, hypothermia, coma and death due to respiratory failure and pulmonary edema.

Treatment

1. Positive pressure respiration.
2. Maintenance of BP.
3. Gastric lavage with potassium permagnate ($KMnO_4$) to remove unabsorbed drug.
4. Specific antidote is naloxone (0.4–0.8 mg IV repeated every 10–15 min).

Uses of Morphine

1. **Analgesic:** It is a most potent analgesic. It affords symptomatic relief of severe pain, *e.g.*, acute myocardial infarction, fractures, burns, pulmonary embolism, terminal stages of cancer, acute pericarditis, spontaneous pneumothorax and postoperative pain. Morphine is given with atropine to relieve renal and biliary colic. Epidural morphine can be used to produce epidural analgesia.
2. **As pre-anaesthetic medication:** It is not preferred as they have certain disadvantages, *e.g.*, depress respiration, induce vomiting, may interfere with pupillary response to anaesthesia and postoperative urinary retention and constipation may occur. Pethidine is preferred over morphine.
3. **Acute left ventricular failure:** Morphine is used to alleviate the dyspnoea of LVF and pulmonary edema. The relief may be due to:
   a. Peripheral vasodilatation and decreased TPR leading to shifting of blood from pulmonary to peripheral circulation, thereby reducing cardiac workload.
   b. Reduction in the work of the heart due to decreased fear and apprehension. Reduced anxiety decreases sympathetic stimulation which in turn decreases cardiac work.
   c. Alteration in the patient's reaction to impaired respiratory function.
4. **Diarrhea.**
5. **Cough.**

Precautions and Contraindications

1. Avoid in patients with respiratory insufficiency, COPD, bronchial asthma.
2. In extremes of age, elderly with BHP, hepatic disease.
3. Head injury: Morphine increases CSF pressure by retaining CO_2 and thereby increases the intracranial tension and vomiting, miosis and mental clouding seen with morphine interfere with diagnosis and assessment of progress in head injuries.
4. In hypovolaemic shock.
5. Hypothyroidism.
6. Undiagnosed acute abdomen (biliary colic).

Other Opioids

Heroin or diamorphine or diacetyl morphine is converted to morphine in the body. It has higher lipid solubility because of which euphoric effects are faster and greater resulting in higher abuse potential, so not used therapeutically.

Levorphanol is similar to morphine but it is longer acting.

Codeine is a naturally occurring opium alkaloid. Codeine depresses the cough centre in sub-analgesic doses.

Papaverine is devoid of opioid and analgesic activity.

Noscapine is a naturally occurring opium alkaloid. In therapeutic doses, it has no significant actions on the CNS except for anti-tussive effects. In large doses it may cause bronchoconstriction due to the release of histamine.

Dextromethorphan: It acts centrally to elevate the threshold for coughing for which it is as effective as codeine.

Tramadol is recently developed synthetic codeine analog. It is an effective centrally acting analgesic, but it is a weak opioid agonist. It inhibits reuptake of NA and 5-HT and thus activates monoaminergic spinal inhibition of pain. Respiratory depression is mild. It is a drug of dependence. It may precipitate seizures. It should be avoided in patients on MAO inhibitors. It is effective in mild to moderate pain.

Tramadol is used in acute and chronic pain, like postoperative pain and neuralgias.

Pethidine

It is chemically unrelated with morphine, it interacts with opioid receptors and its actions are blocked by naloxone.

When compared to morphine:

- Pethidine is 1/10th as potent as morphine and effective orally.
- The onset of action is more rapid and duration of action is shorter.
- It does not suppress cough effectively.
- It produces corneal anaesthesia.
- It is not a good antitussive.
- It is less constipating.
- It may cause dysphoria, it also has anticholinergic effects.
- In toxic doses, pethidine sometimes produces CNS stimulation with tremors, restlessness and convulsions instead of sedation.

- Retention of CO_2 produces cerebral vasodilatation and increase ICT.

Pethidine is used as an analgesic in visceral pain and also for other indications of morphine. Given during labour, pethidine produces less respiratory depression in the newborn. It does not interfere with uterine contractions and labour and is therefore preferred to morphine for obstetric analgesia. It is also used as pre-anaesthetic medication.

Fentanyl

- It is about 100 times more potent than morphine as an analgesic.
- Fentanyl is highly lipid soluble and fast acting, has mild effects on the cardiovascular system and slightly reduces HR and BP. Hence it is found to be safer than other opioids in cardiovascular surgeries. It is not a histamine liberator. It cause muscle rigidity, nausea, vomiting and respiratory depression.
- Unlike morphine, fentanyl does not increase the intracranial pressure.

Uses

1. Neuroleptanalgesia.
2. Epidural fentanyl is used for postoperative and obstetric analgesia.
3. Transdermal patches of fentanyl are available for use in cancer or other chronic pain.

Congeners of fentanyl are sufentanil, alfentanil and remifentanil. They are faster acting and recovery is rapid. They are used for short surgical procedures.

Methadone

It is a synthetic opioid and an effective analgesic. It is effective by oral route. It has a long duration of action. Methadone is about 90% bound to plasma proteins. After repeated administration, it gradually accumulate in tissues and then slowly released from these sites. This probably accounts for its milder withdrawal symptoms. It is used as substitution therapy for opioid dependence.

Dextropropoxyphene is a congener of methadone. It is less constipating, longer acting and has good oral efficacy. Large doses cause CNS stimulation. It also has abuse potential. It is used in mild to moderate pain, with paracetamol.

Mixed Agonist and Antagonists

(Pentazocine, cyclazocine, nalbuphine, buprenorphine, butorphanol and nalorphine)

Pentazocine: It is a k receptor agonist and μ receptor antagonist. Dysphoria can occur due to k receptor stimulation. Sedation and respiratory depression are less marked. Tolerance and dependence develop on repeated use.

Adverse effects include sedation, sweating, dizziness, nausea, dysphoria with anxiety, nightmares and hallucinations which are unpleasant. Biliary spasm and constipation are less severe. Pentazocine increases BP and heart rate and thereby increases cardiac work. It is therefore not suitable in MI. It is also not used in epileptics and patients with psychoses.

Pentazocine is a commonly used opioid analgesic especially in postoperative moderately severe pain and chronic pain.

Nalbuphine (μ-receptor moderate antagonist, k-receptor strong agonist)

Nalbuphine is an agonist antagonist, more potent than pentazocine. It is a good analgesic. Higher doses produce dysphoria. It causes less psychomimetic and cardiovascular effects. It can be used as obstetrical analgesic.

Buprenorphine (μ-receptor partial agonist, k-receptor antagonist)

Buprenorphine is a highly lipid soluble synthetic thebaine congener. It is a partial μ agonist, 25 times as potent as morphine. Though onset of action is slow, duration of analgesia is long. Respiratory depression is less marked. Its effects are not readily reversed by naloxone. It can be used as alternative to methadone for management of opioid withdrawal.

Uses: Chronic pain like in terminal cancer patients (available as sub-lingual preparations).

Nalorphine (μ-receptor antagonist, k-receptor agonist)

Nalorphine is also an agonist antagonist. At low doses, it is a good analgesic. But with increase in dose there is no increase in analgesia.

It causes dysphoria (k agonist) and respiratory depression not used nowadays.

Dezocine is a partial agonist at μ receptors. Its analgesic actions are similar to morphine but respiratory depression does not increase with an increase in dose (ceiling effect).

Opioid Antagonists

Naloxone: It acts as a competitive antagonist to all types of opioid receptors (more potent at μ receptors). It is a pure antagonist. In normal individuals, it does not produce any significant actions. But in opium poisoning, given IV, it promptly antagonizes all the actions of morphine including respiratory depression and sedation and precipitates withdrawal syndrome. It also blocks the action of endogenous opioid peptides. Given orally it undergoes first pass metabolism and is metabolized by the liver. Hence it is given intravenously.

Uses

1. Naloxone is the drug of choice for morphine over dosage (for nalorphine, pentazocine also).
2. It is also used to reverse neonatal asphyxia due to opioids used during labour.
3. It can also be used for the diagnosis of opioid dependence.
4. Naloxone has been found to be beneficial in reversing hypotension.
5. It also partially reverses alcohol intoxication.

Naltrexone

Naltrexone is another pure opioid antagonist. It is more potent than naloxone. It is orally effective and has a longer duration of action.

Naltrexone is used for "opioid blockade" therapy in post addicts so that even if the addicts take an opioid, they do not experience the pleasurable effects and therefore lose the craving. Alcohol craving is also reduced by naltrexone and is used to prevent relapse of heavy drinking.

Nalmefene is given IV and longer acting. It has better bioavailability and is not hepatotoxic. It is used in opioid overdosage.

NON-STEROIDAL ANTI-INFLAMMATORY DRUGS

Non-steroidal anti-inflammatory drugs have analgesic, anti-inflammatory antipyretic and uricosuric properties without addiction liability.

Classification

(A) Nonselective COX Inhibitors (reversible and irreversible inhibitor):

1. *Salicylic acid derivatives:* Aspirin, Sodium salicylate, Diflunisal.
2. *Pyrazolone derivatives:* Phenylbutazone, Azapropazone, Oxyphenbutazone.

3. *Indole acetic acid derivatives:* Indomethacin, Sulindoc.
4. *Aryl acetic acid derivatives:* Diclofenac, Ketorolac, Tolmetin.
5. *Propionic acid derivatives:* Ibuprofen, Fenoprofen, Naproxen, Ketoprofen, Flurbiprofen, Oxaprozin.
6. *Anthranilic acids (Fenamates):* Flufenamic acid, Mefenamic acid, Enfenamic acid, Meclofenamic acid.
7. *Oxicams:* Piroxicam, Tenoxicam, Meloxicam.

(B) Selective COX-2 Inhibitors: Celecoxib, Rofecoxib, Valdecoxib, Etodolac, Etoricoxib, Parecoxib.

(C) Preferential COX-2 Inhibitors (weak COX-1 inhibitor): Nimesulide, Nebumetone.

(D) Analgesic: Antipyretic with poor anti-inflammatory action – Paracetamol, Metamizol, Nefopam.

Another class of cyclo-oxygenase enzyme is also identified recently. Paracetamol is reported to be a selective COX-3 inhibitor. It has poor ability to inhibit COX-1 in the presence of peroxides, which are not produced in hypothalamus.

Mechanism of Action

During inflammation, arachidonic acid liberated from membrane phospholipids, is converted to prostaglandins (PGs). This is catalyzed by the enzyme cyclo-oxygenase (COX). These prostaglandins produce hyperalgesia, as they sensitize the nerve endings to pain (caused by mediators of inflammation like bradykinin and histamine) and lowering the threshold of response to stimuli.

There are two (three?) forms of cyclo-oxygenase enzymes *viz.*, COX-1 and COX-2. COX-1 is found in most of the normal cells (constitutive) and is involved in maintaining tissue homeostasis. COX-2 is induced in the inflammatory cells by cytokines and other mediators of inflammation.

NSAIDs inhibit the PG synthesis by inhibiting the enzyme cyclo-oxygenase.

Aspirin and its derivatives cause irreversible inhibition of COX-1 and COX-2. Anti-inflammatory action is mediated through inhibition of COX-2. Selective COX-2 inhibitors have 50 fold selectivity to COX-2 enzyme (with less selectivity are called preferential COX-2 inhibitors).

Salicylates

Aspirin is taken as prototype.

Pharmacological Actions

1. **Analgesia:** Aspirin inhibits PG synthesis and thereby acts as an analgesic. Pain originating from the integument structures like muscles, bones, joints and pain in connective tissues is relieved. But in vague visceral pain, aspirin is relatively ineffective. The pain is relieved without euphoria and hypnosis. No development of tolerance and dependence occur. It also relieves dysmenorrhoea by decreasing uterine PG levels to provide relief in myomatrium ischemia.
2. **Anti-pyretic action:** It reduces body temperature in fever, but do not cause hypothermia. In fever, pyrogens (IL, TNF-alpha, interferon etc.), circulates in the body and they increases the synthesis of PGE_2 in the hypothalamus, thereby raising its temperature set point. The thermostatic mechanism in the hypothalamus is thus disturbed. Aspirin inhibits PG synthesis in the hypothalamus and resets the thermostat at the normal level bringing down the temperature. Once the temperature returns to normal set point, sweating and cutaneous vasodilatation occur to reduce fever.
3. **Anti-inflammatory action:** At higher doses, aspirin acts as an anti-inflammatory agent. Signs of inflammation are all reduced or suppressed. But, the progression of the disease in rheumatoid arthritis, rheumatic fever or osteoarthritis is not affected. They do not depress the mediators like LTs, PAF and cytokines. Aspirin interferes with the formation of chemical mediators of the kallikrein system. Stabilization of leukocytes, decreases in the adherence of granulocyte to the damaged lysosomal membrane and antagonism of certain actions of kinin may be contributing to its anti-inflammatory action.
4. **Respiration:** In therapeutic doses salicylates increase consumption of oxygen by skeletal muscles and increase in CO_2 production. This increased CO_2 stimulates respiratory centre. Salicylates also directly stimulate the medullary respiratory centre. Both these actions increase the rate and depth of respiration. Plasma CO_2 is washed out leading to respiratory alkalosis. With toxic doses, the respiratory centre is depressed leading to respiratory failure.

5. **Acid base and electrolyte balance:** In anti-inflammatory doses, salicylates resulting in respiratory alkalosis; pH becomes alkaline. This is compensated by increased excretion of HCO_3^- in urine accompanied by Na^+, K^+ and water, pH then returns to normal. This stage is known as compensated respiratory alkalosis.

   With toxic doses, salicylates depress the respiratory centre directly. As a result, more CO_2 is accumulated. Thus plasma CO_2 rises and pH decreases. Since the concentration of HCO_3 is already low due to enhanced renal excretion, the change results in uncompensated respiratory acidosis. This is superimposed by metabolic acidosis caused by accumulation of acids.

   Toxic doses also depresses vasomotor centre, which impairs renal function resulting in an accumulation of strong acids of metabolic origin like lactic, pyruvic and acetoacetic acids.

   The above effects are accompanied by dehydration due to:
   - Water lost in urine with HCO_3^-, Na^+ and K^+.
   - Water lost during hyperventilation, increased sweating and hyperpyrexia (due to increased liberation of energy).

   Thus there is severe dehydration with acidosis.

6. **Metabolic effects:** Increased heat production, hyperpyrexia, increased protein catabolism with resultant amino-aciduria, negative nitrogen balance and mild hypoglycaemia is seen. But in toxic doses, hyperglycemia occurs due to central sympathetic stimulation which increases adrenaline levels.

7. **Gastrointestinal tract:** PGE_2 and PGI_2 inhibit gastric secretion, increase mucous and bicarbonate secretions. Aspirin is a gastric mucosal irritant which leads to epigastric distress, nausea and vomiting. Aspirin also stimulates the CTZ to produce vomiting. Erosive gastritis, mucosal congestion, gastric ulceration and GI bleeding resulting in malena. Occasionally hematemesis can occur particularly in higher doses. All these effects are due to loss of gastro protective effect of prostaglandins.

8. **Cardiovascular system:** In therapeutic doses no significant cardiovascular effects are seen. Large doses cause increases in cardiac output and direct vasodilatation. In toxic doses, it depresses the VMC and thus depresses the circulation.

9. **Uric acid excretion:** In low doses, aspirin increases plasma uric acid levels by decreasing uric acid secretion by the distal tubules. Large doses increase uric acid excretion because it inhibits reabsorption of uric acid by proximal tubule causing uricosuria. But, cannot be used therapeutically because such doses result in prominent adverse effects.
10. **Blood:** In small doses aspirin irreversibly inhibits platelet cyclo-oxygenase and thereby TXA_2 synthesis by the platelets. It therefore interferes with platelet aggregation and prolongs the bleeding time. Aspirin inhibits platelet cyclo-oxygenase in the portal circulation itself and therefore even small doses of aspirin is adequate for its anti-platelet effect.
11. **Local effects:** Salicylic acid when applied locally have keratolytic, mild antiseptic and fungistatic properties.

Pharmacokinetics

Salicylates being acidic drugs are absorbed from the stomach and the upper small intestine. Thus particle size, pH of the GIT, solubility of the preparation and presence of food in the stomach influence the absorption.

They are extensively bound to plasma proteins. Aspirin is deacetylated in the liver (conjugated in liver with glycine and with glucuronic acid), plasma and other tissues to release salicylic acid which is the active form. Elimination is dose dependent. It follows first order kinetics in small doses and zero order kinetics in higher doses. Salicylates are excreted in urine. It slowly enters in brain, freely crosses placenta.

Adverse Effects

Analgesic doses are generally well tolerated but anti-inflammatory doses are usually associated with adverse effects especially when used over a long period.

- *GI tract:* Nausea, epigastric distress, vomiting, erosive gastritis, peptic ulcer.
- *Allergic reactions:* Rashes, urticaria, photosensitivity, rhinorrhoea, angiooedema and asthma. As aspirin inhibits only cyclo-oxygenase pathway, arachidonic acid is available for conversion by lipoxygenase pathway into leukotrienes. Leukotrienes are powerful bronchoconstrictors. Hence aspirin can precipitate bronchial asthma.

- Haemolysis in patients with G-6 PD deficiency (in high doses).
- Nephrotoxicity, hepatotoxicity.
- Reye's syndrome seen in children is a form of hepatic encephalopathy, when aspirin is used to treat viral fever. Hence aspirin is contraindicated in children with viral fever.
- Aspirin when taken at term delays the onset of labour.
- *Salicylism:* Higher doses given for a long time as in treatment of rheumatoid arthritis may cause chronic salicylate intoxication termed 'Salicylism'.

Acute Salicylate Poisoning: It is more common in children.

Treatment is symptomatic and includes:

1. Gastric lavage.
2. IV fluids to correct acid-base imbalance and dehydration.
3. External cooling with alcohol or cold water sponges.
4. Blood transfusion and vitamin K are needed, when bleeding occurs.
5. In severe cases, forced alkaline diuresis with sodium bicarbonate and a diuretic like furosemide is given along with IV fluids.

Precautions and Contraindications

Peptic ulcer, liver diseases, bleeding tendencies and viral fever in children contraindicate the use of aspirin/salicylates. Aspirin should be avoided in pregnancy because it can cause premature closure of the ductus arteriosus in the fetus, increases risk of PPH and causes prolongation of gestation. Aspirin should be stopped one week before elective surgery.

Therapeutic Uses

1. As analgesic, anti-inflammatory and anti-pyretic.
2. *Rheumatoid arthritis:* Osteoarthritis.
3. Post myocardial infarction and post stroke: Aspirin in a low dose inhibits platelet aggregation and this may lower the incidence of reinfarction. Low dose aspirin is also given to patients with angina pectoris.
4. Acute rheumatic fever.
5. *Miscellaneous uses:*
   a. In pre-eclampsia by suppressing TXA_2.
   b. Low doses is associated with a lower incidence of colon cancer, polyposis.

c. Closure of PDA in the newborn by inhibiting PG, if this fails to occur at birth.
d. In Alzheimer's disease to slow down cataract progression and niacin induced cutaneous flush and pruritis.

6. *Local:* Salicylic acid is used as a keratolytic, fungistatic and mild antiseptic.

Drug Interactions

Salicylates compete for protein binding sites and displace drug molecules resulting in toxicity with warfarin, heparin, naproxen, phenytoin and sulfonylurea. Inhibition of platelet aggregation may increase the risk of bleeding with oral anti-coagulants.

In low doses salicylates can counter the uricosuric actions of probenecid by decreasing uric acid excretion.

Other Non-Selective Inhibitors of Cox

Phenylbutazone: It has good anti-inflammatory activity, is more potent, but has poor analgesic and antipyretic effects. It is a uricosuric agent. Phenylbutazone causes retention of Na^+ and water. Thus, leads to edema after 1–2 weeks. It can also precipitate congestive cardiac failure.

It may cause serious hematological complications such as bone marrow depression, aplastic anaemia, agranulocytosis and thrombocytopenia. Because of its toxicity, it is withdrawn from the market in many western countries.

Azapropazone is structurally related to phenylbutazone but is less likely to cause agranulocytosis.

Metamizol is a potent analgesic and antipyretic, but poor anti-inflammatory agent and has no uricosuric properties.

Indomethacin is a potent anti-inflammatory, antipyretic and good analgesic. It inhibits phospholipase A_2 and has some immune suppressive action. It have some CNS toxicities, *e.g.*, hallucination, convulsion, vertigo and confusion. Hypersensitivity reactions like skin rashes, leukopenia and asthma in aspirin sensitive individuals also occur. Indomethacin blunts the diuretic action of furosemide and the anti-hypertensive action of thiazides, furosemide, beta blockers and ACE inhibitors by causing salt and water retention. It is used in:

1. Rheumatoid arthritis.
2. Gout.

3. Ankylosing spondylitis.
4. Psoriatic arthritis.
5. For closure of patent ductus arteriosus.

Diclofenic sodium is an analgesic, antipyretic and anti-inflammatory agent. Its tissue penetrability is good and attains good concentration in synovial fluid which is maintained for a long time. Adverse effects are mild. It is used in:

1. Treatment of chronic inflammatory conditions like rheumatoid arthritis and osteoarthritis.
2. Acute musculoskeletal pain, painful dental lesions.
3. Postoperatively for relief of pain and inflammation. But it is not suitable for IV use.

Ketorolac is another PG synthesis inhibitor having good analgesic and anti-inflammatory properties. It is mostly used parenterally though it can also be given orally, should not be given for more than 5 days.

Ibuprofen is better tolerated than aspirin. Analgesic, antipyretic and anti-inflammatory efficacy is slightly lower than aspirin. Hypersensitivity reaction can occur. It is used in: Soft tissue injuries, fractures, following tooth extraction, to relieve postoperative pain, dysmenorrhoea and osteoarthritis.

Fenamates: They should not be used for more than one week.

Piroxicam: It is long-acting, has good anti-inflammatory, analgesic and antipyretic activity. It is a reversible COX inhibitor. Piroxicam is used for rheumatoid arthritis, osteoarthritis, ankylosing spondylitis, acute musculoskeletal pain and postoperative pain. It can be given once a day. It is also available as local application.

Nabumetone is an anti-inflammatory agent with significant efficacy in rheumatoid arthritis and osteoarthritis. It is long acting.

Coxibs

Celecoxib, rofecoxib and valdecoxib are highly selective COX-2 inhibitors. They have good anti-inflammatory, analgesic and antipyretic properties but do not affect platelet aggregation.

They are better tolerated because of milder gastric irritation due to selective COX-2 inhibitors.

Disadvantages

The coxibs can cause hypertension and edema which can be troublesome in patients with cardiovascular diseases. They can increase the risk of myocardial infarction and stroke because of inhibition of PGI, without inhibiting TXA_2. This results in a pro-thrombotic effect leading to myocardial infarction and stroke.

Nimesulide: It is a weak inhibitor of PG synthesis with a higher affinity for COX-2 than COX-1. It inhibits leukocyte function, prevents the release of mediators and in addition has anti-histaminic and anti-allergic properties. It also reduce superoxide generation, free radical scavenging action, inhibition of PAF synthesis and of metalloproteinase activity in cartilage. It is beneficial in patients who develop bronchospasm with other NSAIDs.

Paracetamol: Paracetamol, a metabolite of phenacetin is found to be safer and effective. Paracetamol has analgesic, good anti-pyretic and weak anti-inflammatory properties. Paracetamol is active on cyclo-oxygenase in the brain which accounts for its antipyretic action. It does not stimulate respiration, has no actions on acid base balance, cellular metabolism, cardiovascular system and platelet function.

Paracetamol is well-absorbed orally and 30% protein bound; it is metabolized by the hepatic microsomal enzymes mainly by glucuronide conjugation (60%) and glutathione conjugation (minor). N-acetyl-p-benzoquinone imine is highly toxic metabolite of paracetamol. With toxic doses, it is not detoxfied and may leads to hepatic and renal toxicity.

Acute paracetamol poisoning occurs in children because their ability to conjugate by glucuronidation is poor. Nephrotoxicity may result in acute renal failure in some.

Treatment of Acute Poisoning

Stomach wash is given. Activated charcoal prevents further absorption. Antidote of paracetamol is N-acetylcysteine. N-acetylcysteine partly replenishes the glutathione stores of the liver and prevents binding of toxic metabolites to the cellular constituents.

TREATMENT OF RHEUMATOID ARTHRITIS AND GOUT

Rheumatoid Arthritis

Rheumatoid arthritis (RA) is a chronic, progressive, autoimmune, inflammatory disease, mainly affecting the joints and the periarticular tissues. The antigen-antibody complexes trigger the pathological process.

Mediators of inflammation released in the joints initiate the inflammatory process and the lesions include vasculitis, followed by synovial edema and infiltration with destruction of articular cartilage due to inflammatory cells. There is local synthesis of prostaglandins, leukotrienes and cytokines (TNF alpha and IL-1).

Drugs Used in the Treatment of Rheumatoid Arthritis (DMARDs)

A. **NSAIDs:** Non-steroidal anti-inflammatory drugs are the first line drugs in RA. NSAIDs afford symptomatic relief but do not modify the course of the disease. They are already discussed in detail.

B. **Disease modifying anti-rheumatoid drugs (DMARDs):**
   1. *Immunosuppressant:* Methotrexate, Cyclosporine, Azathioprine.
   2. Gold, d-Penicillamine.
   3. Chloroquine and hydroxychloroquine.
   4. Sulphasalazine.
   5. Lefluinomide.

C. **Biological response modifiers (BRMs):**
   1. *TNF-alpha inhibitors:* Etanercept, Infliximab, Adalimumab.
   2. *IL-1 antagonist:* Anakinra.

D. **Adjuvant Corticosteroid.**

Disease modifying drugs (DMDs) are also called disease modifying anti-rheumatic drugs (DMARDs). These are the second line drugs and are reserved for patients with progressive disease who do not obtain satisfactory relief from NSAIDs. They are capable of arresting the progress of the disease and inducing remission in these patients.

1. **Immunosuppressants** are reserved for patients with seriously crippling disease with reversible lesions after conventional therapy has failed. **Methotrexate** is a folic acid antagonist. It is potent immunosuppressant and anti-inflammatory. It may cause inhibition of cytokine production; chemotaxis and cell mediated immune response. **Azathioprine** is less commonly used due to its toxicity. **Cyclosporine** inhibits IL-1 and IL-2. It also inhibits macrophages, T-cell interaction and T-cell responsiveness. Also not used routinely.

2. **Gold Salts (Sodium Aurothiomalate, Auranofin)**
   Gold depresses cell mediated immunity. Gold salts concentrate in tissues rich in mononuclear phagocytes; selectively accumulate in the lysosomes of synovial cells and other macrophages in the

inflamed synovium. They alter the structure and functions of the macrophages; depress their migration, inhibit lysosomal enzyme activity and phagocytic activity. They also reduce histamine release. On treatment, a gradual reduction of the signs and symptoms are seen.

Adverse Effects of Gold Salts

Skin and mucous membrane toxicity: Dermatitis, pruritus, stomatitis, pharyngitis, glossitis, gastritis, colitis and vaginitis may occur. Hepatitis, thrombocytopenia, postural hypotension, pulmonary fibrosis, hematuria, glomerulonephritis, encephalitis, peripheral neuritis are some other important adverse effects.

Contraindications: Kidney, liver and skin diseases (as it tend to accumulate); pregnancy and blood dyscrasia.

d-Penicillamine is an analog of the amino acid cysteine and a metabolite of penicillin. It is a chelating agent that chelates copper. Its actions and toxicities are similar to gold but is less effective than gold.

3. **Chloroquine and Hydroxy Chloroquine**
   These are found to be useful in mild non-erosive rheumatoid arthritis. But they are known to depress cell-mediated immunity. They reduce monocyte, IL-1, suppress T. lymphocyte response to mitogens, stabilizes lysosomal enzymes and decrease leukocyte chemotaxis.
4. **Sulfasalazine**
   It is a compound of sulfa-pyridine and 5-amino salicylic acid. This has anti-inflammatory actions though the mechanism is not known. Generation of superoxide radicals and cytokines elaboration by inflammatory cells may be suppressed.
5. **Leflunomide**
   Its active metabolite inhibits autoimmune T cell proliferation and production of auto-antibodies by B cells. Leflunomide is orally effective. It is immunomodulator.

Biological Response Modifiers

TNF$_{alpha}$ Inhibitors

Cytokines, particularly tumour necrosis factor (TNF) play an important role in the process of inflammation. TNF produced by macrophages and activated T cells, acts through TNF receptors to stimulate the release or other cytokines.

Infliximab is a monoclonal antibody which specifically binds to human TNF. When given in combination with methotrexate, it slows the progression of rheumatoid arthritis. It inhibits activated T-cells and macrophage function. Adverse effects of the combination include increased susceptibility to upper respiratory infections, nausea, headache, cough, sinusitis and skin rashes. Long-term use causes development of anti-influximab antibodies.

Etanercept is a recombinant fusion protein that binds to TNF molecules. It is also found to be useful in psoriatic and juvenile arthritis.

Anakinra: It is a recombinant human IL-1 receptor antagonist and is less effective than TNF_{alpha}.

Glucocorticoids have anti-inflammatory and immunosuppressant activity. They produce prompt and dramatic relief of symptoms but do not arrest the progress of the disease. Intra-articular corticosteroids are helpful to relieve pain in severely inflamed joints. Long-term use carries serious adverse effects.

Diet and Inflammation

Diet rich in unsaturated fatty acids decrease morning stiffness, pain and swelling of the joints. Unsaturated fatty acids compete with arachidonic acid for uptake and metabolism.

Pharmacotherapy of Gout

Gout is a familial metabolic disorder characterized by recurrent episodes of acute arthritis due to deposits of monosodium urate in the joints and cartilage. There is an inherent abnormality of purine metabolism resulting in overproduction of uric acid. Uric acid is poorly water soluble, it gets precipitated especially at low pH and get deposited in the cartilages of joints and ears, subcutaneous tissues, bursae and sometimes in kidneys.

There is infiltration of granulocytes which phagocytize the urate crystals and release a glycoprotein that causes joint destruction.

Drugs Used in the Treatment of Gout

I. **In acute attack of gout:** Colchicine, NSAIDs, Prednisolon.

II. **In chronic gout:**

a. *Uric acid synthesis inhibitor:* Allopurinol.

b. *Uricosuric drugs:* Sulfinpyrazone, Benzbromarone, Colchicine, Probenecid.

Colchicine: It is a unique anti-inflammatory agent as it is effective only against gouty arthritis. It is not an analgesic. It has no effect on blood uric acid.

It dramatically relieves pain within a few hours. It increases gut motility by neurogenic stimulation. It is effective as it:

a. Inhibits the migration of granulocytes into the inflamed area.
b. Inhibit the release of glycoprotein.
c. It binds to microtubules and arrests cell division in metaphase.

Colchicine is rapidly absorbed orally, metabolized in the liver and undergoes enterohepatic circulation.

Adverse effects are dose related. Nausea vomiting, diarrhea and abdominal pain are the earliest side effects and may avoid by giving colchicine intravenously. In high doses hemorrhagic gastroenteritis, nephrotoxicity, CNS depression, muscular paralysis and respiratory failure can occur. It is used in acute gout as well as for the prophylaxis of recurrent episodes of gouty arthritis (but not recommended for chronic therapy).

NSAIDs afford symptomatic relief in the treatment of gout. Indomethacin, naproxen, piroxicam are the most commonly used agent in acute gout. NSAIDs are not recommended for long-term use due to their toxicity.

Corticosteroids: They are reserved for refractory cases, not responding or tolerating NSAIDs. They are given by intra-articular injection.

Allopurinol is an analog of hypoxanthine and inhibits the biosynthesis of uric acid. Purine nucleotides are degraded to hypoxanthine. Allopurinol and its metabolite alloxanthine both inhibit the enzyme xanthine oxidase and thereby prevent the synthesis of uric acid.

Allopurinol is 80% absorbed orally.

Adverse effects are mild. Hypersensitivity reactions include fever and rashes. Gastrointestinal irritation, headache, nausea and dizziness may occur.

Drug Interactions: The anti-cancer drugs 6-mercaptopurine and azathioprine are metabolized by xanthine oxidase, so the dose of these anti-cancer drugs should be reduced. It can potentiate the effect of warfarin and theophylline by inhibiting their metabolism. It should be used with caution during pregnancy.

Allopurinol is used in:

1. Chronic gout and secondary hyperuricaemia (due to cancer chemotherapy) tophi are gradually reabsorbed and the formation of renal stones are prevented.
2. In kala-azar.
3. During the treatment of blood dyscrasias where cell destruction creates high level of uric acid crystals.

Probenecid blocks tubular reabsorption of uric acid and thereby promotes its excretion. It is well-absorbed and well-tolerated. Adverse effects include gastrointestinal irritation and skin rashes.

Probenecid is indicated in chronic gout and secondary hyperuricemia. Probenecid may also precipitate acute attacks of gout due to fluctuating uric acid levels.

Sulfinpyrazone has actions and adverse effects similar to probencid. It is used in chronic gout. It has additive effect on the probenecid.

Benzbromarone acts by inhibiting renal tubular reabsorption of uric acid. It is used as an alternative in patients allergic to other drugs. Benzbromarone can also be used in combination with allopurinol and is more effective.

TREATMENT OF PARKINSONISM

Drugs Used in Parkinsonism

Parkinsonism is a chronic, progressive, motor disorder characterized by rigidity, tremors and bradykinesia. Other symptoms include excessive salivation, abnormalities of posture and gait, seborrhea and mood changes.

In idiopathic parkinsonism, there is degeneration of nigrostriatal neurons in the basal ganglia resulting in dopamine deficiency. Thus balance between inhibitory dopaminergic neurons and excitatory cholinergic neurons is disturbed.

Anti-parkinsonian drugs can only help to alleviate the symptoms and improve the quality of life. The strategies in the treatment is:

(i) To enhance dopamine activity.
(ii) To depress cholinergic over activity; or
(iii) Combination of both.

Classification

Drugs used in parkinsonism can be classified as:

I. Drugs that increase dopamine levels

a. *Dopamine precursor:* Levodopa.

b. *Drugs that facilitate the release of dopamine:* Amantadine.
c. *Dopaminergic agonists:* Bromocriptine, Lisuride, Ropinirole, Pramipexole, Pergolide, Cabergoline, Piribedil.
d. *Monoamine oxidase (MAO) inhibitors:* Selegiline.
e. *Catechol-o-methyl transferase (COMT) inhibitors:* Tolcapone, Entacapone.
f. *Peripheral decarboxylase inhibitor:* Carbidopa, Benserazide.

II. Drugs influencing cholinergic system

a. *Central anti-cholinergic:* Benztropine, Biperidine, Trihexyphenidyl (Benzhexol), Ethopropazine.
b. *Antihistamines:* Diphenhydramine, Orphenadrine, Promethazine, Chlorphenoxamine.

Dopamine Precursor

Levodopa

Dopamine is of no therapeutic value because it does not cross the blood brain barrier. Levodopa is a prodrug which is converted to dopamine in the body. It crosses the BBB and is taken up by the surviving nigrostriatal neurons.

There is an overall improvement in all the symptoms. Large amounts of levodopa are converted to dopamine in the periphery which brings about other actions.

- Dopamine stimulates the CTZ to induce vomiting.
- It causes postural hypotension, tachycardia and arrhythmias. Tolerance develops to these effects after few weeks.
- Dopamine suppresses the prolactin secretion, increase growth hormone secretion (not in patient with parkinsonism).

Carbidopa and Benserazide

Carbidopa and benserazide are peripheral dopa decarboxylase inhibitors. They prevent the formation of dopamine in the periphery. They are effective orally. They do not cross the BBB and hence allow levodopa to reach the CNS. The combination is synergistic and therefore levodopa is always given with carbidopa/benserazide as fixed dose combination.

Advantages of the Combination

1. Dose of L-dopa can be reduced by 75%.
2. Response to L-dopa appears earlier.

3. Side effects like vomiting and tachycardia are largely reduced.
4. Pyridoxine does not interfere with treatment.

Pharmacokinetics

Levodopa is rapidly absorbed from the small intestine. Presence of food delays absorption. Some amino acids in the food compete with levodopa for absorption and transport to the brain. It undergoes first pass metabolism in the gut and the liver. Its $t_{½}$ is 12 hours.

Adverse Reactions

1. Nausea, vomiting, anorexia, postural hypotension, palpitation and occasionally arrhythmias can occur. Tolerance develops to these effects after some time. These peripheral effects can be prevented by concurrent administration of domperidone, which is a peripheral dopamine antagonist.
2. *Dyskinesia:* Abnormal involuntary movements like facial tics, grimacing, choreoathetoid movements of the limbs may develop after few months of use and require reduction in the dose of levodopa.
3. Fluctuation in response to levodopa can occur after 2–5 years of use. It is known as 'on off' phenomenon where the patient swings alternately from periods of good response to severe disabling disease.
4. *Behavioral effects:* Hallucination, mania, insomnia, anxiety, nightmare and depression. These effects are more common in elderly.
   Levodopa is the most effective drug in idiopathic parkinsonism but is not useful in drug induced parkinsonism.

Contraindications

Levodopa is contraindicated in patients with psychosis, peptic ulcer, glaucoma, malignant melanoma, IHD, arrhythmias.

Drug Interactions

1. Pyridoxine enhances peripheral decarboxylation of levodopa and thus reduces its availability to the CNS (as dopa-decarboxylase is a pyridoxine dependent enzyme).
2. Phenothiazines and metoclopramide are DA antagonists. They reverse or abolish therapeutic effects of levodopa.
3. Reserpine and other anti-hypertensive also abolish the effect of L-dopa (by depleting monoamines).

Drugs that Release Dopamine

Amantadine is an antiviral drug. It enhances the release of DA in the brain and diminishes the reuptake of DA. The response starts early and its adverse effects are minor. Amantadine is used in mild cases of parkinsonism. It can also be used along with levodopa as an adjunct.

Dopamine Receptor Agonists

Bromacriptine and pergolide are ergot derivatives having dopamine agonistic activity at D_2, receptors. Bromocriptine is also a partial agonist or antagonist at D_2 receptor while pergolide is an agonist at both D_1 and D_2 receptors. The newer agents ropinirole and pramipexole are selective D_2, agonists, are better tolerated, quickly attain therapeutic levels and adverse effects are milder except that they may cause some sleep disorders. Ropinirole also has moderate affinity for opioid receptors in vitro. They are useful in the treatment of 'on off' phenomenon.

Adverse effects include nausea, vomiting, hallucinations and skin eruptions, syncope (careful monitoring of BP is required).

Drugs that Inhibit DA Metabolism

MAO Inhibitor

Selegiline (Deprenyl) is a selective MAO-B inhibitor. MAO-B is present in DA containing regions of the CNS. Selegiline prolongs the action of levodopa by preventing its degradation. Selegiline may delay the progression of parkinsonism.

Adverse effects include nausea, postural hypotension, confusion, hallucinations and involuntary movements.

COMT Inhibitors

Tolcapone and entacapone inhibit the peripheral metabolism of levodopa thereby increasing its bioavailability. Tolcapone crosses the BBB and enhances the availability of levodopa in the brain. Adverse effects are nausea, orthostatic hypotension, confusion and hallucinations. Tolcapone can also cause hepatotoxicity.

COMT inhibitors are used as add on drugs in parkinsonism.

Anticholinergic Drugs

The cholinergic overactivity is overcome by anticholinergic drugs. Tremors, seborrhoea and sialorrhoea are reduced more than rigidity. Atropine derivatives like benztropine, trihexyphenidyl are used. Antihistamines also have beneficial effects in parkinsonism because of their anticholinergic properties.

Anticholinergics are used as (i) adjunct to levodopa, (ii) drugs of choice in drug-induced parkinsonism.

Drug-induced parkinsonism: Drugs like reserpine, metoclopramide and phenothiazines can induce parkinsonism.

Treatment: Withdrawal of the drug usually reverses the symptoms. When drugs are needed, one of the anticholinergics is effective. Levodopa or other dopamine agonists are not effective because symptoms occurs due to blocked of DA receptors by drugs like metoclopramide and phenothiazines not due to deficiency of dopamine.

MULTIPLE CHOICE QUESTIONS

Q. 1 Which of the following chemicals does not satisfy the criteria for a neurotransmitter role in the CNS?

(A) Acetylcholine (B) Glycine
(C) Substance P (D) Nitric oxide

Q. 2 Neurotransmitters cause:

(A) Increase chloride conductance to cause inhibition
(B) Increase potassium conductance to cause excitation
(C) Increase sodium conductance to cause inhibition
(D) Increase calcium conductance to cause inhibition

Q. 3 Which receptor shares the same potassium channel at the 5- $HT1_A$ receptor?

(A) Delta opioid receptor (B) Dopamine D_2 receptor
(C) $GABA_B$ receptor (D) Muscarinic M_1 receptor

Q. 4 In strychnine poisoning, convulsions occurs because of antagonistic effects at receptors for:

(A) Aspartate (B) GABA
(C) Glutamate (D) Glycine

Q. 5 The minimal alveolar concentration of an inhalational anaesthetic is a measure of its:

(A) Potency
(B) Therapeutic index
(C) Diffusibility
(D) Oil: water partition coefficient

Q. 6 Which of the following agent cause less cardiac toxicity?

(A) Halothane (B) Propofol
(C) Isoflurane (D) Chloroform

Q. 7 Which of the following agent cause massive hepatic necrosis?

(A) Ether (B) Isoflurane
(C) Halothane (D) Enflurane

---

1 (D) 2 (A) 3 (C) 4 (D) 5 (A) 6 (C) 7 (C)

Q. 8 In terms of minimum alveolar concentration, the most potent anaesthetic agent is:

(A) Nitrous oxide (B) Halothane
(C) Enflurane (D) Ketamine

Q. 9 Which of the following is a sign of deep anaesthesia?

(A) Increase in lacrimal secretion
(B) Presence of swallowing
(C) Fall in blood pressure
(D) Resistance to passive inflation of lungs

Q. 10 "Second gas effect" is exerted by which of the following agent when co-administered with halothane?

(A) Nitrogen (B) Cyclopropane
(C) Nitrous oxide (D) Helium

Q. 11 The anesthetic action of thiopentone sodium is characterized by:

(A) Good muscle relaxation
(B) Poor analgesia
(C) Sensitization of heart to epinephrine
(D) No postoperative residual CNS depression

Q. 12 Dissociative anaesthesia is produced by:

(A) Ketamine (B) Propofol
(C) Fentanyl + droperidol (D) Halothane

Q. 13 All of the following are true for propofol *except:*

(A) It has rapid onset of action
(B) Recovery is rapid and patient can ambulate sooner
(C) It has no effect on blood pressure
(D) Post operative vomiting is uncommon

Q. 14 Factors that influence the action of local anaesthetic do not include:

(A) Acetyl cholinesterase activity in the area
(B) Amount of local anaesthetic injected
(C) Blood flow through the tissue in which the injection is made
(D) Tissue pH

---

8 (B) 9 (C) 10 (C) 11 (B) 12 (A) 13 (C) 14 (A)

Q. 15 Vasoconstrictors reduce the systemic absorption of all of the following local anaesthetic agent *except:*

(A) Procaine (B) Prilocaine
(C) Lignocaine (D) Mepivacaine

Q. 16 All of the following are long acting local anaesthetic agents *except:*

(A) Procaine (B) Tetracaine
(C) Bupivacaine (D) Ropivacaine

Q. 17 Which of the following local anaesthetic agent is more likely to produce methemoglobinemia?

(A) Prilocaine
(B) Lidocaine
(C) Mepivacaine
(D) Procaine

Q. 18 Characteristic features of the amide linked local anaesthetic (LA) are:

(A) They are not good surface anaesthetics
(B) They have a shorter duration of action
(C) They are degraded in the plasma
(D) Does not show cross-sensitivity with ester linked LA

Q. 19 The duration of spinal anaesthesia depends on each of the following *except:*

(A) Which local anaesthetic agent is used
(B) Concentration of the local anaesthetic used
(C) Posture of the patient
(D) Whether epinephrine has been added to the LA

Q. 20 Epidural anaesthesia differs from spinal anaesthesia in that:

(A) Epidural anaesthesia produced less cardiovascular complications
(B) Headache is more common after epidural anaesthesia
(C) Blood concentration of LA are lower after epidural anaesthesia
(D) Greater separation between sensory and motor blockade can be obtained with epidural anaesthesia

---

15 (B) 16 (A) 17 (A) 18 (D) 19 (C) 20 (D)

Q. 21 Which of the following is best describes the mechanism of action of benzodiazepine (BZD)?

(A) Activate $GABA_B$ receptors in the spinal cord
(B) Increase the frequency of opening of chloride ion channels that are coupled to $GABA_A$ receptors
(C) Inhibit GABA transaminase to increase brain levels of GABA
(D) Stimulate the release of GABA from nerve ending in the brain

Q. 22 Lorazepam, a BZD is preferred in elderly as pre-anaesthetic medication because:

(A) It is a selective anxiolytic
(B) Actively secreted in the renal proximal tubule
(C) Conjugated extra hepatically
(D) Eliminated via the lungs

Q. 23 The most frequent type of drug interaction that occurs in patients using BZD is:

(A) Additive CNS depression
(B) Antagonism of sedative or hypnotic action
(C) Induction of liver drug metabolizing enzymes
(D) Competition for plasma protein binding

Q. 24 Inverse agonist of benzodiazepine receptor is:

(A) Phenobarbitone
(B) Flumazenil
(C) Gabapentin
(D) Beta-carboline

Q. 25 Hypnotic doses of diazepam produces the following action:

(A) Tachycardia
(B) Constipation
(C) Hyperalgesia
(D) Decreased nocturnal gastric secretion

Q. 26 Which of the following drug antagonizes diazepam action non-competitively?

(A) Adenosine (B) Flumazenil
(C) Bicuculline (D) Valproic acid

---

21 (B) 22 (C) 23 (A) 24 (D) 25 (D) 26 (C)

Q. 27 Which of the following statement is not true of zopiclone?

(A) It is a non benzodiazepine hypnotic with similar efficacy and safety as that of BZD
(B) It does not produce rebound sleep disturbances on discontinuation
(C) It does not act by potentiating GABA
(D) It is used to wean off insomnias from regular benzodiazepine use

Q. 28 Select the correct statement about flumazenil:

(A) It is a CNS stimulant used as an antidote for BZD poisoning
(B) It is a CNS depressant but block the action of diazepam
(C) It has no CNS effect of its own but blocks the depressant effects of BZD and barbiturates
(D) It has no CNS effect of its own but block the depressant effects of diazepam as well as stimulant effect of beta carboline

Q. 29 Barbiturates nowadays are primary used as:

(A) Hypnotic (B) Sedative
(C) Antiepileptic (D) Pre anaesthetic medication

Q. 30 Barbiturates exert all of the following actions *except:*

(A) Anti convulsant (B) Analgesic
(C) Anti anxiety (D) Respiratory depressant

Q. 31 The effect of sedative hypnotic on the pattern of normal sleep includes all of the following *except:*

(A) Latency of sleep onset is decreased
(B) Duration of REM sleep is decreased
(C) Duration of stage 2 NREM sleep is increased
(D) Nocturnal peaks in GH are abolished

Q. 32 Which of the following is true about action of ethyl alcohol?

(A) It exerts anticonvulsant action followed by lowering of seizures threshold
(B) Lowers pain threshold
(C) Increases confidence and reduce number of errors
(D) Increases heat production and helps to keep warm in cold weather

---

27 (C) 28 (D) 29 (C) 30 (B) 31 (D) 32 (D)

Q. 33 Moderate doses of alcohol produces all of the following effects *except:*

(A) Flushing (B) Tachycardia
(C) Diuresis (D) Rise in body temperature

Q. 34 The combination of ethanol and disulfiram result in nausea and hypotension as a result of accumulation of:

(A) Acetaldehyde (B) Acetate
(C) Methanol (D) Pyruvate

Q. 35 Chronic alcohol abuse can cause all of the following types of anaemia *except:*

(A) Megaloblastic anaemia (B) Iron deficiency anaemia
(C) Hemolytic anaemia (D) Pernicious anaemia

Q. 36 All of the following drugs are useful in alcohol withdrawl syndrome *except:*

(A) Clonidine (B) Diazepam
(C) Methadone (D) Propranolol

Q. 37 The most probable mechanism of anti-convulsant action of phenytoin is:

(A) Facilitation of GABAergic inhibitory transmission
(B) Hyper polarization of neurons
(C) Interaction with Ca^{2+} channels to promote Ca^{2+} influx
(D) Prolongation of voltage sensitive neuronal Na^{+} channel inactivation

Q. 38 Which of the following adverse effect of phenytoin is related to high plasma drug concentration?

(A) Ataxia (B) Hirsutism
(C) Gum hyperplasia (D) All of the above

Q. 39 Which anti-epileptic drug is also effective in manic depressive illness?

(A) Ethosuximide (B) Primidone
(C) Phenobarbitone (D) Carbamazepine

33 (D) 34 (A) 35 (C) 36 (C) 37 (D) 38 (A) 39 (D)

Q. 40 Mechanism of action of sodium valproate as an anti-epileptic drug includes:

(A) Prolong neuronal Na^+ channel inactivation
(B) Attenuate 'T' type Ca^{2+} current in neurons
(C) Inhibit degradation of GABA by GABA transaminase
(D) All of the above

Q. 41 The preferred drug for suppressing febrile convulsion is:

(A) Intramuscular phenobarbitone
(B) Rectal diazepam
(C) Intravenous phenytoin
(D) Oral sodium valproate

Q. 42 Gabapentin is effective as it:

(A) Have $GABA_A$ agonist action
(B) Act as precursor of GABA
(C) Act by enhancing GABA release
(D) Act by GABA independent mechanism

Q. 43 The preferred drug for status epilepticus is:

(A) Intravenous diazepam
(B) Intravenous phenytoin sodium
(C) Intramuscular phenobarbitone
(D) Rectal paraldehyde

Q. 44 Concomitant administration of which anti-epileptic drug is most likely to elevate the plasma concentration of other anti-epileptic drugs?

(A) Carbamazepine (B) Phenobarbitone
(C) Phenytoin (D) Valproic acid

Q. 45 Which statement about vigabatrin is true?

(A) It blocks neuronal uptake of GABA
(B) It is drug of choice in absence seizures
(C) Visual field defects occur in upto one third of patients
(D) Life threatening skin disorders may occur

Q. 46 Withdrawal of which anti-epileptic is less likely to cause problems?

(A) Clonazepam (B) Phenytoin
(C) Ethosuximide (D) Phenobarbitone

---

40 (D) 41 (B) 42 (C) 43 (A) 44 (D) 45 (C) 46 (C)

Q. 47 Concomitant administration of which of the following anti-epileptic drug can precipitate absence status with clonazepam?

(A) Sodium valproate (B) Phenytoin
(C) Phenobarbitone (D) Carbamazepine

Q. 48 Drug of choice for epilepsy in pregnancy is:

(A) Carbamazepine (B) Phenobarbitone
(C) Sodium valproate (D) Phenytoin

Q. 49 Which statement concerning the adverse effects of anti-psychotic drug is accurate?

(A) Acute dystonic reaction occur infrequently with olanzepine
(B) Blurring of vision and urinary retention are common side effects of haloperidol
(C) Retinal pigmentation is a dose dependent toxic effect of clozapine
(D) The choreo-athetoid movements caused by conventional anti-psychotic drugs are reduced by anti-muscarinic agents

Q. 50 The major difference between typical and atypical anti-psychotic is that:

(A) The latter cause minimal or no increase in prolactin
(B) The former cause tardive dyskinesia
(C) The former are available as parenteral preparation
(D) The later cause substantial sedation

Q. 51 Actions of chlorpromazine include the following *except:*

(A) Indifference to external stimuli
(B) Postural hypotension
(C) Hypoprolactinemia
(D) Local anaesthetic activity

Q. 52 Which of the following adverse effect of neuroleptic drug is correlated with its potency?

(A) Sedation
(B) Extrapyramidal motor disturbance
(C) Postural hypotension
(D) Lowering of seizure threshold

---

47 (A) 48 (B) 49 (A) 50 (B) 51 (C) 52 (B)

Q. 53 Which anti-psychotic drug most likely to cause ocular toxicity in long term use is?

(A) Thioridazine (B) Haloperidol
(C) Pimozide (D) Flupenthixol

Q. 54 Which of the following statements is not true about anti-psychotic drugs?

(A) They only control symptoms of schizophrenia without affecting the basic disorders
(B) Combination of two or more anti-psychotic drug is more efficacious than any single drug
(C) In treating psychosis high potency drugs are preferred over low potency drugs
(D) They do not produce dependence

Q. 55 Which anxiolytic BZD, has additional anti-depressant (mild) property?

(A) Oxazepam (B) Alprazolam
(C) Lorazepam (D) Chlordizepoxide

Q. 56 Which of the following is non-sedative anxiolytic?

(A) Buspiron (B) Meprobamate
(C) Alprazolam (D) Hydroxyzine

Q. 57 Which monoamine oxidase (MAO) inhibitor does not produce cheese reaction?

(A) Moclobemide (B) Isocarboxazid
(C) Phenelzine (D) Tranycypromine

Q. 58 Tricyclic anti-depressant abolish the anti-hypertensive action of the following drug:

(A) Enalapril (B) Clonidine
(C) Atenolol (D) Diltiazem

Q. 59 The advantage of selective serotonin reuptake inhibitor (SSRI) (Fluoxetine) over tricyclic anti-depressant drugs includes all of the following *except:*

(A) It is less likely to produce cardiac arrhythmias
(B) It infrequently produces sedative and anticholinergic side effect
(C) It block neuronal uptake of biogenic amines
(D) It can elevate mood of apparently non-depressed patients suffering from chronic somatic illness

---

53 (A) 54 (B) 55 (B) 56 (A) 57 (A) 58 (B) 59 (C)

Q. 60 Tricyclic anti-depressants (TCADs) are effective in all *except:*
(A) Bulimia (B) Phobic states
(C) Schizophrenia (D) Obsessive compulsive disorder

Q. 61 All is true about lithium *except:*
(A) It has a sedative action in normal individual
(B) It controls mania
(C) It is also effective in unipolar depression
(D) In refractory cases, it can be combined with TCADs

Q. 62 Which of the following drug is effective in mania and in bipolar illness?
(A) Haloperidol (B) Clomipramine
(C) Carbamazepine (D) Diethyl carbamazine

Q. 63 Prolonged lithium therapy can cause:
(A) Gout (B) Parkinsonism
(C) Goiter (D) Diabetes insipidus

Q. 64 Which statement about lithium is correct?
(A) Excessive intake of sodium chloride enhances the toxicity of lithium
(B) Lithium does not cross placental barrier
(C) The elimination rate of lithium is equivalent to that of creatinine
(D) Dose of the lithium need to be reduced in patients taking thiazide

Q. 65 Tianeptine is a:
(A) 5-HT reuptake enhancer
(B) MAO inhibitor
(C) GABA inhibitor
(D) Norepinephrine reuptake inhibitor

Q. 66 Which of the following drug is safe and effective in bipolar depression during pregnancy?
(A) Valproic acid
(B) Olanzapine
(C) Lithium
(D) Carbamazepine

---

60 (C) 61 (A) 62 (C) 63 (D) 64 (D) 65 (A) 66 (B)

Q. 67 Which of the following anti-psychotic does not cause extra pyramidal dysfunction or hemopoietic toxicity?

(A) Chlorpromazine (B) Haloperidol
(C) Ziprasidone (D) Fluphenazine

Q. 68 Fentanyl patches used as analgesic may cause:

(A) Respiratory depression
(B) Diarrhoea
(C) Relaxation of skeletal muscles
(D) Hypertension

Q. 69 Opioid analgesic are either contraindicated or must be used with caution in following situations:

(A) Hepatic disease (B) Biliary tract surgery
(C) Hypothyroidism (D) All of the above

Q. 70 Genetic polymorphism in drug metabolism to be responsible for variation in analgesic effect to which of the following opioid?

(A) Codeine (B) Buprenorphine
(C) Methadone (D) Propoxyphene

Q. 71 Which statement about nalbuphine is accurate?

(A) It activates μ receptors
(B) It is non-sedating
(C) It cause respiratory depression
(D) Response to naloxone in overdose of nalbuphine may be unreliable

Q. 72 Which statement about dextromethorphan is correct?

(A) It activates 'kappa' receptors
(B) It has no abuse liabilities
(C) It produces analgesia equivalent to pentazocine
(D) It causes less constipation than codeine

Q. 73 Which statement about propoxyphene is correct?

(A) It produces analgesia equivalent to oxycodone
(B) It causes seizures in overdose
(C) Cause dose limiting diarrhoea
(D) It is antagonist at 'μ' receptors

67 (C) 68 (A) 69 (D) 70 (A) 71 (D) 72 (D) 73 (B)

Q. 74 The difference between morphine and aspirin as an analgesic is:

(A) Morphine has a higher ceiling
(B) Morphine covers both perception as well as psychic processing of the pain
(C) Visceral and ischemic pain is relieved better than somatic inflammation pain with morphine
(D) All of the above are correct

Q. 75 Morphine causes fall in blood pressure by following mechanism *except:*

(A) Vasomotor centre depression
(B) Direct cardiac depression
(C) Direct reduction of vascular tone
(D) Histamine release

Q. 76 Which of the following is not true about morphine?

(A) Its glucuronide metabolite is an active analgesic
(B) Its active metabolite penetrates blood brain barrier better than morphine
(C) Its oral parenteral activity ratio is 1:4
(D) It undergoes enterohepatic cycling

Q. 77 The antidote of choice for morphine poisoning is:

(A) Nalorphine (B) Nalbuphine
(C) Naloxone (D) Naltrexone

Q. 78 Morphine is contraindicated in head injury because:

(A) It does not relieve the pain of head injury
(B) It is liable to cause addiction
(C) It can cause constipation
(D) It can raise intracranial tension

Q. 79 Which of the following is not true of pethidine?

(A) In equi-analgesic doses it cause less respiratory depression than morphine
(B) It is less constipating
(C) It is poor anti-tussive
(D) In overdose it often produce excitatory effects

74 (D) 75 (B) 76 (B) 77 (C) 78 (D) 79 (A)

Q. 80 Which of the following opioid is more potent than morphine?

(A) Pethidine (B) Fentanyl
(C) Tramadol (D) Dextropropoxyphene

Q. 81 Which analgesic act through both opioid as well as spinal mono aminergic mechanism?

(A) Tramadol (B) Alfentanil
(C) Ethoheptazine (D) Dextropropoxyphene

Q. 82 The correct statement about pentazocine is:

(A) It causes bradycardia and fall in blood pressure
(B) Its subjective effects are pleasurable at low doses, but turn unpleasant in higher doses
(C) It induces vomiting frequently
(D) It substitute for morphine in dependent subjects

Q. 83 Which of the following is true of buprenorphine?

(A) It is an agonist antagonist type of opioid analgesic
(B) Its subjective effects are different from those of morphine
(C) Naloxone is largely ineffective in reversing its effect
(D) It produces mydriasis

Q. 84 Which of the following statement is true about endogenous opioid peptides?

(A) They activate only μ opioid receptors
(B) They do not occur in peripheral tissue
(C) They mediate stress induced analgesia
(D) Naloxone fails to antagonize their action

Q. 85 Which of the following action is not mediated by 'μ_1' receptors?

(A) Supra-spinal analgesia (B) Reduced intestinal motility
(C) Dependence (D) Euphoria

Q. 86 The characteristic feature of cyclo oxygenase-2 (COX-2) enzyme is:

(A) It is not inhibited by indomethacin
(B) It is inducible
(C) It generates cytoprotective prostaglandin in gastric mucosa
(D) It is found only in fetal tissue

80 (B) 81 (A) 82 (B) 83 (C) 84 (C) 85 (B) 86 (B)

Q. 87 Metabolic effects of high doses of aspirin includes all *except:*

(A) Increased CO_2 production
(B) Hepatic glycogen depletion
(C) Metabolic acidosis
(D) Compensated respiratory alkalosis

Q. 88 Aspirin is contraindicated in pregnant women at near term because:

(A) Labour may be delayed or prolonged
(B) Blood loss during delivery may be more
(C) Foetus may suffer premature closure of ductus arteriosus
(D) All of the above

Q. 89 Phenylbutazone should be used only in patient not responding other NSAIDs because:

(A) It has lower anti-inflammatory efficacy than other NSAIDs
(B) It has potential to cause agranulocytosis
(C) It has weak analgesic action
(D) It alters the protein binding and metabolism of many drugs

Q. 90 The NSAIDs contraindicated in drivers and machine operator is:

(A) Phenylbutazone
(B) Naproxen
(C) Indomethacin
(D) Diclofenac sodium

Q. 91 Which NSAIDs is more appropriate for pain of musculo-skeletal disorder?

(A) Ibuprofen (B) Tolmetin
(C) Indomethacin (D) Phenybutazone

Q. 92 What is the true about nimesulide?

(A) It exerts anti-inflammatory action by several other mechanism in addition to cyclo oxygenase inhibition
(B) It is preferred for long-term use in rheumatoid arthritis
(C) It is contraindicated in aspirin intolerant asthma patients
(D) All of the above

---

87 (C) 88 (D) 89 (B) 90 (C) 91 (A) 92 (A)

Q. 93 N-acetyl cysteine is beneficial in acute paracetamol poisoning because:

(A) It reacts with paracetamol to form a non-toxic complex
(B) It inhibits the generation of the toxic metabolite of paracetamol
(C) It is a free radical scavenger
(D) It replenishes hepatic glutathione which in turn bind the toxic metabolite of paracetamol

Q. 94 Which of the following statement is correct about gold therapy of rheumatoid arthritis?

(A) It is indicated only in rapidly progressing disease not controlled by NSAIDs
(B) It is indicated when both NSAIDs and prednisolon failed
(C) NSAIDs must be discontinue when gold therapy started
(D) In severe case intramuscular gold act rapidly

Q. 95 Which statement is true about disease modifying drugs used in rheumatoid arthritis (DMARDs)?

(A) Beneficial effects occur after 2-3 months of therapy
(B) Recurrence of disease does not occur after remission
(C) They are to be used life long
(D) Concurrent use of more than one disease modified drug is not recommended

Q. 96 Among disease modifying anti-rheumatic drugs (DMARDs), the fastest symptom relief obtained by:

(A) Methotrexate (B) Auranofin
(C) Penicillamine (D) Sulfasalazine

Q. 97 The most important dose limiting adverse effect of colchicine is:

(A) Sedation (B) Kidney damage
(C) Diarrhoea (D) Muscle paralysis

Q. 98 Drug which is used in chronic gout but is not uricosuric?

(A) Probenecid (B) Phenylbutazone
(C) Allopurinol (D) Sulfinpyrazone

Q. 99 The most effective single drug in parkinsonism is:

(A) Bromocriptine (B) Selegeline
(C) Levodopa (D) Biperiden

---

93 (D) 94 (A) 95 (A) 96 (A) 97 (C) 98 (C) 99 (C)

Q. 100 The major advantage of carbidopa in parkinsonism is that it:

(A) Crosses the BBB
(B) Inhibits monoamine oxidase-A (MAO-A) enzyme
(C) Inhibits L-amino acid decarboxylase enzyme
(D) Inhibits MAO-B enzyme

Q. 101 Which of the following combination should not be used in parkinsonism?

(A) Levodopa + Anticholinergic
(B) Levodopa + Amantadine
(C) Levodopa + Bromocriptine
(D) Amantadine + Anticholinergic

Q. 102 Which anti-parkinsonian drug act by inhibiting the degradation of dopamine in the brain?

(A) Carbidopa (B) Amantadine
(C) Selegiline (D) Bromocriptine

Q. 103 Which anti-parkinsonian drug should be used with caution in elderly male?

(A) Levodopa (B) Benztropine
(C) Ropinirole (D) Selegeline

Q. 104 The drug which abolishes the therapeutic effect of levodopa but not that of levodopa + carbidopa is?

(A) Metoclopramide (B) Pyridoxine
(C) Isoniazid (D) Chlorpromazine

Q. 105 The drug of choice for hyperkinetic children is:

(A) Methylphenidate (B) Nikethamide
(C) Caffeine (D) Clonazepam

Q. 106 Indications of piracetam includes all of the following *except:*

(A) Apnea in preterm infant
(B) Learning defects in children
(C) Confusional states in the elderly
(D) Memory impairment following ECT

---

100 (C) 101 (D) 102 (C) 103 (B) 104 (B) 105 (A) 106 (A)

ANSWERS

Ans. 1 **(D)** Nitric oxide synthetase is the enzyme which generates nitric oxide. It is found in some neurons in the CNS. However, a role for NO in synaptic transmission in the CNS has not been established.

Ans. 2 **(A)** Activation of chloride or potassium ion channels often generates inhibitory post synaptic potentials (IPSP). Activation of sodium and inhibition of potassium in channels generate excitatory post synaptic potential (EPSP).

Ans. 3 **(C)** $GABA_B$ receptors and $5\text{-}HT1_A$ receptors share the same potassium ion channels with a G-protein involved in the coupling mechanism. The spasmolytic drug baclofen is an activator of $GABA_B$ receptors in the spinal cord.

Ans. 4 **(D)** Activation of both $GABA_A$ and glycine receptors present on neurons in the spinal cord leads to membrane hyperpolarization via increase in chloride ion conductance. In the case of glycine, its inhibitory action at the level of the spinal cord is opposed by strychnine.

Ans. 5 **(A)** The potency of inhaled anaesthetic is quantified by the MAC, which is the minimum concentration of anaesthetic that is required to prevent movements in 50% of patients in response to surgical skin incision.

Ans. 6 **(C)** Isoflurane has a very stable molecule that undergoes minimal metabolism, so less fluoride is produced. Hence the chance of organ toxicity (nephrotoxicity, hepatotoxicity) is less. It does not sensitize myocardium as with halothane, so chances of cardiac toxicity is also less (enflurane is also not cardio toxic but causes epilepsy and nephrotoxicity, so not used nowadays).

Ans. 7 **(C)** Halothane is metabolized by oxidation into a tissue toxic metabolite, trifluoroethanol and bromide ion which causes transient hepatitis. Repeated administration of halothane can cause severe hepatic necrosis.

Ans. 8 **(B)** Among the given list halothane is more potent. Its MAC value is (0.75%). Smaller the MAC value, more potent is anaesthetic, as anaesthetic with higher lipid solubility have lower MAC value. Methoxyflurane is most potent (MAC is 0.16%) anaesthetic but because of its toxicity it is not used nowadays.

Ans. 9 (C) Blood pressure begins to fall as anaesthesia deepens. All the secretion are completely abolished, all the muscles are flaccid (complete relxations), followed by severe depression of vital medullary centre (if anaesthesia is more deep) and respiratory failure.

Ans. 10 (C) In the initial part of induction, diffusion gradient from alveoli to blood is high, so the large quantity of anaesthetic enters. Loss of alveolar gas volume and sucking is there when high doses of nitrous oxide are used. When another potent anaesthetic agent, halothane is used, it also delivered to blood at the rate higher than minute volume, so the induction is faster. This is known as 'second gas effect'. Reverse will occur when nitrous oxide is discontinued after prolonged administration. It readily diffuses into alveoli and dilutes the alveolar air. This results into hypoxia, known as diffuse hypoxia.

Ans. 11 (B) Thiopental sodium is a poor analgesic, and muscle relaxants, causes respiratory depression. It also depresses myocardium directly and causes hypotension and arrhythmias.

Ans. 12 (A) Ketamine causes complete analgesia with amnesia and sedation and induce a state known as dissociative anaesthesia, as patient is dissociated from the surrounding.

Ans. 13 (C) Propofol (combined with lignocaine to make injection less painful) causes rapid, smooth and pleasant induction with low incidence of excitatory voluntary movements. Recovery also rapid with minimum incidence of vomiting (it is antiemetic). It causes dose dependent cortical depression and has anti-convulsant activity. But it produces marked fall in BP and bradycardia during induction as it decreases peripheral resistance.

Ans. 14 (A) Local anaesthetic is poor substrate for acetyl cholinesterase, which have no role in termination of action of LA. Pseudo cholinesterase hydrolyses ester type of LA, so unusually sensitivity to procaine is observed in the patients having genetic defect in its activity.

Ans. 15 (B) Prilocaine does not cause vasodilatation and can be used without epinephrine, so it is a good choice in patient, in whom epinephrine is contraindicated.

Ans. 16 (A) Tetracaine, Bupivacaine, Ropivacaine, Dibucaine are long acting, Cocaine, Lignocaine, Mepivacaine, prilocaine are intermediate acting and Procaine, Benzocaine and Chloroprocaine are short acting (last two are better and safe to be used as surface anaesthetic agent).

Ans. 17 (A) Prilocaine has low incidence of CNS toxicity but its metabolite has potential to cause methemoglobenemia.

Ans. 18 (D) The characteristic features of amide LA are: they produce intense and long lasting anaesthesia (surface anaesthetics), bind to alpha-1 acid glycoprotein, not hydrolyzed by plasma esterase, rarely cause hypersensitivity reaction and does not show cross-sensitivity with ester LA.

Ans. 19 (C) The duration of action of spinal anaesthesia depends on drug and its concentration, use of hyperbaric/hypoboric solution and addition of epinephrine but least affected by posture of the patient.

Ans. 20 (D) With epidural anaesthesia, motor paralysis occur 4-5 segments caudal especially with lower concentration of drug. Greater separation between sensory and motor block is obtained by use of 0.25% bupivacaine which is valuable for obstetric purpose and for the post operative pain relief.

Ans. 21 (B) BZD exerts most of their effect by increasing the inhibitory effects of GABA interacting with component $GABA_A$ receptor chloride channels. They do not affect metabolism or release and they are not GABA receptor agonist.

Ans. 22 (C) The elimination of most BZD involves their metabolism by liver enzymes including cytochrome P-450. Lorazepam metabolized extra hepatically and produce no active metabolite and is less likely to cause CNS effects as entry is low in the brain.

Ans. 23 (A) Additive CNS depression is most common drug interaction with BZD, with concomitant use of alcohol, opioid analgesics, anti-convulsants and phenothiazines.

Ans. 24 (D) Beta carboline is an inverse agonist of BZD which produce signs of anxiety and convulsion (effects opposite to BZD).

Ans. 25 (D) Hypnotic doses of BZD affect respiration or cardiac action, causes analgesia (Diazepam) and has no effect on bowel movement. It causes decrease in nocturnal gastric acid secretion and prevent stress ulcer.

Ans. 26 (C) Bicuculline is an antagonist to $GABA_A$ receptors and causes convulsion. It antagonizes BZD action in a non-competitive manner.

Ans. 27 (C) Zolpidem, Zopiclone Eszopiclone and zalepion are non-BZD hypnotics, Zopiclone is long acting and does not alter REM sleep, no rebound insomnia, and it is used for short term insomnia. They have their action by acting on GABA receptor.

Ans. 28 (D) Flumazenil compete with BZD agonist (diazepam) as well as inverse agonist (Beta carboline) for the BZD receptor and reverse their depressant and stimulant effects respectively.

Ans. 29 (C) Due to adverse effect and availability of better drugs (BZD) barbiturates are no more used as sedative hypnotics (pre anaesthetic medication). But they are still useful as anti-epileptic agent.

Ans. 30 (B) Barbiturate unlike diazepam does not possess analgesic activity.

Ans. 31 (D) Nocturnal peaks in GH are not abolished, as it occur during 3rd and 4th stage of NREM, but not during REM sleep.

Ans. 32 (D) Alcohol in moderate doses, dilate skin vessels by depressing the vasomotor centre and causes flushing and feeling of warmth. This effect prevents normal cutaneous vasoconstriction on exposure to cold. Hence it may be harmful, as body may lose more heat.

Ans. 33 (D) Flushing, tachycardia and diuresis are the common effect with alcohol, though it gives the warmth sensation but not increase in body temperature (as mentioned above).

Ans. 34 (A) Disulfiram inhibits aldehyde dehydrogenase and block the oxidation of acetaldehyde which is a metabolite to ethyl alcohol. This act on cardiovascular system and have symptoms, *e.g.*, palpitation, perspiration, vomiting, nausea, flushing and fall in B.P.

Ans. 35 (C) Chronic alcoholics develop various nutritional deficiencies which may lead to anaemia (due to B_6, B_{12}, and iron deficiency) polyneuritis. Hemolytic anaemia is not due to nutritional deficiency.

Ans. 36 (C) Characteristic features of alcohol withdrawal syndrome are usually managed by diazepam. The intensity of symptoms may reduce by clonidine and propranolol. Methadone has no role in this situation.

Ans. 37 (D) Phenytoin block Na^+ channels and inhibits the generation of repetitive action potential. In higher doses, it also reduces the influx of Ca^{2+}.

Ans. 38 (A) Overdose toxicity of phenytoin includes nystagmus, ataxia, CNS depression, lethargy and blurred vision. It may cause cardiovascular collapse and death in still higher doses. While gum hyperplasia, megaloblastic anaemia, hirsutism are chronic toxicity (not dose dependent).

Ans. 39 (D) Carbamazepine can be used.

Ans. 40 (D) Sodium valproate (valproic acid) is broad spectrum anti-epileptic. It blocks Na^+ channels, increase GABA activity, decrease the release of glutamate in the brain and block T-type Ca^{2+} channels.

Ans. 41 (B) Diazepam is preferred drug given rectally in children.

Ans. 42 (C) Gabapentin and Pregabalin are GABA analogues which readily cross BBB and increase the synthesis and release of GABA to increase its concentration in brain.

Ans. 43 (A) Intravenous diazepam is first drug of choice in the treatment of status epilepticus. It acts rapidly. Parenteral phenobarbitone, phenytoin or other drugs are given in non-responding patient, as they act slowly.

Ans. 44 (D) Carbamazepine, phenobarbitone, phenytoin are enzyme inducers, so decreases the plasma concentration and efficacy of other drugs. Sodium valproate is enzyme inhibitor so decreases the metabolism of other drugs, and increases plasma concentration.

Ans. 45 (C) Vigabatrin is an inhibitor of GABA transaminase and thus increases GABA level in the brain. It is used in the treatment of simple and complex partial seizures. It causes irreversible visual field defect due to peripheral retinal atrophy. No skin lesion occurs with vigabatrin.

Ans. 46 (C) Ethosuximide inhibits the low threshold 'T' type Ca^{2+} channels. It is used in absence seizures. Withdrawal is not a problem as it is not used for prolonged period and can afford to withdrawal in six months.

Ans. 47 (A) Concurrent administration of clonazepam with sodium valproate is contraindicated. Though it is not CNS depressant but potentiate the CNS depressant effect of phenobarbitone and benzodiazepines (clonazepam).

Ans. 48 (B) Phenobarbitone is the safe drug to be used during pregnancy. Magnesium sulphate IV can be used in PET.

Ans. 49 (A) Olanazapine has minimal dopamine receptor blocking action and unlikely to cause acute dystonia. Muscarinic blocker exacerbates tardive dyskinasia.

Ans. 50 (B) Unlike classical neuroleptics (D_2 blocker) atypical drugs have their action mediated through 5-HT_{2A}, D_4 and D_2 receptor blockade, so EPS does not occur. They can be given parenterally.

Ans. 51 (C) Chlorpromazine causes elevation of serum prolactin and may cause inhibition of ovulation. It can produce amenorrhea, galactorrhea and loss of libido. It also blocks release of growth hormone.

Ans. 52 (B) EPS occur due to blockade of D_2 receptor. More potent the drug, more blockade and more adverse effect will occur.

Ans. 53 (A) Thioridazine having marked central anti-cholinergic effects. Cardiac arrhythmia and interference with male sexual function is common. It causes eye damage, which limits its use.

Ans. 54 (B) Combination of anti-psychotic is not very effective. Highly potent drugs are preferred over the low potency drugs.

Ans. 55 (B) Alprazolam is a high potency anxiolytic BZD, having some mood elevating action in mild depression.

Ans. 56 (A) Buspiron, Ipsapirone and Gepirone are non GABAnergic drugs. They have their effect by acting as partial agonist at brain 5-HT_{1A} receptor. Buspiron has no muscle relaxant, anti-convulsant or hypnotic action. All other are sedative hypnotics.

Ans. 57 (A) Moclobemide is a selective, reversible inhibitor of MAO-A with short duration of action. Because of competitive enzyme inhibitor, tyramine is able to displace catecholamines, but potentiating the presser response to ingested amine is weak, so dietary restriction is not required.

Ans. 58 (B) TCADs abolish the anti-hypertensive effect of guanethidine and clonidine by preventing their transport into adrenergic neurons.

Ans. 59 (C) They mainly and selectively block the 5-HT reuptake and have less marked anti-muscarinic, anti-histaminic effect with less sedation, with fewer cardiovascular effects. They may cause agitation and mania.

Ans. 60 (C) TCADs are effective in depression, anxiety, panic disorders, phobias, bulimia, migraine, obsessive-compulsive disorder but not in schizophrenia.

Ans. 61 (A) Lithium doses not cause sedation, while controlling psychomotor overactivity (as compared to chlorpromazine which causes sedation).

Ans. 62 (C) Carbamazepine is used as an alternative to lithium in manic disorder. Other drugs, *i.e.*, sodium valproate, lamotrigine, gabapentin, topiramate (anti-epileptic), olanzepine (anti-psychotic) are also effective alternative to lithium.

Ans. 63 (D) Long-term use of lithium may cause nephrogenic diabetes insipidus. It inhibits ADH stimulated adenylate cylase and cAMP. Collecting duct become impermeable to water, which is retained in collecting duct and then excreted.

Ans. 64 (D) High urinary levels of sodium inhibit renal tubular reabsorption of lithium, thus decreasing its plasma level. Lithium clearance is decreased by distal tubule diuresis (with thiazide) because natriuresis stimulates a reflex increase in the proximal tubule reabsorption of sodium and lithium and cause toxicity.

Ans. 65 (A) Tianeptine is an antidepressant which increase 5-HT uptake. It is neither sedative nor stimulant.

Ans. 66 (B) Olanzapine can be used during pregnancy as all other drugs are teratogenic.

Ans. 67 (C) Ziprasidone and olanzapine both act on 5-HT_2 receptor which causes less EPS and hemopoietic toxicity.

Ans. 68 (A) Fentanyl patches (transdermal) can increase arterial PCO_2 because of depression of the brainstem respiratory center.

Ans. 69 (D) Contraindication (use with caution) of opioid analgesics are hypotension, hypothyroidism, head injury, hypertrophy of prostate, hepatic damage, bronchial asthma, biliary colic and in babies (newborn). It may cause respiratory depression.

Ans. 70 (A) Codein, hydrocodone and oxycodone are metabolized by the cytochrome P-450 and variation in analgesic response to these drugs has been attributed to geno-typic polymorphism.

Ans. 71 (D) Nalbuphine is mixed agonist antagonist. When depression occurs with overdose of this drug, reversal with naloxone is unpredictable. It is antagonist at μ receptor, less likely to cause respiratory paralysis and may cause sedation.

Ans. 72 (D) Dextromethorphan is cough suppressant. It does not possess analgesic activity (but anti-tussive) and causes less constipation.

Ans. 73 (B) Propoxyphene is related with methadone, but having low analgesic, anti-tussive activities, and probably less constipating. Delirium and convulsions may occur in overdose.

Ans. 74 (D) Morphine has a high ceiling (dose dependent analgesia and euphoria is there), more effective in visceral pain and have no anti-inflammatory effect.

Ans. 75 (B) Morphine does not have direct effect on myocardium. Fall in BP is due to histamine release, depression of vasomotor centre and decrease in tone of blood vessels (direct action).

Ans. 76 (B) Morphine-6 glucuronide is an active metabolite which is more potent than morphine, but it does not cross BBB rapidly (similar to that of morphine).

Ans. 77 (C) Naloxone is a pure antagonist, used IV in the treatment of acute morphine poisoning. Naltrexone is also pure antagonist but effective orally, so used in post addict in opioid dependence.

Ans. 78 (D) Morphine causes miosis and increased ICT which may worsen the situation in head injury. It may mask the prognosis in case of head injury.

Ans. 79 (A) In equianalgesic doses it causes equivalent respiratory depression, sedation and euphoria.

Ans. 80 (B) Fentanyl, a pethidine congener is more potent than morphine as analgesic as well as in causing respiratory depression.

Ans. 81 (A) Tramadol act centrally and relieve pain by acting on both opioid receptors as well as by inhibiting reuptake of NA and 5-HT. Thus activate monoaminergic spinal inhibition of pain.

Ans. 82 (B) Unpleasant effects, *e.g.*, dysphoria and psychotomimetic effects limits the use of pentazocine. Abuse liability is also low.

Ans. 83 (C) Buprenorphine is μ receptor partial agonist more potent than morphine. It binds with μ receptors with high affinity and dissociates very slowly, so respiratory depression is not readily reversed by naloxone, but it may be alternative to methadone for management of opioid withdrawal.

Ans. 84 (C) Naloxone blocks placebo, acupuncture and stress induced analgesia, suggesting the involvement of opioid peptide in these response.

Ans. 85 (B) Supraspinal analgesia, euphoria, physical dependence is mediated by μ_1 receptors, while spinal analgesia, respiratory depression and decrease gut motility are mediated through μ_2 receptors.

Ans. 86 (B) COX-1 enzyme is constitutively expressed, *i.e.,* always present in most of the cells while COX-2 is inducible in inflammation cells by inflammatory stimuli, *i.e.,* endotoxin, kinin and TNF_{alpha}.

Ans. 87 (C) Metabolic acidosis is not caused by high doses with aspirin. It is observed with toxic doses (See text for details).

Ans. 88 (D) Prolongation of gestation by NSAIDs has been reported in humans. Indomethacin has been used off-label to terminate pre-term labour. This has been associated with premature closure of ductus arteriosus, and impaired fetal circulation in utero. It may increase the risk of PPH. Indomethacin is used in PDA after birth.

Ans. 89 (B) Phenylbutazone, and its active metabolite oxyphenbutazone, though very potent drug, but because of toxicity, *i.e.,* peptic ulcer and bone marrow depression not used commonly.

Ans. 90 (C) Indomethacin may cause frontal headache, dizziness, mental confusion, hallucination, depression and psychosis. It is contraindicated in machinery operators, drivers, psychiatric patient and during pregnancy.

Ans. 91 (A) Ibuprofen among all is safest and conventional NSAID.

Ans. 92 (A) Nimesulide exerts its anti-inflammatory action by inhibiting COX-2 and PG synthesis, reducing generation of superoxide by neutrophils, inhibition of PAF synthesis, TNF alpha release, free radical scavenging and inhibition of metalloproteinase activity in cartilage.

Ans. 93 (D) N-acetyl cystein replenish the glutathione stores in liver and prevent the binding of the toxic metabolite.

Ans. 94 (A) DMARDs are toxic, so their use should be weighed against their potential adverse effect (which may be serious). So early and mild cases are still treated with NSAIDs.

Ans. 95 (A) In advance cases, two or more drugs can be used together. They cannot be used for longer period due to their toxicity. They lose their efficacy with time and relief of symptoms may take time (from few weeks to months).

Ans. 96 (A) Methotrexate causes rapid relief of symptom among all (4–6 weeks).

Ans. 97 (C) Colchicine causes dose related toxicity, which includes nausea, vomiting, watery or bloody diarrhoea and abdominal cramps.

Ans. 98 (C) Allopurinol is xanthine oxidase inhibitor, an enzyme which is responsible for synthesis of uric acid.

Ans. 99 (C) Levodopa is first drug of choice in the treatment of parkinsonism.

Ans. 100(C) Levodopa is a dopamine precursor, when used is metabolized by dopa decarboxylase enzyme before it reaches to brain. So less concentration reaches in the brain and high doses are required to achieve optimum effect. Carbidopa is decarboxylase inhibitor; which inhibit the metabolism of L-dopa in periphery, so more L-dopa reaches in the brain.

Ans. 101(D) Amantidine and anticholinergic combination should not be used as amantidine is used in milder cases while anticholinergic only improve cholinergic effects, *e.g.*, tremors, excessive salivary secretions, but hypokinesia is affected least. So the combination of these is not very beneficial.

Ans. 102(C) Selegiline is a selective MAO-B inhibitor, so decrease the metabolism of dopamine.

Ans. 103(B) Benztropine, an anticholinergic should be used with caution in elderly as it may cause impairment of memory and confusional state, urinary retention and other atropine like adverse effects.

Ans. 104 (B) Pyridoxine abolishes therapeutic effect of levodopa by enhancing peripheral decarboxylation which can be minimized by combination of levodopa and carbidopa.

Ans. 105 (A) Methylphenidate is used in ADHD, as it improves behavior and learning.

Ans. 106 (A) Piracetam is cyclic GABA derivative but has no GABA like activity and called 'nootropic'. It improves learning memory, cognitive impairment and dementia in elderly. It is also effective in mental retardation in children. But not for apnoea where doxapram is used.

8

HORMONES AND HORMONE ANTAGONISTS (ENDOCRINOLOGY)

The pituitary gland, under the influence of the hypothalamus secretes many hormones which either control the secretion of other glands or directly act on the target tissues. Hormone is a substance of intense biological activity that is produced by specific cells in the body and then transported to act as target cell through circulation. These are peptides and act by binding to specific receptors present on the target cells.

HYPOTHALAMUS AND ANTERIOR PITUITARY HORMONES

Hypothalamic Hormones

Hypothalamus produces many releasing and inhibiting hormones. These includes:

1. Growth hormone releasing hormone (GHRH), which stimulates anterior pituitary to secrete growth hormone.
2. Somatostatin which is growth hormone release-inhibiting hormone present in the hypothalamus, parts of the CNS, pancreas and in gastrointestinal tract. It inhibits the secretion of growth hormone, TSH and prolactin by pituitary and insulin and glucagon by pancreas. Octreotide is the synthetic analog of somatostatin which is longer acting and useful in acromegaly.
3. Thyrotropin releasing hormone (TRH) secreted by the hypothalamus stimulates the release of TSH from the anterior pituitary.
4. Corticotropin releasing factor (CRF) releases ACTH from the anterior pituitary. It is used in diagnostic tests in Cushing's disease.
5. Gonadotropin releasing hormone (GnRH, LH-RH/FSH-RH) secreted in a pulsatile manner and regulates the secretion of gonadotropins FSH and LH. It is used in diagnostic tests in hypogonadism. Nafarlelin is long acting GnRH agonist more potent than GnRH and used in assisted reproduction and endometriosis.

Anterior Pituitary Hormones

Growth Hormone (GH): The secretion of growth hormone is regulated by GHRH and somatostatin (GHRIH). GH deficiency in children results in dwarfism while excessive production results in gigantism in children and acromegaly in adults. It is used in:

- *GH deficiency:* Replacement therapy in pituitary dwarfism, Turner syndrome (with GH deficiency in children). It can also be used in adults with GH deficiency.
- Chronic renal failure; and
- Catabolic states like severe burns and AIDS, bed-ridden patients, osteoporosis etc.
- Nowadays recombinant human GH (rhGH), *e.g.*, somatropin and somatrem is used.

Corticotrophin (Adrenocorticotropic hormone, ACTH): It controls the synthesis and release of glucocorticoids, mineralocorticoids, and androgens from the adrenal cortex. It is used primarily for diagnosis of disorders of pituitary adrenal axis. For therapeutic purpose, corticosteroids are preferred.

Thyroid stimulating hormone (TSH, Thyrotropin) stimulates the production and secretion of thyroid hormones and thus regulates thyroid function. It has no therapeutic value.

Gonadotropins: Follicle stimulating hormone (FSH) and luteinising hormone (LH)–produced by the anterior pituitary regulate gonadal function. In men they promote spermatogenesis. It is used in:

1. Gonadotropin deficiency in males (Hypogonadism).
2. Undescended testes.
3. Amenorrhoea and infertility in females.
4. In vitro fertilization.

Prolactin (PRL): Prolactin has mammotropic and lactogenic effects. It also play an important role in regulating immune system. This also promotes the growth and development of breast during pregnancy. It stimulates milk production along with other hormones like estrogens and progestin. Deficiency results in lactation failure while excess prolactin results in galactorrhoea. Suckling is the principal stimulus for prolactin secretion.

Posterior Pituitary Hormones

Oxytocin: Its primary role is in milk ejection and in initiation of labour and parturition.

Vasopressin (Anti-diuretic Hormone): Its role is discussed with diuretics.

INSULIN AND ORAL HYPOGLYCEMIC AGENTS

Diabetes mellitus is a metabolic disorder characterized by hyperglycemia, glycosuria, hyperlipidemia, negative nitrogen balance and sometimes ketonemia. Due to thickening of capillary basement membrane, increase in vessel wall matrix and cellular proliferation, risk of vascular complications like atherosclerosis, peripheral vascular disease neuropathy and retinopathy increased. Diabetes mellitus can be divided into:

1. Type I or insulin dependent diabetes mellitus (IDDM).
2. Type II or non-insulin dependent diabetes mellitus (NIDDM).
3. Type III diabetes due to other causes, *e.g.*, drug induced, chronic pancreatitis.
4. Type IV or Gestational diabetes mellitus (during 2nd or 3rd trimester of pregnancy).

Insulin

The islets of Langerhans are composed of 4 types of cells, beta cells secrete insulin, alpha cells secretes glucagon, delta (D) cells secretes somatostatin and PP or F cells secrete pancreatic polypeptide.

Natural insulin is a polypeptide synthesized from the precursor proinsulin. It has two peptide chains A chain (with 21 amino acids) and B chain (with 30 amino acids) linked by disulphide bridge which is essential for its biological activity. Insulin is stored in granules in the beta cells of islet cells of the pancreas. The secretion is regulated by factors like food, hormones and by autonomic nervous system. During biotransformation, disulfide bond is reduced, and A and B chains are separated. Plasma half life of insulin is 5–9 min.

Actions of Insulin

The major target organs of insulin are liver, adipose tissue and skeletal muscle. Insulin regulate blood sugar level by acting on these organs and affecting carbohydrate protein and lipid metabolism.

1. **Carbohydrate metabolism:** Insulin stimulates the uptake and metabolism of glucose in the peripheral tissues especially in skeletal muscles and adipose tissue, inhibit gluconeogenesis and glycogenolysis by liver. It lowers the blood glucose concentration by increasing peripheral utilization of glucose and by glycogen synthesis.
2. **Lipid metabolism:** Insulin inhibits lipolysis in adipose tissue and promotes the synthesis of triglycerides. Insulin indirectly enhances lipoprotein lipase activity and decrease lipolysis resulting in increased clearance of VLDL and chylomicrons.
3. **Protein metabolism:** Insulin facilitates amino acid uptake and protein synthesis and inhibits protein breakdown in all tissues and have anabolic effect.

Mechanism of Action: Insulin acts by binding to specific receptors located on the cell membrane of all cells. Insulin receptor is made up of two alpha and two beta subunits. Insulin binds to alpha subunit of these receptors present on the surface of target cells. This binding stimulates tyrosine kinase activity in the beta subunit. This in turn activates a cascade of phosphorylation and dephosphorylation reactions which stimulate or inhibit the enzymes involved in the metabolic actions of insulin.

Side Effects

1. Hypoglycemia is the most common side effect of insulin therapy.
2. Allergy: This is due to the contaminating proteins. Urticaria, angioedema and rarely anaphylaxis can occur. It is rare with purified preparations and human insulin.
3. Lipodystrophy: Atrophy of the subcutaneous fat at the site of injection.
4. Insulin presbiopia.
5. Insulin neuropathy.
6. Obesity.
7. Insulin resistance: When insulin requirement seem to exceed 100 IU/day due to development of antibodies.

Preparations of Insulin

All preparations are given SC. Only regular insulin can be given IV in emergencies. Doses are calculated by monitoring blood glucose and glycosylated hemoglobin levels (HbA_{1c}). 6% value of HbA_{1c} is equal to 110 mg/dL of blood sugar.

(A) Conventional Insulins

a. *Short and Rapid acting:* Regular, Semilente (insulin Zn suspension).
b. *Intermediate acting:* Lente insulin, Isorphane and Natural protamine Hagedorn (NPH) insulin.
c. *Long acting:* Ultra lente insulin, Protamine zinc insulin.

(B) Highly Purified Insulins

a. *Single peak insulin:* Regular, Lente.
b. *Monocomponent insulin:* Regular, Lente.
c. *Human insulin:* Regular, Lente, Isophane (short acting).
d. *Insulin analogs:* Insulin lispro, Insulin aspart, Insulin glulisine, all are ultra short acting. Insulin glargine is long acting. Insulin analogs have been synthesized by genetic engineering, absorbed 3 times faster than human insulin. Blood glucose control is better than with regular insulin.
e. *Insulin mixtures:* Combination of 20-50% regular with 80-50% NPH insulin.

Disadvantages of the Conventional Preparations

1. They are allergenic.
2. They are not very stable.

Highly purified insulin is mostly porcine insulin purified by more developed purification techniques including gel filtration and ion exchange chromatography. Human insulin is produced by recombinant DNA technology.

Highly purified insulin and human insulin have the following advantages over conventional insulin:

1. They are less antigenic.
2. More stable.
3. Lesser chances of resistance: Insulin resistance is said to be present when the insulin requirement is increased to > 200 U/day. It is due to the formation of antibodies to insulin which partly neutralize it. This is rare with purified preparations and human insulin.
4. Lesser chances of lipodystrophy.

Indications for Highly Purified Human Insulin are:

1. Allergy to conventional preparations.
2. Insulin resistance.

3. Lipodystrophy at the site of injection.
4. Pregnancy.

Drug Interactions

1. Beta adrenergic blockers mask tachycardia, which is the important warning symptom of hypoglycemia, by inhibiting compensatory mechanisms acting through $beta_2$ receptors.
2. Salicylates precipitate hypoglycemia by enhancing both insulin secretion and beta cell sensitivity to glucose.
3. Thiazides, furosemide, OCP increase BSL by decreasing effectiveness of insulin.

Indications of Insulin Therapy

Insulin is effective in all types of diabetes mellitus.

1. IDDM.
2. NIDDM – Patients who have onset before 30–35 years.
3. All diabetes with complication, *e.g.*, ketoacidosis CCF etc.
4. During surgical procedure.
5. Diabetic pre coma and coma.
6. Primary or secondary failure to oral hypoglycemic therapy.
7. Pregnancy.

Management of Diabetic Ketoacidosis

1. Diagnosis must be confirmed by IV glucose (50 ml of 50%) to differentiate to hypoglycemia.
2. IV fluids (to control electrolyte imbalance and to correct dehydration).
3. Regular insulin.
4. Potassium chloride.
5. Correction of acidosis: Sodium bicarbonate is added to fluid.
6. Phosphate.
7. Antibiotics.
8. Other measures of good nursing care, treatment of cause etc.

Newer Insulin Delivery Systems

1. Insulin syringe.
2. Insulin pump.
3. Inhaled insulin.
4. Portable pen injections.
5. Biodegradable microspheres.

Oral Hypoglycemic Agents

They are mainly used in the treatment of T2DM.

Classification of Oral Hypoglycemic Agents

1. **Sulfonylureas**
   a. *1st generation:* Tolbutamide, Chlorpropamide, Acetohexamide, Tolazamide.
   b. *2nd generation:* Gibenclamide (glyburide), Glipizide, Gliclazide, Glimepiride.
2. **Biguanides:** Phenformin, Metformin.
3. **Meglitinide:** Repaglinide, Nateglinide.
4. **Thiozolidinediones (PPAR gamma agonist):** Troglitazone, Rosiglitazone, Pioglitazone.
5. **Alpha glucosidase inhibitors:** Acarbose, Miglitol, Voglibose.
6. **Analogue of glucagon like peptide-1 (GLP-1),** *e.g.,* Liraglutide, Exenatide.
7. **Inhibitors of dipeptidyl-peptidase-4 (DPP-4),** *e.g.,* Saxagliptin, Sitagliptin, Linagliptine.
8. **Sodium glucose co-transporter-2 (SGLT-2) inhibitors:** Dapaglifozin, Serglifozin, Remoglifozin.

Sulfonylurea and meglitinides are insulin secretagogues while biguanide and thiozolidindiones (PPAR gamma agonist) are known as insulin sensitizers.

Sulfonylureas

Mechanism of Action: Sulfonylureas reduce the blood glucose level by:

1. Stimulating the release of insulin from the pancreatic beta cells (both production and secretion).
2. Increasing the sensitivity of peripheral tissues to insulin.
3. Decreasing the elevated FFA.
4. Suppressing hepatic gluconeogenesis and glycogenoloysis and increase affinity/concentration of insulin receptors.

Sulfonylurea binds to specific receptors on pancreatic beta cells and inhibits efflux of potassium. They block the ATP sensitive K^+ channels. This reduced K^+ conductance and causes depolarization and Ca^{++} -influx leading to increased insulin secretion. Thus some functional beta cells are essential for the action of sulfonylurea. They also suppress glucagon level. Glimepiride additionally increases the sensitivity of peripheral tissue to insulin and have antioxidant activity.

Tolbutamide is short acting and is therefore associated with lesser risk of hypoglycemia; hence it is safer in the elderly diabetics. Second generation agents are more potent, have fewer side effects and drug interactions. But they can cause hypoglycemia because of which they should be used cautiously particularly in the elderly.

Pharmacokinetics: Sulfonylureas are well-absorbed orally, extensively bound to plasma proteins and have low volume of distribution. They are metabolized in liver and some are excreted in the urine. Hence they should be used cautiously in patients with renal or liver dysfunction. They crosses placental barrier.

Adverse Effects: Hypoglycemia is the most common adverse effect. Nausea, vomiting, jaundice and allergic reactions can occur. Patients on sulfonylurea may have an increase in the rate of cardiovascular death.

Uses

1. NIIDM.
2. With insulin in insulin resistant DM.

Contraindications

1. Pregnancy 2. IDDM 3. Hepatic and renal dysfunction (use with caution).

Drug Interactions

1. *Drugs that augment hypoglycemic effect:*
   - NSAIDS, warfarin and sulfonamides displace sulfonylurea from protein binding sites.
   - Alcohol, chloramphenicol and cimetidine inhibit metabolism excretion.
2. *Drugs that decrease the action of sulfonylurea:*
   - Diuretics and corticosteroids increase blood glucose levels by suppressing insulin release.
   - Enzyme inducers by increasing metabolism.

Biguanide (Anti-Hyperglycemic Agents)

They do not stimulate insulin release but remain ineffective in the absence of insulin, so presence of some insulin is essential for their action. They:

- Suppress hepatic gluconeogenesis and reduce hepatic glucose output.
- Inhibit glucose absorption from the intestines (with other hexoses, amino acids and Vitamin B_{12}).

- Stimulate peripheral uptake of glucose in tissues in the presence of insulin by enhancing anaerobic glycolysis.

  They increase binding of insulin to insulin receptor and cause weight reduction–due to anorexia. Thus, preferred in obese diabetics, either alone or with sulfonylurea. They do not cause hypoglycemia.

Adverse Effects

1. Lactic acidosis can occur.
2. Long-term use may interfere with Vitamin B_{12} absorption.
3. Nausea, diarrhea, metallic taste (transient).

They are contraindicated in renal, hepatic and cardiac diseases, and in alcoholics.

Indications

1. Obese with NIDDM.
2. Secondary failure to sulfonylurea.
3. In brittle IDDM with fluctuation in BSL.
4. To treat hirsutism in polycystic ovarian syndrome.

Meglitinide Analogue

Repaglinide and nateglinide are insulin secretogogues, they enhance the release of insulin by blocking the ATP dependent K^+ channels in the pancreatic beta cells. Both drugs can cause hypersensitivity reactions and hypoglycemia.

Meglitinides can be used in type 2 diabetes mellitus either alone or with biguanide. They provide rapid but less sustained secretion of insulin, so chances of late phase hypoglycemia are less. Adverse effects include dizziness, nausea and flu-like symptoms.

Thiazolidinediones (TZDs)

Thiazolidinediones are agonists at the PPAR gamma receptors (gamma sub type of peroxisome proliferators activated receptors). They activate the PPAR gamma receptors and induce the synthesis of genes which enhance insulin action and promote glucose utilization in peripheral tissue.

- TZDs increase insulin mediated glucose transport into muscle and adipose tissue by enhancing the synthesis and translocation of specific forms of the glucose transport proteins.
- They reduce hepatic gluconeogenesis.

- Once a day administration is required.
- Low potential for hypoglycemia.
- Increase HDL cholesterol and decrease TG.
- No clinically significant drug interactions known so far.
- They are effective orally and metabolized by Cytochrome P-450.
- TZDs are used as adjuvant to sulfonylurea or biguanide in type II diabetes mellitus.
- They decrease HbA_{1c} levels.

Disadvantages

- 6–12 weeks of treatment are required to establish maximum therapeutic effect.
- May cause weight gain and anaemia.
- May cause edema and precipitate or worsen CCF.
- Liver function should be monitored regularly.
- Troglitazone causes severe hepatotoxicity and therefore is not used now.

Alpha Glucosidase Inhibitors

Acarbose, voglibose and miglitol competitively inhibit the enzymes alpha glucosidases present in the intestinal brush border and thereby prevent the absorption of carbohydrates. Monosaccharide like glucose and fructose are absorbed from the intestines, while disaccharides and oligosaccharides are broken down into monosaccharide before being absorbed. This 'breaking down' is done by the enzyme alpha glucosidases, alpha amylase present in the intestinal wall. Glucosidase inhibitors inhibit the hydrolysis of disaccharides and decrease carbohydrate absorption. They also inhibit gluco amylase and sucrase.

- Alpha glucosidase inhibitors reduce the glucose absorption from upper intestines thereby reducing postprandial blood glucose levels.
- Alpha glucosidase inhibitors do not cause hypoglycemia.
- They may cause gastrointestinal disturbances including abdominal distention, flatulence and diarrhoea because of undigested carbohydrates.
- They can be used alone in patients with predominantly postprandial hyperglycemia or in combination with other oral anti-diabetics or insulin.

Newer Agents

GLP-1 Analogue and DPP-4 Inhibitors

- GLP-1 analogue-liraglutide and exenatide and DPP-4 inhibitor saxagliptin etc. are the new anti-diabetic agents to be used in T2DM. These agents targeting incretin hormones, glucagon like peptide-1 (GLP-1) and glucose dependent insulinotropic peptide (GIP). They stimulate insulin output from pancreatic beta-cells and suppress pancreatic alpha cell secretion and glucagon.
- Dipeptidyl peptidase (DPP-4) inhibitors inhibit the inactivation of incretin hormone by inhibiting DPP-4 enzyme thereby enhancing and prolonging the activity of GLP-1 and GIP and attenuating P.P. glucose excursion.
- GLP-1 analogue exenatide and liraglutide reduces plasma glucose level by increasing insulin secretion, reduces P.P. glucagon secretion, delays gastric emptying, improve beta-cell function and reduces appetite. These agents may be an effective treatment options for use in patients with T2DM.
- *SGLT-2 inhibitors:* They decrease the amount of glucose reabsorption from the proximal tubule and increase its excretion in urine. SGLT-2 system is exclusively present in the proximal tubules of the kidney. They cause weight loss. They also possess anti-diuretic effect, so have beneficial effect in patients with hypertension. They improve insulin resistance and not induce insulin secretion, so chances of hypoglycemia are not there. The main adverse effect is increased risk of urinary bacterial/fungal infection due to glucosuria and risk of Na^+ loss. They are at present in clinical trial phase IV.

Treatment of Diabetes Mellitus

The aim of treatment is to keep the blood sugar within normal limits and prevent complications of diabetes. Mild NIDDM may be controlled by diet, exercise and weight reduction. When not controlled, an oral hypoglycemic should be given. Most NIDDM patients may require insulin some time later in life. IDDM type I diabetes mellitus is treated with insulin.

Glucagon

Glucagon is synthesized in the alpha (A) cells of the pancreatic islets of

Langerhans; like insulin, the secretion of glucagon is regulated by nutrients chiefly glucose, paracrine hormones and autonomic nervous system. Sympathetic stimulation, fasting, high protein diet stimulates glucagon secretion while hyperglycemia and somatostatin inhibits its release.

Glucagon increases blood glucose level by glycogenolysis and gluconeogenesis in the liver. It evokes insulin release and conversion of stored fat and amino acids into glucose in liver. Glucagon increases the heart rate and force of contraction. It also relaxes the intestinal smooth muscles. Glucagon can be used in the emergency treatment of severe hypoglycemia due to insulin.

THYROID HORMONES AND ANTI-THYROID DRUGS

Thyroid Hormones

Thyroid gland secretes three hormones:

Thyroxine (T_4), Triiodothyronine (T_3) and Calcitonin. T_4 is a less active precursor of T_3.

Synthesis, Storage and Secretion: The thyroid hormones are synthesized and stored in the thyroid follicles. The principle source of iodine is diet. The main steps involved in the synthesis of thyroid hormones are as follows:

1. Uptake of plasma iodide by thyroid follicular cells (iodine trapping).
2. Oxidation of iodide to I^+ (iodinium ions) by a thyroperoxidase enzyme.
3. Iodine atom get attached with tyrosine molecule present in TG (organification of iodine). Tyrosine molecule contain one atom of iodine monoiodotyrosine (MIT) and two atom of iodine diiodotyrosine (DIT).
4. Coupling: Pairs of MIT and DIT are coupled to form T_3 (MIT+DIT) and T_4 (DIT+DIT). TG containing iodinated tyrosine residues are stored in the follicles.
5. T_4 and T_3 are released into the circulation, when needed.

The thyroid secretion is regulated by TSH, secreted by the anterior pituitary and TRH from the hypothalamus.

Thyroid hormones are essential for normal growth, development, function and maintenance of all body tissues. Thyroid hormones have important metabolic functions. They increase metabolic rate, enhance carbohydrate and protein metabolism and stimulate lipolysis and metabolism of cholesterol to bile acids. Hypercholesterolemia is a feature of hypothyroidism. They facilitate erythropoiesis. They are also essential for normal functioning of the skeletal muscles, cardiovascular system, reproductive system GIT, kidney and CNS. They have calorigenic action. Congenital deficiency results in cretinism.

Mechanism of Action: Thyroid hormones act on thyroid receptors which are nuclear receptors like the steroid receptors. T_3 enters into the cells, bind to the receptor and cause synthesis of specific mRNA. This in turn activates gene transcription and regulates protein synthesis.

An acute increase in the supply of iodide leads to increase in iodine content. This immediately inhibits the iodine trapping and responsiveness to TSH is diminished. Thus release of thyroid is auto regulated.

Adverse effects include tachycardia, palpitation, tremors, weight loss and heat intolerance.

Uses

1. Replacement therapy in Cretinism, Hypothyroidism and Myxoedema.
2. Nontoxic goiter (endemic or sporadic).
3. Thyroid carcinoma.
4. Hyperthyroidism (Graves' disease).
5. Miscellaneous – Refractory anaemias, infertility, menstrual disorders and non-healing ulcers.

Anti-Thyroid Drugs

Hyperthyroidism is due to an excess of circulating thyroid hormones. Graves' disease, an autoimmune disorder, is the most common cause. Hyperthyroidism is characterized by increased BMR, tachycardia, heat intolerance hyperreflexia etc. Diffuse goiter and IgG antibodies that activate TSH receptors are present in Graves' disease. Anti-thyroid drugs may act by interfering with the synthesis, release or actions of thyroid hormones.

Anti-Thyroid Drugs

A. *Thiomide derivatives:* Propylthiouracil, Methimazole, Carbimazole.
B. *Radioactive iodine.*
C. *Iodides:* Lugol's iodine.
D. *Iodinated contrast media:* Oral ipodate and ipanoic acid, Diatrizoate (Intravenous).

A. Thioamide Derivatives

They reduce the synthesis of thyroid hormones by:

a. Inhibiting thyroid peroxidase which is required for intrathyroidal oxidation of I^-.
b. Inhibiting iodination of tyrosine residues; and
c. Coupling of iodotyrosine residues.

Propylthiouracil also inhibits peripheral conversion of T_4 to T_3 by inhibiting DID-I enzyme. T_3 and T_4 levels fall. Large doses may stimulate release of TSH resulting in thyroid enlargement. Propylthiouracil is faster acting while carbimazole is longer acting.

Pharmacokinetics: They are effective orally; about 75% propylthiouracil is firmly bound to plasma proteins, they are widely distributed in the body. Carbimazole and methimazole cross the placenta and are secreted in the milk. They are metabolized in the liver.

Adverse effects are allergic reactions, jaundice and headache. Agranulocytosis is a rare but serious adverse effect. Loss or graying of hair in hypothyroidism is due to over treatment.

Uses

1. Definitive therapy of hyperthyroidism, *e.g.*, Graves' disease and toxic modular goiter
2. *Preoperatively:* Hyperthyroid patients are made euthyroid with anti-thyroid drugs prior to surgery. Carbimazole is preferred.
3. *Hyperthyroidism in pregnancy:* Propylthiouracil is the preferred drug as it poorly crosses the placental barrier in lactating mothers.
4. Thyroid storm is sudden, severe exacerbation of thyrotoxicosis and can be life threatening. It is precipitated by factors like stress, infections, trauma surgery etc. Propylthiouracil, oral/rectal, potassium iodide, IV hydrocortisone, tepid sponging, sedation, IV fluids and supportive therapy are needed immediately. Many of the symptoms of hyperthyroidism are due to sympathetic over-activity as there is increased tissue sensitivity to catecholamine in hyperthyroidism. **Beta adrenergic blockers** like propranolol relieve symptoms like palpitation, tremors, nervousness, sweating and myopathy. They only afford symptomatic relief and are used as adjuvant in hyperthyroidism and thyrotoxic crisis. It also impairs the conversion of T_4 to T_3 which may add to the beneficial effect.

B. Radioactive Iodine (^{131}I)

Radioactive iodine given orally as a solution is rapidly absorbed and is concentrated by the thyroid in the follicles. It emits both gamma and beta rays. The gamma rays pass through the tissue while beta particles penetrate only 0.5 to 2 min of the tissue due to which it destroys only the thyroid tissue without damaging the surrounding structures. They destroy some of the thyroid follicles and produce fibrosis, impair the ability of remaining follicle to replicate.

^{131}I has a half-life of 8 days but the radioactivity is present upto 2 months. It is given as a single dose. Clinically the effect is seen after 1–2 months.

Radioactive Iodine (3–10 m curie) is used:

1. In the patients >35 years of age in the treatment of hyperthyroidism.
2. Thyroid carcinoma.
3. Small dose is used for diagnostic purpose in thyroid function tests.
4. In patients allergic to anti-thyroid drugs.

Advantages of ^{131}I over thyroidectomy are:

(i) Administration is simple, highly effective and convenient.
(ii) Surgery and its associated risks can be avoided.
(iii) Less expensive when compared to surgery.

The disadvantages are:

(i) It take long time (3 months) for its maximum response.
(ii) Have the risk of hypothyroidism, which may develop after a few months or years. So not recommended for children, women of child-bearing age and during pregnancy.
(iii) Risk of developing thyroid carcinoma.
(iv) Cannot be used as therapeutic trial.

C. Iodides

They inhibit the release of thyroid hormones and when given in thyrotoxic patients the symptoms subside in 1–2 days. They shut off the release of preformed thyroid hormone and cause thyroid constipation. Iodides are administered orally as Lugol's iodine or as potassium iodide solution. Lugol's iodine is 5% iodine in 10% potassium iodide. Iodine is converted into iodides in the intestine which is then absorbed.

Adverse effects include allergic reactions like skin rashes, conjunctivitis, swelling of the lips and salivary glands, fever and lymphadenopathy. Chronic overdose can cause iodism with metallic taste, excessive salivation, lacrimation, burning sensation in the oral cavity and throat, running nose, sore throat, cough, headache and rashes. It crosses placental barrier and may cause goitrous cretinism in fetus.

Uses

1. Preoperative preparation for thyroidectomy. 10-14 days prior to surgery.
2. Thyroid storm.
3. Prophylaxis to prevent endemic goiter.
4. Antiseptic and expectorant

D. Iodinated Contrast Media

Iodinated contrast media, *e.g.*, ipodate and ipanoic acid (oral) and diatrizoate (IV), inhibit 5'-deiodinase (DID-I and DID-II) enzymes and therefore prevent the conversion of T_4 and T_3 in the liver, kidney, pituitary gland and brain. They cause dramatic improvement in subjective and objective symptoms of hyperthyroidism, when used with thioamides. They are less toxic than iodine (reserved for short term treatment of patients with severe thyrotoxicosis).

ADRENOCORTICOIDS

Adrenal glands consist of two different zones. Corticosteroids are hormones produced in the cortex of the adrenal gland and include glucocorticoids, mineralocorticoids and a small amount of androgens. Cortisol is the major glucocorticoid while aldosterone is the major mineralocorticoid. The secretions of the adrenal cortex are under the control of ACTH secreted by the anterior pituitary and this is in turn regulated by CRF and plasma corticosterone levels. This is termed as hypothalamic pituitary adrenal (HPA) axis.

Glucocorticoid Actions

1. **Carbohydrate, Protein and Fat Metabolism:** Glucocorticoids promote gluconeogenesis and glycogen deposition in the liver and inhibit peripheral utilization of glucose by decreasing cellular uptake resulting in increased blood glucose levels. They enhance

protein breakdown and nitrogen is excreted leading to negative nitrogen balance (anti-anabolic effect). They promote lipolysis and causes redistribution of fats. Fat is mobilized from extremities and deposited over the face, neck and shoulder and this fat deposition in excess glucocorticoid activity is described as 'moon face', 'fish mouth' and 'buffalo hump', respectively.

2. **Anti-inflammatory and Immunosuppressive Effects:** Glucocorticoids suppress the development of inflammatory response to all types of stimuli, *e.g.*, chemical, mechanical and immunological. They inhibit both early (pain, heat, edema etc.) and late manifestations of inflammation, inhibition of late response like capillary proliferation, collagen deposition, fibroblastic activity and scar formation. They may delay wound healing. They inhibit migration and depress the function of the leucocytes and macrophages and inhibit the release of chemical mediators. In addition glucocorticoids also induce the synthesis of a lipocortin, which inhibits phospholipase A_2, thereby decreasing the production of prostaglandins and leukotrienes.
   Glucocorticoids thus suppress cell-mediated immunity by inhibiting genes that code for IL and TFN-alpha, prevent manifestations of allergy and prevent homograft rejection. Large doses also inhibit antibody production.
3. **Other Actions**
   - They have important physiological role in development of lungs in neonates.
   - Glucocorticoids reduce capillary permeability, thereby reducing fluid exudation and maintain the tone of arterioles. They have a positive inotropic effect on the heart.
   - They are essential for normal muscular activity and for normal glomerular filtration.
   - Glucocorticoids enhance the secretion of gastric acid and pepsin in the stomach and causes peptic ulceration.
   - Glucocorticoids inhibit absorption and enhance the renal excretion of calcium. They antagonize the effect of vitamin D on calcium absorption. Bone resorption takes place (specially vertebrae and ribs).
   - Glucocorticoids have a lympholytic effect which is very prominent in lymphomas, it increases number of RBCs, platelets and neutrophills in circulation.

- Glucocorticoids also have a weak mineralocorticoid action and cause retention of salt and water and excretion of potassium.
- CNS: They cause mild euphoria, followed by insomnia, anxiety and depression.

Mechanism of Action

Corticosteroids bind to specific receptors (transcortin) in the cytoplasm and activate them. The drug receptor complex is then transported into the nucleus where it binds to specific sites on DNA (glucocorticoid response element GRE) and induces the synthesis of specific mRNA. By this they regulate the synthesis of new proteins that bring about the hormone effects. They also induce formation of lipocortin-1.

Pharmacokinetics

Glucocorticoids are well absorbed orally. Hydrocortisone undergoes high first pass metabolism. It is 95% bound to plasma proteins (corticosteroid binding globulin CBG or transcortin). They are metabolized in the liver by oxidation and reduction followed by conjugation. Metabolites are excreted by the kidneys.

Adverse Effects of Glucocorticoids

Adverse effects of glucocorticoids are depend on dose, duration of therapy and the relative potency of additional mineralocorticoid effects. Whenever possible, they should be used topically to avoid systemic effects. Single doses are harmless while short courses are well tolerated. Prolonged use is associated with toxicity.

Adverse effects include: Cushing's syndrome, hyperglycemia, susceptibility to infections, osteoporosis, avascular necrosis, peptic ulceration, mental disturbances, cataract, delayed wound healing, muscle wasting and myopathies. Less common adverse effects include raised intracranial pressure, convulsions, hypercoagulability of the blood and menstrual disorders and HPA axis suppression. Prolonged use may cause edema; hypokalemia, hypertension, thinning of skin, hirsutism etc.

Uses: Used as replacement therapy in:

1. Acute adrenal insufficiency.
2. Chronic adrenal insufficiency (Addison's disease).
3. Congenital adrenal hyperplasia.

Used in the Treatment of (as Pharmacotherapy) in:

1. Rheumatoid arthritis and osteoarthritis.
2. Rheumatic carditis.
3. Acute gout.
4. Allergic disease like angioneurotic edema, hay fever, serum sickness, contact dermatitis, urticaria, drug reactions and anaphylaxis.
5. Bronchial asthma.
6. Collagen diseases like polyarthritis nodosa, lupus erythematosus, polymyositis, Wegener's granulomatosis and other rheumatoid disorders.
7. Eye diseases: Allergic conjunctivitis, uveitis, optic neuritis and other inflammatory conditions.
8. Renal diseases like nephrotic syndrome are treated with steroids.
9. Gastrointestinal diseases: Inflammatory bowel disease like ulcerative colitis are treated with steroid.
10. Liver diseases like autoimmune chronic active hepatitis and alcoholic hepatitis.
11. Hematologic disorders like purpura and hemolytic anemia.
12. Cerebral edema.
13. Malignancies: Steroids are used in the treatment of acute lymphocytic leukemia and Hodgkin's lymphomas.
14. Lung diseases like aspiration pneumonia and prevention of infant respiratory distress syndrome.
15. Organ transplantation: For prevention and treatment of graft rejection.
16. Others: Sarcoidosis, pneumocystis carinii pneumonia (in patients with AIDS), in haemolytic anaemia.

Steroids should be used with caution in peptic ulcer, hypertension, viral and fungal infections, diabetes mellitus, ocular infections particularly viral infections, osteoporosis, psychoses, epilepsy, CCF, glaucoma, renal failure.

Metyrapone, trilastane, aminoglutethimide and ketoconazole inhibit the synthesis of adrenal steroids by inhibiting certain enzymes involved in steroid synthesis. They are used in Cushing's syndrome and some prostatic and breast cancers.

Mineralocorticoids

The most important natural mineralocorticoid is aldosterone, synthesized in zona glomerulosa of the adrenal cortex. Small amounts of desoxycorticosterone are also released. Mineralocorticoids promote sodium and water retention by distal renal tubules with loss of potassium. Adverse effects include weight gain, edema, hypertension and hypokalemia. Fludrocortisone has predominantly mineralocorticoid properties and is used for replacement therapy in aldosterone deficiency as in Addison's disease. Although aldosterone is the principal natural mineralocorticoid, it is not used therapeutically since it is not effective orally.

ESTROGENS, PROGESTINS AND HORMONAL CONTRACEPTIVES

Estrogens

The estrogens are produced by the ovaries, placenta and in small amounts by the adrenals and testes. The major estrogens are estradiol, secreted by ovary synthesized in the graffian follicle. Estradiol is converted to estrone and estriol by the liver and other tissues.

Natural estrogens are: Estradiol, Estrone, Estriol (weaker estrogen).

Synthetic estrogens are: Ethinyl estradiol, Mestranol, Tibolone, Quinesterol.

Synthetic non-steroidal estrogens are: Stilbesterol, Dienestrol.

Estrogen binds strongly to sex hormone binding alpha 2 globulin (SH-BG) and to serum albumin (low affinity). There are two types of estrogen receptors ER alpha and ER beta:

ER alpha: Predominates in female reproduction tract (uterus, vagina), breast, blood vessels and hypothalamus.

ER beta has wide distribution in ovaries and prostate. This receptor–estrogen complex binds to DNA and stabilizes a multi protein complex (RNA polymerase) necessary for initiation of RNA synthesis.

Actions: Estrogens are required for:

1. The normal development of maturation of the female reproductive tract.
2. Development of secondary sexual characters in the female.
3. Stimulation of pre ovulatory endometrium.
4. Vasodilatation of capillaries.

5. Metabolic effects. Estrogens inhibit the resorption of bone and maintain the bone mass. They promote the fusion of epiphyses. They are weak diabetogenic.
6. For the maintenance of normal structure of the skin and blood vessels in women.
7. Estrogens decrease plasma LDL cholesterol and raise HDL cholesterol and triglycerides and have cardioprotective effect.
8. Effect on blood coagulation: Estrogens enhance the coagulability of the blood.

Exogenous estrogen produces proliferative changes in endometrium (in women with deficient ovarian function) and retention of sodium and water. It is carcinogenic, anti-androgenic and increases coagulability.

Pharmacokinetics: Natural estrogens are metabolized rapidly during first pass to the liver hence are not effective orally. They have a short $t_{1/2}$. They are largely bound to plasma proteins. Synthetic estrogens are orally effective and are long acting due to enterohepatic circulation.

Adverse Effects: Nausea, breast tenderness, migraine headaches bleeding irregularities, thromboembolic phenomenon, hyperpigmentation, hypertension and cholestasis may be seen. In men gynaecomastia and feminization can occur. Increased incidence of endometrial and breast cancers are reported on long term estrogen therapy.

When given to a pregnant lady estrogens may:

- Increase risk of vaginal and cervical cancers in female child.
- Genital abnormalities in male child.

Uses

1. **Replacement therapy**
   a. *In primary amenorrhea hypogonadism:* Estrogen started at 11–13 years of age stimulates the development of secondary sexual characters and menstruation.
   b. *Postmenopausal syndrome:* Due to decreased estrogen production at menopause, hot flushes, anxiety, fatigue, sweating, muscle and joints pain are common. Osteoporosis, genital atrophy, skin changes, increased risk of cardiovascular disease and psychological disturbances may be seen. Estrogens given in low doses as hormone replacement therapy (HRT) are highly effective in reversing most of the changes. Ethinyl estradiol is preferred for HRT.

2. Senile vaginitis, hirsutism, acne.
3. **Osteoporosis:** Estrogens restore calcium balance and need to be given for a long time.
4. Oral contraceptives.
5. **Dysmenorrhoea:** Estrogens combined with progestins suppress ovulation and such anovulatory cycles are painless.
6. Dysfunctional uterine bleeding.
7. Carcinoma prostate is an androgen dependent tumor. Estrogens antagonize the action of androgens, suppress androgen production and are useful for palliative therapy.

Contraindications: Estrogen dependent tumors, liver disease, thromboembolic disorders, pregnancy, diabetes, undiagnosed uterine bleeding.

Selective Estrogen Receptor Modulators (SERMs) and Anti-Estrogens

SERMs are non-steroidal synthetic agents whose agonist or antagonist activities on estrogen receptors are tissue selective.

They act as an agonist, antagonist or partial agonist depending on the site, *e.g.*, Tamoxifen, Doloxifen, Toremifen, Fulvestrant, Clomiphene, Ormeloxifene (Centchroman).

Tamoxifen: It acts as:

- Agonists at bone, lipid, brain and liver.
- Antagonists at breast, pituitary and endometrium, blood vessels.
- Partial agonist at genitourinary epithelium, in bone remodeling and cholesterol metabolism.

It inhibits the proliferation of tumor cells in the breast, stimulates the proliferation of the endometrium. It reduces bone resorption and decreases total cholesterol.

Side effects include hot flushes, nausea, vomiting, vaginal dryness, cataract and skin rashes. Tamoxifen increases the risk of endometrial cancer and thromboembolism.

It is used in breast cancer in postmenopausal women with estrogen receptor positive tumors.

Raloxifene used in women with postmenopausal osteoporosis. It has anti-resorptive effects on the bone. It reduces bone loss and may even help to gain bone mass. Raloxifene also lowers LDL.

Adverse effects include hot flushes, leg cramps and an increased risk of deep vein thrombosis and pulmonary embolism.

Toremifene has actions similar to tamoxifen and is indicated in the treatment of metastatic breast cancer in postmenopausal women.

Ormiloxifene is estrogen antagonist and used in the treatment of dysfunctional uterine bleeding (DUB).

Clomiphene Citrate

Clomiphene citrate binds to the estrogen receptors and acts as a competitive inhibitor of endogenous estrogens. Like tamoxifen, it is also a partial agonist. Clomiphene opposes the negative feedback of endogenous estrogens on the hypothalamic-pituitary axis resulting in increased gonadotropin secretion FSH and LH secretion thereby induces ovulation.

Side effects include ovarian hyper stimulation resulting in multiple pregnancy, ovarian cysts, hot flushes, headache and skin rashes, weight gain and vertigo.

Uses

1. Infertility: It is given orally, 50 mg daily for 5 days starting from 5th day of the cycle; course is repeated till ovulation occurs.
2. In vitro fertilization.

Estrogen Synthesis Inhibitors

Aromatase inhibitors like formestane, exemestane, anastrozole, letrozole and vorazole block the production of estrogens and are used in the treatment of breast cancer.

Progestins

Progesterone is the natural progestin synthesized in the ovary and placenta. It is also synthesized by the testis and adrenals where it acts as a precursor of various steroid hormones. They convert the estrogen primed endometirum to secretary one and maintain pregnancy.

Actions

1. **Uterus:** The secretary changes in the endometrium like increased tortuosity of the glands are due to progesterone. In pregnancy, decidual changes in the endometrium take place under the influence of progesterone. It prepare the endometrium for implantation.

2. **Cervix:** The watery cervical secretions are changed to a viscid scanty secretion by progesterone.
3. **Vagina:** Vaginal epithelium changes to that seen in pregnancy.
4. **Mammary gland:** Along with estrogen, progesterone is responsible for the development of alveolar (acinar) system of the breast and prepares the gland for lactation.
5. **Body temperature:** Increase in the body temperature by 1°C during luteal phase beginning at ovulation is due to progesterone.

Progesterone Preparation

1. **Progesterone analogue:** Hydroxy progesterone acetate, Medroxy progesterone acetate, Megestrol, Nomegestrol.
2. **19-Nortestosterone derivatives:** Norethindrone, Norgesteral Levonorgestrel, Desogestrel, Norgestimate, Gestodene (newer drugs).

Adverse Effects: Headache, breast engorgement, rise in body temperature, edema, acne, breakthrough bleeding, irritability and mood swings may be seen. Progesterone is teratogenic.

Contraindication: Depression and pregnancy.

Uses

1. Contraception.
2. Hormone replacement therapy.
3. Ovarian suppression.
4. Threatened or habitual abortion.
5. Endometrial carcinoma.
6. Dysfunctional uterine bleeding.

Antiprogestins

Mifepristone binds to the progesterone receptor and blocks the actions of progesterone. It causes termination of pregnancy directly by blocking progesterone support to endometrium. This causes decidual breakdown; blastocyst gets detached, HCG and progesterone secretions fall. This in turn increases prostaglandin levels and stimulate uterine contractions. It also softens the cervix and facilitates expulsion of the blastocyst.

Adverse effects include prolonged bleeding, abdominal cramps, vomiting and diarrhea.

Uses

1. Termination of pregnancy.
2. Post coital contraceptive.
3. For softening of cervix.
4. For induction of labour.

Hormonal Contraceptives

Oral Pill

1. **Combined pill** contains low doses of an estrogen and a progestin. Ethinyl estradiol or mestranol are the estrogens used. Newer progestins like desogestrel and norgestrel are used as progestin. They cause least side effects. The pill is started on the 5th day of the menstrual cycle, taken daily for 21 days followed by a gap of 7 days during which bleeding occurs. This is **monophasic** regimen. Oral contraceptives are also available as **biphasic** or **triphasic** preparations. This reduces the amount of hormones needed and more closely mimics menstrual cycle.

Mechanism of Action of Combined Pills

Combined pills act by multiple mechanisms.

- *They prevent ovulation:* By negative feedback on the hypothalamus, progesterone decreases GnRH pulses and thereby LH release which is essential for ovulation.
- Estrogens suppress FSH release by negative feedback on the pituitary. As a result the ovarian follicle fails to develop.
- Progesterone also inhibits estrogen-induced midcycle LH surge.
- Progesterone renders the cervical mucous thick and unfavorable for sperm penetration.
- Oral contraceptives (OCs) alters the uterine endometrium making it not favorable for implantation.

Adverse Effects

- Headache, migraine headache in some women, nausea, vomiting, edema, breast tenderness, amenorrhea and irregular menstrual cycles may be commonly seen.
- Weight gain, acne, mood swings and hirsutism may occur.

- Cardiovascular effects increase the risk of MI and venous thromboembolism, increase the coagulability of blood, hypertension.
- Incidence of cervical, breast and other cancers increases.
- Cholestatic jaundice and gallstones.
- OCs may impair glucose tolerance.

Contraindications to Combined Pill

- Thromboembolic and cerebrovascular disease, breast cancers, liver disease. OCs should be used with caution in diabetes, hypertension, convulsive disorders, edema and CCF.

Benefits of Combined Pills

- Effective and convenient method of contraception.
- Reduced risk of ovarian cancers (ovarian stimulation by gonadotropins).
- Reduced risk of endometrial cancers.
- Reduced incidence of pelvic inflammatory disease and ectopic pregnancy.
- Less menstrual blood loss, less iron deficiency; premenstrual tension and dysmenorrhea are less intense.

2. **Mini pill:** A low dose progestin is taken daily without a gap, efficacy is lower, menstrual cycles may be irregular and is not popular.
3. **Post coital contraceptives:** High dose of combination of oestrogen and progestins is now preferred. The pill should be started within 72 hours of coitus and has an efficacy of 90–98%. Ulipristal (SPRM) in a single dose is effective. Mifepristone in high doses is also effective and used within 72 hours of unprotected coitus.

Depot Preparations of contraceptives are given as:

1. **Progestin injections**
   - i. Depot medroxyprogesterone acetate (DMPA 150–400 mg) or Norethisterone enanthate (NET EN 200 mg).
   - ii. Implants: They are implanted under the skin. Norplant capsules implanted subcutaneously in the forearm or upper arm work for 5 years. They contain levonorgestrel.

Disadvantages (i) Amenorrhea is frequent (ii) Permanent sterility may occur.

2. Combined injectable contraceptives (estradiol + 17 hydroxy progesterone).
3. Transdermal patch containing a progestin and an estrogen is applied once a week for 3 weeks and the next week withdrawal bleeding occurs.
4. Vaginal rings.

Centchroman (Ormeloxifene) is a non-steroidal oral contraceptive. It has anti-estrogenic and anti progestogenic activity and may act by preventing implantation. Success rate claimed is 97–99% and is devoid of the side effects of hormonal contraceptives. It is well tolerated.

Androgens

Androgens are produced chiefly in the testes and small amounts in the adrenal cortex. Testosterone is the most important natural androgen. Secretion is regulated by gonadotrophins and GnRH.

Physiological Actions: Testosterone is essential for the development of secondary sexual characters and sex organs in males. It is necessary for normal spermatogenesis and is important for maintaining sexual function in men. Testosterone promotes bone growth, enhances the muscle mass, protein synthesis and positive nitrogen balance. It has anabolic actions. In females they cause hirsutism, frontal baldness and suppression of ovulation.

Mechanism of action is similar to other steroids. Androgens bind to androgen receptors on the target cells, the complex moves to the nucleus where it stimulates protein synthesis.

Adverse Effects: Masculinization and acne in females, hepato-toxicity, increased libido and precocious puberty can occur in young boys. Suppression of spermatogenesis (due to inhibition of LH and FSH), gynaecomastia (in men), salt and water retention, polycythemia and erythrocytosis also occur.

Uses

1. Replacement therapy in male/female hypogonadism.
2. In senile osteoporosis and carcinoma of the breast in premenopausal women.
3. Treatment of anaemia.

Anabolic Steroids

Anabolic steroids are synthetic androgens with higher anabolic and low androgenic activity. These are believed to enhance protein synthesis and increase muscle mass. Methandienone, Nandrolone, Oxandrolone and Stanozolol are some anabolic steroids available.

Uses

1. Catabolic states.
2. Senile osteotiorosis.
3. Growth stimulation in children.
4. Other uses: Chronic renal failure to reduce nitrogen load on the kidneys.
5. Abuse in athletes.

Anti-Androgens

Cyproterone acetate is a derivative of progesterone. It competitively binds to androgen receptors and thus blocks the actions of androgens. Cyproterone was used to treat severe hypersexuality in males, in carcinoma prostate and in female hirsutism but now rarely used. **Flutamide** is a potent competitive antagonist at androgen receptors. It is used with GnRH/ leuprolide in the treatment of carcinoma prostate and hirsutism.

Danazol: It has weak androgenic, anabolic and progestational activity. It suppresses gonadotrophin secretion from the pituitary. It is used in endometriosis in women and precautious puberty in boys.

Finasteride inhibits the enzyme 5-alpha reductase and thus inhibits the conversion of testosterone to its active metabolite dihydrotestosterone. It is used in benign prostatic hypertrophy to reduce the prostate size. Dutasteride, turosteride, bexlosteride and izonsteride are other new 5-alpha reductase inhibitor.

Biculutamide, nilutamide, flutamide are androgen receptor antagonist used in the treatment of prostatic carcinoma.

Drugs Used in Male Sexual Impotence

Several drugs have been tried including testosterone, yohimbine, papavarine and antidepressants. The recent introduced drug **Sildenafil** (Viagra) has been a success in a large percentage of them.

Sildenafil is the first agent to be effective orally for the treatment of erectile dysfunction. Sildenafil inhibits the enzyme phosphodiesterase in the penis and thus prolongs the action of cyclic GMP. This causes relaxation of smooth muscle in the corpus cavernosum and vasodilatation, both resulting in cavernosal engorgement and penile erection.

Adverse Effects and Precautions: Due to vasodilatation, headache, dizziness and nasal stuffiness can occur. It potentiates the hypotensive action of nitrates and is contraindicated in patients on nitrates and in patients with coronary artery disease, elderly men above 60 years need less dose.

Alprostadil is a PGE, analogue, injected directly into the cavernosa or placed inside the urethra. Its use is associated with low incidence of priapism and fibrosis.

DRUGS AFFECTING BONE AND PARATHORMONE

Agents Affecting Bone Mineral Turnover

Calcium and phosphorus are the most important minerals of the bone. Calcium and phosphorus metabolism is chiefly regulated by Vitamin D and parathormone. Other hormones that influence calcium and phosphorus metabolism are calcitonin, growth hormone, insulin, thyroid hormone, prolactin, glucocorticoids and sex hormones.

Calcium

Calcium is essential for tissue excitability, muscular excitation-contraction coupling, secretion from glands, myocardial contractility and formation of bones and teeth. It also maintains the integrity of mucous membranes and cell membrane. Calcium is essential for normal blood coagulation. Calcium is absorbed from the small intestines by a carrier mediated active transport which is controlled by a calcium binding protein.

Adverse Effects: Oral calcium is well tolerated but may produce constipation, abdominal bloating and rarely intestinal obstruction.

Uses

1. To prevent and treat calcium deficiency. Calcium supplements are given orally in children (rickets), pregnant and lactating women and in postmenopausal osteoporosis.
2. As an antacid calcium carbonate is used.
3. For placebo effect IV calcium is used in weakness, pruritis and some dermatoses.

Phosphate

Phosphates play a vital role in various enzymatic reactions, which are important for the structure and function of the cells. It is important constituents of teeth and bones. Hypophosphatemia results in muscle weakness and abnormal bone mineralization.

Parathyroid Hormone (Parathormone, PTH)

Parathormone is a peptide secreted by the parathyroid gland. PTH is regulated by plasma Ca^{++} concentration. Low plasma Ca^{++} stimulates PTH release, while high levels inhibit secretion. PTH maintains plasma calcium concentration by mobilizing calcium from the bone, promoting reabsorption of Ca^{2+} from the kidneys and by stimulating the synthesis of calcitriol which in turn enhances calcium absorption from the intestines.

Hypoparathyroidism is characterized by low plasma calcium levels with its associated manifestations.

PTH is not therapeutically used.

Vitamins

Vitamins are organic compounds essential for normal metabolism in the body. They are supplied in the diet. A balanced diet supplies adequate amounts of vitamins to fulfil the daily requirement. The requirement is increased during periods of rapid growth, pregnancy and lactation. Vitamin deficiencies result in characteristic signs and symptoms.

Vitamin D

Vitamin D is a fat soluble vitamin. It is converted to active metabolites in the body which regulate plasma calcium levels and various functions of the cells.

Source

- Diet from plants, fish, liver, fish liver oils.
- Cholecalciferol is synthesized in the skin from 7-dehydrocholesterol.

Actions

- Calcitriol stimulates calcium and phosphate absorption in the intestine by binding to its receptors present on gut.
- Mobilizes calcium from bone by promoting osteoclastic activity.
- Both calcitriol and calcifediol increases reabsorption of Ca^{++} from kidney tubules (weaker as compared to PTH).

Vitamin D deficiency results in low plasma calcium and phosphate levels due to inadequate intestinal absorption, with abnormal mineralization of the bone; causes rickets in children and osteomalacia in adults.

Daily Requirement: 400 IU (10 mg).

Adverse Reactions: High doses of Vitamin D used for long periods result in hypervitaminosis D, manifesting as generalized decalcification of the bones, hypercalcemia, hyperphosphatemia resulting in weakness, drowsiness, nausea, abdominal pain, thirst, renal stones and hypertension.

Uses

1. For prophylaxis to prevent Vitamin D deficiency. In the breastfed infants, from the first month onwards oral Vitamin D supplements are needed.
2. Nutritional rickets and osteomalacia, senile osteoporosis.
3. Hypoparathyroidism.
4. Renal tubular defect with Vitamin D resistant/dependent rickets and osteomalacia.

Calcitonin

Calcitonin is a peptide hormone secreted by the para follicular 'C' cells of the thyroid gland. Secretion is regulated by plasma Ca^{++} concentration, *i.e.*, high plasma Ca^{++} stimulates calcitonin release. The chief effects of calcitonin are to lower serum calcium and phosphate by its actions on the bone and kidney. It inhibits osteoclastic bone resorption, it reduces both calcium and phosphate reabsorption in the kidney. So, it is useful in the treatment of Paget's disease, hypercalcaemia and osteoporosis.

In general the effects are opposite to that of PTH.

Other hormones that regulate bone turnover are glucocorticoids and estrogens. Glucocorticoids antagonize Vitamin D stimulated intestinal calcium absorption and enhance renal calcium excretion. Estrogens reduce bone resorption by PTH and also enhance calcitriol levels. Commonly used calcitonin preparation is synthetic salmon calcitonin.

Bisphosphonates (BPNs)

Bisphosphonates are analogs of pyrophosphate. They inhibit bone resorption. Bisphosphonates get incorporated into bone matrix. They inhibit osteoclastic resorption of bones by binding to the hydroxyapatite crystals of bone resulting in reduced bone resorption and promotion of bone remodeling by an increase in bone density. These includes: Alendronate, Etidronate, Pamidronate, Residronate etc.

Uses

1. Paget's disease.
2. Hypercalcemia.
3. Osteoporosis.
   Raloxifene is a non-hormonal agent (SERM) useful in women for the prevention of postmenopausal osteoporosis.

MULTIPLE CHOICE QUESTIONS

Q. 1 Action of growth hormone include the following *except:*

(A) Increased protein synthesis
(B) Increased fat utilization
(C) Increased carbohydrate utilization
(D) Glucose intolerance

Q. 2 Indications of somatostatin include:

(A) Macroprolactinoma (B) Zollinger Ellison syndrome
(C) Constipation (D) Bleeding esophageal varices

Q. 3 All statements are true about octreotide *except:*

(A) It is active orally
(B) It suppresses growth hormone secretion
(C) It is used for variceal bleeding
(D) It is useful in secretary diarrhea

Q. 4 All are short acting insulin *except:*

(A) Lispro (B) Aspart
(C) Glulisine (D) Glargine

Q. 5 Which one of the following drugs promotes the release of endogenous insulin?

(A) Metformin (B) Pioglitazone
(C) Glipizide (D) Acarbose

Q. 6 Important action by which insulin control blood sugar level (BSL) is:

(A) Increased conversion of amino acids into glucose
(B) Increased gluconeogenesis
(C) Increased glucose transport into cells
(D) Inhibition of lipoprotein lipase

Q. 7 The most likely complication of insulin therapy is:

(A) Hyponatremia (B) Hypertension
(C) Hypoglycemia (D) Pancreatitis

---

1 (C) 2 (D) 3 (A) 4 (D) 5 (C) 6 (C) 7 (C)

Q. 8 Which of the following type of insulin does not contain zinc?

(A) Lente insulin (B) Isophane insulin suspension
(C) Regular human insulin (D) Semi lente insulin

Q. 9 All of following conditions decreases the insulin requirement in diabetic *except:*

(A) Vigorous exercise
(B) Consumption of alcohol
(C) Development of renal disease
(D) Pregnancy

Q. 10 Which insulin preparation is preferred in diabetic ketoacidosis?

(A) Regular insulin (B) Lente insulin
(C) Isophane insulin (D) Monocomponent insulin

Q. 11 The advantage of human insulin over bovine insulin are:

(A) They are more potent
(B) They have a faster kinetics of absorption and elimination
(C) They have longer biological half life
(D) They penetrate blood brain barrier more efficiently

Q. 12 Which of the following drugs is taken during the first part of meal for the purpose of delaying the absorption of dietary carbohydrate?

(A) Acarbose (B) Glipizide
(C) Pioglitazone (D) Exendatide

Q. 13 Which one of the following statement about biguanide is not true?

(A) It do not stimulate insulin release
(B) It decrease hepatic glucose production
(C) Renal dysfunction is not a contraindication for their use
(D) They can be given in combination with sulfonylurea

Q. 14 All of the following are true regarding oral hypoglycemic agent *except:*

(A) They are effective only after total pancreatectomy
(B) Metformin causes lactic acidosis
(C) They causes release of insulin from beta cells
(D) They are useful in obese maturity onset diabetes

---

8 (C) 9 (D) 10 (A) 11 (B) 12 (A) 13 (C) 14 (A)

Q. 15 Sulfonylurea act through all of the following mechanisms *except:*

(A) Stimulate insulin release
(B) Facilitate insulin secretion from beta cells
(C) Increases peripheral insulin release
(D) Increase glucagon secretion

Q. 16 The hypoglycemic action of sulfonylurea is likely to be attenuated by the concurrent use of:

(A) Hydrochlorothiazide (B) Propranolol
(C) Chloramphenicol (D) Aspirin

Q. 17 Which of the following drug tends to reverse insulin resistance by increasing cellular glucose transport?

(A) Glibenclamide (B) Pioglitazone
(C) Acarbose (D) Prednisolon

Q. 18 All of the following are true statements regarding rapaglinide *except:*

(A) They have rapid and short lasting effect
(B) They should be avoided in hepatic disease
(C) They are used to control post prandial hyperglycemia
(D) They can be effective as mono therapy in T2DM

Q. 19 Carbimazole is associated with all *except:*

(A) Agranulocytosis (B) Loss or graying of hair
(C) Joint pain (D) Neck swelling

Q. 20 Drug which causes hypothyroidism is:

(A) Carbamazepine (B) Lithium
(C) Sulphur (D) Methotrexate

Q. 21 Which anti-thyroid drug can be used safely in pregnancy?

(A) Propylthiouracil (B) Radioactive iodine
(C) Carbimazole (D) Methimazole

Q. 22 Methimazole reduces serum concentration of T_3 primarily by:

(A) Accelerating the peripheral metabolism of T_3
(B) Inhibiting the secretion of TSH
(C) Inhibiting the uptake of iodine by cells in the thyroid
(D) Preventing the addition of iodine to tyrosine residues on thyroglobulin

---

15 (D) 16 (A) 17 (B) 18 (D) 19 (D) 20 (B) 21 (A) 22 (D)

Q. 23 An useful adjuvant in the treatment of thyroid storm is:

(A) Propranolol (B) Betamethasone
(C) Epinephrine (D) Radioactive iodine

Q. 24 Overdose with exogenous T_4 causes:

(A) Angina (B) Lethargy
(C) Dry puffy skin (D) Bradycardia

Q. 25 In elderly, with hypothyroidism, initially small doses of T_4 are prescribed to avoid:

(A) Overstimulation of heart
(B) Seizures
(C) A flare of exophthalmoses
(D) Acute renal failure

Q. 26 Which of the following is an indication of radioactive iodine?

(A) Large retrosternal goiter
(B) Young child with thyrotoxicosis
(C) Thyrotoxicosis in young female
(D) Elderly with cardiac disease

Q. 27 All of the following are advantages of glucocorticoids given in thyrotoxicosis *except:*

(A) They inhibit peripheral conversion of T_4 to T_3
(B) They have inhibitory effect on T_4 release from thyroid gland
(C) They antagonize cellular hormonal effects of thyroxine
(D) They treat co-existing adrenal exhaustion simultaneously

Q. 28 Myxoedematous coma is treated by all *except:*

(A) Hypertonic saline
(B) Parenteral hydrocortisone
(C) Oral/parenteral thyroxine
(D) Rapid warming of body surface

Q. 29 Action of thyroxine include all of the following *except:*

(A) Rise in blood sugar level
(B) Reduction in plasma cholesterol level
(C) Fall in plasma free fatty acid level
(D) Induction of negative nitrogen balance

23 (A) 24 (A) 25 (A) 26 (D) 27 (C) 28 (D) 29 (C)

Q. 30 Thyroxine should not be used for:

(A) Nontoxic goiter (B) Endemic cretinism
(C) Myxoedema coma (D) Papillary carcinoma of thyroid

Q. 31 Lugol's iodine is used in hyperthyroidism:

(A) As a long term definitive mono therapy
(B) Pre-operatively for 10-15 days
(C) Post operatively for 10-15 days
(D) As adjuvant to carbimazole for long term therapy

Q. 32 Which one of the following is true of adrenal suppression due to prolonged steroid therapy?

(A) It is not associated with atrophy of the adrenal glands
(B) It does not occur in patients receiving inhaled steroid
(C) It should be expected in any one receiving >5 mg prednisolon daily for prolonged period
(D) Following cessation, the stress response normalizes after 8 weeks

Q. 33 All of the following manifest as adverse effects with steroid given in anti-inflammatory dosage *except:*

(A) Diabetes mellitus (B) Hyperkalemia
(C) Osteoporosis (D) Sodium and water retention

Q. 34 Prolonged use of steroids may cause:

(A) Decrease in bone matrix protein
(B) Hypoglycemia
(C) Hypotension
(D) Early healing of wound

Q. 35 Hypernatremia is caused by:

(A) Prednisolon (B) Fludrocortisone
(C) Hydrocortisone (D) Dexamethasone

Q. 36 Pharmacological effects of exogenous glucocorticoid include:

(A) Increased muscle mass
(B) Increased excretion of salt and water
(C) Inhibition of leukotriene synthesis
(D) Improved wound healing

---

30 (B) 31 (B) 32 (B) 33 (B) 34 (A) 35 (B) 36 (C)

Q. 37 Gradual tapering of the glucocorticoid is needed after prolonged use to allow recovery of:

(A) Depressed release of insulin from pancreatic beta cells
(B) Normal osteoblast function
(C) The control of water excretion by vasopressin
(D) The hypothalamic pituitary adrenal system

Q. 38 In patients having severe acute adrenal insufficiency the rational combination of drug given is:

(A) Aldosterone and fludrocortisone
(B) Cortisol and fludrocortisone
(C) Triamcinolone and dexamethasone
(D) Dexamethasone and metyrapone

Q. 39 A drug that blocks the glucocorticoid receptor is:

(A) Aminoglutethimide (B) Beclomethasone
(C) Mifepristone (D) Spironolactone

Q. 40 Which steroid is used for acquired respiratory distress syndrome (ARDS) in neonates?

(A) Betamethasone (B) Cortisol
(C) Prednisolone (D) Dexamethasone

Q. 41 Use of topical steroid is contraindicated in:

(A) Herpes simplex keratitis (B) Interstitial keratitis
(C) Phlectynular conjunctivitis (D) Vernal conjunctivitis

Q. 42 The estrogen that is used in most combined hormonal contraceptive is:

(A) Ethinyl estradiol
(B) Estron
(C) Diethyl stilbestrol (DES)
(D) Norgesterol

Q. 43 Combined oral contraceptive should be avoided in females who has:

(A) Evidence of hirsutism
(B) History of pelvic disease
(C) History of gastroesophageal reflux disease (GERD)
(D) History of epilepsy

---

37 (D) 38 (B) 39 (C) 40 (A) 41 (A) 42 (A) 43 (D)

Q. 44 Large doses of androgens in male increase the risk of:

(A) Anaemia (B) Hirsutism
(C) Cholestatic jaundice (D) Testicular enlargement

Q. 45 Diethyl stilbestrol (DES) should never be used in pregnant as it is associated with:

(A) Deep vein thrombosis
(B) Feminization of the external genitalia of male offspring
(C) Infertility and development of vaginal cancer in female offspring
(D) Virilization of the external genitalia of female offspring

Q. 46 The unique property of selective estrogen receptor modulator (SERM) is that they:

(A) Act as agonists in some tissue and antagonist in other
(B) Have both estrogenic and progestational agonist activity
(C) Inhibit the aromatase enzyme required for estrogen synthesis
(D) Produce estrogenic effects without binding to estrogen receptors

Q. 47 All of the following are advantages of using raloxifene over estrogen in post menopausal women *except:*

(A) They reduces fracture rates
(B) They avoid endometrial hyperplasia
(C) They reduces incidence of venous thrombosis
(D) There is no increase in incidence of breast carcinoma

Q. 48 Which of the following is the most potent androgen?

(A) Dehydroepiandrostenedione (DHEA)
(B) Testosterone
(C) Dihydrotestosterone (DHT)
(D) Androstenedione

Q. 49 All statements are true *except:*

(A) Clomiphene have antiestrogenic effect
(B) Danazole increases release of both LH and FSH
(C) Cyproterone is a potent antiandrogen
(D) Tibolone has estrogenic, progestational as well as weak androgenic activity

---

44 (C) 45 (C) 46 (A) 47 (C) 48 (A) 49 (B)

Q. 50 Gynaecomastia is caused by:

(A) Spironolactone (B) Rifampicin
(C) Thiazide (D) Propranolol

Q. 51 Which of the following is an androgen receptor blocking drug?

(A) Tamoxifen (B) Nilandron
(C) Mifepristone (D) Cyproterone acetate

Q. 52 All are true about the action of oral contraceptive pills (OCPs) *except:*

(A) They inhibit ovulation
(B) They decreases incidence of endometrial carcinoma
(C) They interfere with implantation
(D) They interfere placental functioning

Q. 53 The treatment for a case of virilizing adrenal hyperplasia is:

(A) Estrogen
(B) Antiandrogen
(C) Adrenocorticotropic Hormone (ACTH)
(D) Cortisone

Q. 54 Which of the following is true of anabolic steroid?

(A) They are testosterone congeners having anabolic but no androgenic activity
(B) They are androgens with relatively selective anabolic activity
(C) They are suitable for long term therapy in children
(D) All of the above

Q. 55 Danazole is used for all of the following disorders *except:*

(A) Amenorrhoea
(B) Endometriosis
(C) Fibrocystic breast disease
(D) Precocious puberty in male children

Q. 56 Estrogen exert all of the following actions *except:*

(A) Cornification of vaginal epithelium
(B) Proliferation of endometrium
(C) Maturation of graffian follicle
(D) Anabolism

---

50 (A) 51 (D) 52 (D) 53 (D) 54 (B) 55 (A) 56 (C)

Q. 57 Which of the following is true about tibolone?

(A) It is an anti-estrogen used for palliative treatment of carcinoma breast
(B) It is an estrogenic + progestational steroid used for hormone replacement therapy (HRT) in post menopausal women
(C) It is an anti-androgen used for male pattern baldness
(D) It is a non-steroidal estrogen used topically or senile vaginitis

Q. 58 All of the following statements are true about tamoxifen *except:*

(A) It is used for palliative treatment of carcinoma breast
(B) It can be used in both pre and post menopausal women
(C) It causes endometrial proliferation due to its agonistic action
(D) It increases prolactin levels

Q. 59 Progestin alone can be used in:

(A) Threatened abortion
(B) Premenstrual tension
(C) Dysfunctional uterine bleeding
(D) Hormonal replacement therapy

Q. 60 Which of the following can be used as a single dose post-coital contraceptive pill?

(A) Danasol (B) Medroxyprogesterone
(C) Clomiphene (D) Mifepristone

Q. 61 The most undesirable adverse effect of injectable depot contraceptive preparation is:

(A) Nausea and vomiting
(B) Venous thrombosis
(C) Hypertension
(D) Disruption of cyclical menstrual bleeding

Q. 62 Biphosphonates act by:

(A) Increasing the osteoid formation
(B) Increasing the mineralization of osteoid
(C) Decreasing the osteoclast mediated resorption of bone
(D) Decreasing the parathyroid hormone secretion

---

57 (B) 58 (D) 59 (A) 60 (D) 61 (D) 62 (C)

Q. 63 Bromocriptin is not used in:

(A) Induction of ovulation (B) Galactorrhoea
(C) Post pill amenorrhea (D) Luteal phase defect

Q. 64 A drug that is added to calcium supplementation to prevent rickets in children is:

(A) Cholecalciferol (B) Calcitriol
(C) Sevelmer (D) Plicamycin

Q. 65 The active metabolite of Vitamin D acts through a nuclear receptor to:

(A) Decrease the absorption of calcium from bone
(B) Increase parathormone (PTH) formation
(C) Increase the absorption of calcium from GIT
(D) Increase renal production of erythropoietin

Q. 66 The drug that lowers the parathormone (PTH) concentration is:

(A) Calcitriol (B) Risedronate
(C) Galliumnitrate (D) Cholecalciferol

Q. 67 Which of the following corticosteroid has least glucocorticoid activity?

(A) Dexamethasone (B) Triamcinolone
(C) Betamethasone (D) Fludrocortisones

Q. 68 All statements are true about metformin *except:*

(A) It increases the absorption of the glucose
(B) It should be avoided in hepato-renal failure
(C) It lowers triglyceride
(D) It causes lactic acidosis

Q. 69 Drug of choice in hyperprolectinemia due to pituitary adenoma who is not a good operative candidate is:

(A) Methysergide (B) Bromocriptine
(C) Ergometrine (D) Aprotinin

Q. 70 Glyburide act through:

(A) Increase insulin secretion
(B) Decrease glucocorticoid levels
(C) Decrease tissue sensitivity to insulin
(D) Decrease insulin half-life

---

63 (A) 64 (A) 65 (C) 66 (A) 67 (D) 68 (A) 69 (B) 70 (A)

Q. 71 The drug having significant mineralocorticoid activity is:

(A) Triamcinolone (B) Fludrocortisone
(C) Betamethasone (D) Dexamethasone

Q. 72 The anti-thyroid drug carbimazole act by inhibiting:

(A) Synthesis of thyroglobulin protein
(B) Proteolysis of thyroglobulin
(C) Oxidation of iodide
(D) Iodide trapping

Q. 73 Which of the following agent is approved for treatment of diabetic neuropathy?

(A) Phenytoin (B) Carbamazepine
(C) Valproic acid (D) Gabapentin

Q. 74 Which of the following is an orally active ovulation inducing agent?

(A) Menotropin (B) Mifepristone
(C) Danazol (D) Clomiphene citrate

Q. 75 Which of the following is not a legitimate indication for the use of anabolic steroid?

(A) To enhance the physical ability of sportsmen
(B) To treat senile osteoporosis
(C) To treat anaemia
(D) During convalescence from prolonged illness

Q. 76 Transdermal estradiol differ from oral estrogen therapy in that it:

(A) Causes less induction of hepatic synthesis of clotting factor
(B) Does not inhibit FSH secretion
(C) Does not affect vaginal cytology
(D) All of the above

---

71 (B) 72 (C) 73 (D) 74 (D) 75 (A) 76 (A)

ANSWERS

Ans. 1 **(C)** Actions of GH include increased protein synthesis and positive nitrogen balance, decrease in glucose uptake and increase release of glucose (diabetogenic effect) and lipolysis.

Ans. 2 **(D)** Somatostatin is a growth hormone releasing inhibiting hormone (GHRIH). It inhibits secretion of GH, TSH, insulin and gastrin hormone. It can be used in bleeding esophageal varies. But because of short half life and lack of specificity, octreotide, a long acting analogue of somatostatin, is used. It controls the symptoms of carcinoid syndrome, gastrinoma, secretary diarrhea (associated with IBS and diabetes), bleeding esophageal varices, insulinoma etc.

Ans. 3 **(A)** Octreotide is given by S.C. route (not orally).

Ans. 4 **(D)** Insulin lispro, aspart, glulisine and glarigine, all are insulin analogue, produced by using DNA recombinant technology. These agents have greater stability and consistency. Lispro, aspart and glulisine are short acting, and needs to be injected immediately before or after the meals. They have low incidence of late post prandial hypoglycemia. Insulin glargine on other hand is a long acting insulin, onset of action is delayed but relatively low levels of insulin are maintained for upto 24 hours.

Ans. 5 **(C)** Glipizide, a second generation sulfonylurea promotes insulin release by closing potassium channels in pancreatic beta cells.

Ans. 6 **(C)** Insulin controls blood sugar level by increasing glucose uptake and glycogen synthesis by inhibiting glucogenolysis and gluconeogenesis, by inhibiting proteolysis and release of amino acids and by inhibiting lipolysis.

Ans. 7 **(C)** Hypoglycemia is the most common and the most serious complication of insulin therapy, which must be treated promptly, otherwise it may lead to irreversible neurological defect. Other adverse reactions of insulin therapy are allergy, local reactions and dependent edema due to Na^+ retention.

Ans. 8 **(C)** Isophane insulin suspension, lente insulin and semi lente insulin all contain zinc, to stabilize the insulin preparations. The insulin molecule self aggregate to form hexamers around zinc ions. Regular human insulin is produced by recombinant technology, and indicated in patients having allergy to bovine preparations.

Ans. 9 (D) Hypoglycemia is a common adverse effect of insulin. Common causes of hypoglycemia are too large dose and failure to eat. Vigorous exercise, ingestion of alcohol and aged diabetics may also precipitate hypoglycemia, so dose of the insulin to be adjusted accordingly.

Ans. 10 (A) In diabetic ketoacidosis, regular insulin is used to correct the metabolic abnormalities. This is given by infusion. Other drugs given in diabetic ketoacidosis are, IV fluids to correct dehydration, potassium chloride, sodium bicarbonate, phosphate and antibiotics.

Ans. 11 (B) Highly purified insulin preparations and monocomponent insulin are more stable, cause less insulin resistance or lipodystrophy. Human insulins are more water soluble and has a slightly more rapid absorption when given subcutaneously. They have slightly shorter duration of action with earlier and more defined peak.

Ans. 12 (A) To be absorbed, carbohydrates must be converted into monosaccharide by the action of alpha-glucosidase enzyme in the GIT. Acarbose inhibits alpha-glucosidase and during digestion delays the uptake of carbohydrates.

Ans. 13 (C) Biguanides, *e.g.*, metformin and phenformin cause little or no hypoglycemia. They do not stimulate beta pancreatic cells. They suppress hepatic gluconeogenesis and glucose output from liver. They also retard absorption of glucose from intestine. Combination of sufonylurea is indicated when monotherapy is ineffective. Biguanides are contraindicated in hypotensive states, cardiovascular, respiratory, hepatic and renal disease and in alcoholics because of increased risk of lactic acidosis.

Ans. 14 (A) Oral hypoglycemic of sulfonylurea group, act by releasing the preformed insulin from beta cells. They will be ineffective after total pancreatectomy. Oral hypoglycemic metformin (preferred in obese diabetic patients) causes lactic acidosis.

Ans. 15 (D) Sulfonylurea act on sulfonylurea receptors present on beta pancreatic cell membrane and causes depolarization. The rate of insulin release in response to glucose is increased, *i.e.*, they stimulate insulin secretion. They also reduce glucagon secretion by increasing insulin and somatostatin release.

Ans. 16 (A) The drugs which have opposite action or suppress insulin and thus decrease hypoglycemic effect of sulfonylurea are enzyme inducers (phenytoin, rifampicin), steroids thiazides, furosemide and oral contraceptives. While salicylates, propranolol, chloramphenicol, alcohol, warfarin, lithium and theophylline enhance action of sulfonylurea and may precipitate hypoglycemia.

Ans. 17 (B) Thiozolidinediones, *e.g.*, Rosiglitazone and Pioglitazone are selective agonist for peroxisome proliferator activated receptor gamma (PPAR gamma). They reverse the insulin resistance by stimulating $GLUT_4$ expression, thus entry of glucose into muscle and fat is improved. Adipocyte turnover and differentiation may also be affected. Improve glycaemic control results in lowering of circulating HbA_{1C} and insulin level in diabetes mellitus (T2 DM).

Ans. 18 (D) Rapaglinide and Nateglinide are meglitidine analogue. They normalize glucose excursion after meals and control post prandial hyperglycemia. They have rapid but short lasting insulin release. They are used to supplement metformin/ long acting insulin and must be avoided in hepatic disease.

Ans. 19 (D) Carbamazole is an anti-thyroid drug used to control thyrotoxicosis in both toxic nodular goiter and Graves' disease. When given during pregnancy risk of fetal hypothyroidism and goiter is there. Propylthiouracil is preferred during pregnancy because of its less transfer to foetus. The common adverse effects are, *i.e.*, intolerance, loss or graying of hair, vasculitis, joint pain, cholestatic jaundice, agranulocytosis etc. but not neck swelling.

Ans. 20 (B) Lithium causes hypothyroidism.

Ans. 21 (A) Propylthiouracil is preferred during pregnancy and lactation.

Ans. 22 (D) Anti-thyroid drugs, *e.g.*, propylthiouracil, methimazole, carbimazole, act by inhibiting iodination of tyrosine residue in thyroglobulin, coupling of iodotyrosine residue to form T_3 and T_4. But they do not interfere with trapping of iodide. Goiter is due to increased TSH release as a result of reduction of feedback inhibition.

Ans. 23 (A) Beta-blockers are very useful in hyperthyroidism and thyroid storm, as they not only control the symptoms (due to blockade of sympathetic overactivity) but also reduce the peripheral conversion of T_4 and T_3.

Ans. 24 (A) Rapid correction of hypothyroidism in patients with ischemic heart disease may precipitate angina. Other adverse effects include tachycardia, palpitation, arrhythmias, tremors, weight loss, headache, insomnia and heat intolerance.

Ans. 25 (A) Overstimulation of heart may occur. So the treatment should be started with small dose (see Ans. 24 also).

Ans. 26 (D) Radioactive iodine (^{131}I) is preferred in hyperthyroidism due to Graves' disease or small toxic nodular goiter. It is contraindicated in young pregnant females, in children. But it is preferred after 25 years of age, in elderly with CHF angina or if any other contraindications to surgery is present.

Ans. 27 (C) Corticosteroids (hydrocortisone), followed by oral prednisolone is given in thyrotoxicosis because they help to tide over crisis, cover adrenal insufficiency and inhibit conversion of T_4 to T_3 in periphery.

Ans. 28 (D) Treatment of myxoedema coma includes alpha thyroxine (T_4) (loading dose) hydrocortisone to cover adrenal insufficiency, respiratory and cardiac support and correction of hyponatraemia and hypoglycemia.

Ans. 29 (C) Thyroid hormones have marked effect on lipid, carbohydrate and protein metabolism. They causes rise in plasma free fatty acid and causes lipogenesis and increases cholesterol metabolism. They also stimulate carbohydrate metabolism which causes hyperglycaemia and diabetic like state. T_3 have catabolic effect and more proteins are used as energy source.

Ans. 30 (B) Endemic cretinism is due to extreme deficiency of iodine, so thyroxine may not be very useful. Other uses of thyroxine are adult hypothyroidism, thyroid nodule and myxoedema coma.

Ans. 31 (B) Lugol's iodine (5% iodine in 10% potassium iodide) is used preoperatively (before thyroidectomy) to make the gland firm, less vascular and easier to operate on. It is also used in thyroid storm and for prophylaxis of endemic goiter.

Ans. 32 (B) Suppression of HPA axis with steroid therapy depends on both dose and duration of therapy. Atrophy of adrenal cortex also occurs. It is very common when patient receive 20-25 mg/day of steroid for prolonged period. Stoppage of exogenous steroid may cause withdrawal symptoms which include malaise, fever, anorexia, postural hypotension etc. To minimize HPA axis suppression, measures like using short acting steroids for shorter period, alternate day therapy and if indicated local (inhaled, ocular, nasal, rectal) preparation must be used.

Ans. 33 (B) Sodium and water retention, hypokalemia (not hyperkalemia), edema (mineralocorticoid effects) may occur with steroids but rare nowadays due to highly selective preparation. Other adverse effects includes osteoporosis, suppression of HPA axis, hyperglycemia, myopathies, peptic ulceration, susceptibility to infection, psychiatric disturbances etc.

Ans. 34 (A) Prolonged use of steroids causes hyperglycemia, hypertension and delayed healing of wound. It also causes growth retardation in children. They causes protein breakdown and amino acid mobilization from peripheral tissue and causes muscle wasting, loss of osteoid from bone and thinning of skin, decrease in bone matrix protein and make the patient prone to traumatic fracture (of vertebrae). Resorption of bones occurs through an increase in parathyroid hormone release and inhibitory effect on osteoblasts.

Ans. 35 (B) Fludrocortisone is a potent mineralocorticoid, so causes Na^+ and water retention. All other three are having potent glucocorticoid activity.

Ans. 36 (C) Exogenous glucocorticoids exhibit anti-inflammatory effect by inducing the production of lipocortin. They also block the production of arachidonic acid and thus inhibit synthesis of PG, PAF and leukotrienes which are important mediators of inflammation. They also block the release of IL from lymphocytes. They decrease the production of collagenase and stromelysin and thus prevent collagen destruction, but after prolonged therapy they decrease the production of collagen and thus obstruct healing and repair.

Ans. 37 (D) Prolonged and high doses of glucocorticoids cause suppression of HPA axis. Sudden withdrawal may lead to acute adrenal insufficiency in these patients.

Ans. 38 (B) Acute adrenal insufficiency, is characterized by severe hypotension, hyponatremia and hyperkalemia. It is life threatening condition requires vigorous therapy. Large amount of parenteral hydrocortisone, with fluid and electrolytes are required. A mineralocorticoid, *e.g.*, fludrocortisone have beneficial effect (to correct hyponatremia and hyperkalemia) when added to this therapy.

Ans. 39 (C) Mifepristone is a competitive glucocorticoid antagonist. In high doses, it block the feedback regulation of HPA axis and thus increasing endogenous ACTH. It is used in inoperable patients with ectopic ACTH secretion or adrenal carcinoma. Spironolactone, eplerenone and drospirenone are mineralocorticoid antagonists. Metyrapone, aminoglute, thimide, ketoconazole initotone, trilostone etc are steroid synthesis inhibitors.

Ans. 40 (A) Fetal secretion of cortisol helps in maturation of lungs. When high doses of betamethasone are given to mother during labour, it reduces the incidence of ARDS. It has better penetration through placenta as compare to other steroids and its placental binding is less than predinisolone and cortisol. Thus it decreases incidence of neonatal mortality.

Ans. 41 (A) Absolute contraindications of steroid therapy are Cushing's syndrome and herpes ocular infection. Relative contraindications are peptic ulcer, diabetes osteoporosis, epilepsy, cataract and during pregnancy (long term use causes fetal defects).

Ans. 42 (A) Ethinyl estradiol is a synthetic estrogen with good bioavailability and is most commonly used estrogenic component of OCPs, transdermal contraceptive and vaginal ring contraceptive.

Ans. 43 (D) The common contraindication of combined OCP are pregnancy itself (causes congenital deformities), hepatic renal and gallbladder diseases, thromboembolic disorders, undiagnosed vaginal bleeding, diabetes, obesity, epilepsy (as they decrease seizure threshold). It also causes precipitation or worsening of migraine headache.

Ans. 44 (C) The common adverse effects of androgens are virilization, oligospermia, painful erection, precocious puberty, cholestatic jaundice (with methyl testosterone fluxoymesterone and stanozolol), hepatic carcinoma and gynaecomastia due to peripheral conversion of testosterone to estrogen. DHE does not cause as it is not converted into estradiol.

Ans. 45 (C) DES is a non-steroid estrogen agonist and may result in fetal damage that predisposed infertility to female offspring and a rare form of vaginal cancer.

Ans. 46 (A) Selective estrogen receptor modulators are non-steroidal synthetic agents. They produce beneficial estrogenic effects in certain organs/ tissue and prevents some adverse effect by their antagonistic effects. Clomiphene, tamoxifen, doloxifen, toremifen, fulvestrant, raloxifen and ormeloxifen are examples of SERM.

Ans. 47 (C) Raloxifen has estrogenic effect on bone, lipid metabolism and coagulation and anti-estrogenic effect on breast and endometrial tissue. It is used to treat osteoporosis in post menopausal women. It does not relieve hot flushes and increases the risk of deep vein thrombosis due to estrogenic effect on blood coagulation.

Ans. 48 (A) Dehydroepiandrostenedione is the most potent androgen.

Ans. 49 (B) Clomiphene citrate is anti-estrogen to both ER alpha and ER beta receptors and induces Gn hormone and increase LH and FSH release which leads to enlargement of ovaries and ovulation. Danazol is orally active ethisterone having weak androgenic, anabolic and progestational activities. It causes suppression of Gn secretion from pituitary and inhibits testicular/ovarian function. Cyproterone is a potent anti-androgen and competes with dihydrotestosterone for the intracellular androgen receptors.

Ans. 50 (A) Spiranolactone causes gynaecomastia as its adverse effect.

Ans. 51 (D) Cyproterone acetate, danazol, flutamide, bicalutamide are anti-androgen. Ketoconazole, cimetidine and spironolactone, have weak anti-androgenic action as side effect. Progesterone has weak androgen receptor blocking action.

Ans. 52 (D) Third generation contraceptive pills contain desogesterol as progestin and ethinyl estradiol as estrogen in phasic manner. Both estrogen and progestin act synergistically to inhibit ovulation and cause prompt bleeding at the end of cycle (progestin effect). Less chances of developing endometrial carcinoma (estrogen effect) are also there with combination pills. But they do not interfere with placental functioning.

Ans. 53 (D) Cortisone is used in virilizing adrenal hyperplasia.

Ans. 54 (B) Anabolic steroids are synthetic androgens with higher anabolic and low androgenic activity. They includes nandrolone, oxymetholone, stanozolol and methandienone. They increase protein synthesis enhance muscle mass, improve appetite and results into weight gain and a sense of well being.

Ans. 55 (A) Danazole is used in endometriosis, hereditary angioneurotic oedema, fibrocystic breast disease and in menorrhagia (not in amenorrhoea).

Ans. 56 (C) Estrogen causes growth of female sex organs, thickening and cornification of vagina with endometrial proliferation and has anabolic effect similar to testosterone.

Ans. 57 (B) It is a 19 nor steroid used specially for HRT having estrogenic and progestational property with weak androgenic activity. It minimize the menopausal symptoms. It increases the risk of endometrial carcinoma.

Ans. 58 (D) Tamoxifen has potent estrogenic antagonist action on breast cancer and on blood vessels but have partial agonist action on uterus (endometrial proliferation), bone, liver and on pituitary. It is used for breast carcinoma in both pre and post menopausal women. It lowers gonadotropin (Gn) and prolactin levels. It also improves bone mass and lipid profile.

Ans. 59 (A) Progestin alone is used in those patients who have deficiency of progestin. They are effective in preventing premature delivery in high risk pregnancy.

Ans. 60 (D) Mifepristone (single dose taken within 72 hours) can be used as post coital pill. Other post coital (emergency) pill preparations are combination of levonorgesterol and ethinyl estradiol or levonorgesterol alone taken twice with 12 hours gap.

Ans. 61 (D) The most undesirable effects of depot medroxyprogesterone are disruption of menstrual bleeding pattern and total amenorrhea. It is not suitable for adolescent girls and lactating mothers.

Ans. 62 (C) Biphosphonates (BPN) are synthetic pyrophosphate, that inhibits osteoclast-mediated bone resorption. It binds to the hydroxyapatite crystals of the bones and when osteoclast attaches to the bone matrix, they are released from the bone, which are then internalized by endocytosis into the osteoclast to accelerate their apoptosis. They also inhibit the release of IL-G to suppress differentiation of osteoclast precursors. Etidronate is preferred in Paget's disease and for ectopic ossification. Tiludronate orally can be used in osteoporosis. Alendronate, pamidronate and ibandronate are more potent. Risedronate, zolendronate and oxidronate are most potent BPN.

Ans. 63 (A) Bromocriptin is a potent D_2 receptors agonist and a weak D_1 antagonist. It inhibits the secretion of prolactin due to its agonistic action. It is used in hyperprolactinemia (causing galactorrhoea, amenorrhoea and infertility), suppression of lactation (not recommended nowadays), acromegaly and parkinsonism.

Ans. 64 (A) Cholecalciferol, ergocalciferol, calcitriol, alfacalcidol, calcipotriol and doxercacliferol are different Vitamin D preparation. They are added to milk or with multi vitamin preparation in combination to prevent deficiency. Calcitriol and its analogue (last three) poorly bind with Vitamin D and their clearance is faster so not commonly used in deficiency disease but in those where hypercalcemia can be avoided.

Ans. 65 (C) Vitamin D metabolites, *i.e.*, calcifediol or calcitriol act on the intestine and increase Ca^{2+} and PO_4^{-3} absorption by binding to PO_4^{-3} receptors present in gut.

Ans. 66 (A) Calcitriol directly inhibits PTH secretion. It raises proximal tubular reabsorption of both Ca^{2+} and PO_4^{-3} in the kidney which reduces the production of calcitriol by negative feedback.

Ans. 67 (D) Fludrocortisone has minimum glucocorticoid and maximum mineralocorticoid activity.

Ans. 68 (A) It act by decreasing the absorption of glucose from GIT, which increases availability of glucose for its conversion to lactate by enterocytes and causes lactic acidosis as adverse effects.

Ans. 69 (B) Bromocriptine is a dopamine agonist used to treat hyperprolectinemia for suppression of lactation. Aprotinin is used in cardiac surgery to reduce the amount of blood transfusions.

Ans. 70 (A) Sulfonylurea's such as glyburide increase the release of insulin from the pancreas. They may also cause an increase in insulin receptors, which increases tissue sensitivity to insulin.

Ans. 71 (B) Triamcinolone, Betamethasone and Dexamethasone are devoid of any mineralocorticoid activity thus having no adverse effects like fluid retention and hypertension when used. Fludrocortisone on other hand is a potent mineralocorticoid with some glucocorticoid activity as well. It can be used as replacement therapy in Addison's disease in a dose of 50-200 μg daily.

Ans. 72 (C) Antithyroid drugs bind to thyroid peroxidase and prevent oxidation of iodide/idotyrosyl residue thus they cause iodination of tyrosine residue in thyroglobulin and coupling to form T_3 and T_4. They do not interfere with trapping of iodide and do not modify the action of T_3 and T_4 on peripheral tissues or on pituitary.

Ans. 73 (D) Gabapentin, a GABA analogue, binds tightly to alpha and delta type subunits and therefore has been found useful in treating diabetic neuropathy, post hepatic neuralgia trigeminal neuralgia and pain associated with multiple sclerosis.

Ans. 74 (D) Clomiphene citrate is orally active SERM (selective estrogen receptor modulator) with both agonistic and antagonistic activity. It enhanced GnRH and increase FSH and LH secretion and facilitates ovulation and used to treat infertility.

Ans. 75 (A) Anabolic steroids increases proteins synthesis, enhance muscle mass, improve appetite resulting in weight gain and sense of well-being. It also reduces Ca^{2+} ion excretion so used to treat osteoporosis. They also stimulate erythrocyte production. But they are not indicated (though used) in athletes to increase muscle mass.

Ans. 76 (A) The hepatic side effects of estrogen can be minimized by routes that avoid first pass exposure (transdermal, vaginal) as conjugated metabolite enters in the enterohepatic circulation and have high ratio of hepatic and peripheral adverse effects, *e.g.*, thromboembolic disorder and hepatic adenoma on prolonged use.

9

MISCELLANEOUS DRUGS

HAEMATINICS AND ERYTHROPOIETIN

Haematinics

Haematinics such as iron, Vitamin B_{12}, Folic acid, etc. are required for the formation of blood and are used in the treatment of anaemias.

Iron

Iron is an essential element of the body. Its important sources are liver, fish, dry fruits, jaggery, spinach, banana, meat, egg yolk, etc.

The total amount of iron in an adult male is about 4 gm and 2.5 gm in females. Dietary iron exists in ferric form, which is reduced to ferrous iron with the help of HCl in the stomach. Absorption of most of the iron takes place in the duodenum and upper jejunum.

Factors Affecting Iron Absorption

Iron absorption is **facilitated** by acidic pH of the stomach, ascorbic acid and cysteine, which reduces the ferric iron to ferrous form. Iron deficiency states also increase the absorption of iron. Iron absorption is **inhibited** by excess of phosphates, oxalates and phytates. Milk, antacids and tetracycline reduce iron absorption by forming insoluble complexes.

Preparations of Iron

- *Oral preparations:* Ferrous sulphate, ferrous gluconate, ferrous fumarate etc.
- *Adverse effects* of oral iron are nausea, vomiting, epigastric discomfort, dyspepsia, metallic taste, constipation or diarrhoea and staining of teeth (mainly with liquid preparation).

Parenteral Preparations

1. **Iron sorbitol citric acid complex (Jectofer):** It is given intramuscularly, but never intravenously. It is contraindicated during pregnancy.

2. **Iron dextran (Imferon):** It is the most commonly used parenteral preparation and can be administered intravenously or intramuscularly.
3. **Sodium ferric gluconate:** Recently approved preparation for I.V. use, has a much lower risk of anaphylactic reaction than iron dextran.

Indications for Parenteral Iron Therapy

1. Intolerance to oral iron.
2. Severe malabsorption (failure to absorb iron adequately due to ulcerative colitis).
3. Non-compliance to oral iron.
4. Severe anaemia in the late stages of pregnancy.
5. Along with erythropoietin in patients with renal disease.

Adverse Effects of Parenteral Iron

The injections are painful, may cause abscess formation and discoloration of the skin at the site of injection. The systemic side effects are headache, pyrexia, nausea, vomiting, arthralgia, lymphadenopathy and urticaria. Anaphylactic reaction may also occur.

Therapeutic Uses of Iron

1. *To treat iron deficiency anaemia*
   - During pregnancy.
   - Chronic blood loss.
   - Due to nutritional iron deficiency.
   - Due to poor absorption of iron from the gut.
2. *Prophylaxis:* During pregnancy and lactation.

Acute Iron Poisoning

It is seen frequently in infants and young children. Iron poisoning is very rare in adults. Sign and symptoms of poisoning are vomiting, abdominal pain, hematemesis, diarrhea, cyanosis, dehydration, convulsion, cardiac collapse and death.

Treatment

a. *General measures:* Induce vomiting, gastric lavage.

b. *Specific therapy:* Desferrioxamine, a potent iron chelating agent is administered by I.V. infusion or intramuscularly depending on the severity of poisoning. It binds with iron in the blood and facilitates its excretion.

c. *Supportive measures:* Maintain airway, breathing, circulation, fluid and electrolyte and acid-base balance.

VITAMINS

Vitamin B_{12}

Vitamin B_{12} is water soluble vitamin and acts as a coenzyme in certain metabolic pathways. The coenzyme forms are methylcobalamin (methyl B_{12}) and 5'deoxyadenosyl cobalamin. Methylcobalamin is necessary for the conversion of homocysteine to methionine, for the conversion of methyl malonyl CoA to succinyl CoA, in nucleic acid metabolism and protein synthesis.

The ingested vitamin B_{12} form complexes with intrinsic factor (IF) in the stomach, which is secreted by gastric parietal cells. This so formed vitamin B_{12}: IF complex reaches the terminal ileum, where it binds to specific receptors, and vitamin B_{12} gets absorbed into the blood in combination with beta-globulin, *e.g.*, transcobalamine II (TC II). Excess vitamin B_{12} is transported to liver for storage. Vitamin B_{12} is excreted in bile and undergoes enterohepatic cycling. Deficiency of vitamin B_{12} leads to arrest of maturation of cells in the bone marrow and defective myelination of large nerve fibers in the spinal cord leads to sub acute combined degeneration, a neurological syndrome.

Sources: Liver, kidney, fish, egg yolk and pulses.

Daily requirement: 1-3 microgram/day (during pregnancy 3-5 microgram).

Preparations

Vitamin B_{12} is available for oral and parenteral administration. Cyanocobalamin, hydroxocobalamin and methylcobalamin are some preparations.

Deficiency of vitamin B_{12} occurs due to pernicious anaemia, gastric disease, malabsorption and nutritional deficiency.

Uses

1. Pernicious anaemia: It is due to auto immune destruction of the gastric parietal cells that synthesize IF. In pernicious anaemia, oral vitamin B_{12} is not absorbed because of the deficiency of IF. They always require parenteral vitamin B_{12}. Cyanocobalamin with intrinsic factor is the preparation of choice and is given through I.M./S.C. (but never intravenously). The dose of cobalamin is 30–100/μg/day for 10 days initially, 100 μg once a week for 8 weeks followed by 100 μg every month for life long. Folic acid also combined with vitamin B_{12} in neurological complications.

2. Tobacco Amblyopia

Folic Acid

Folic acid is a combination of glutamic acid, para amino benzoic acid and pteridine nucleus. It is abundantly found in fresh green leafy vegetables, liver, yeast, kidney, fruits, etc. Most of the dietary folic acid is found as polyglutamates, but these are not absorbed unless they form mono glutamate by the action of intestinal enzyme folate reductase. It is reduced to dihydro folic acid (DHFA) and then gets methylated. In the blood, it is transported to various tissues as N-methyl tetrahydrofolic acid. It is bound with albumin and is stored mainly in liver. The stores are exhausted in about 3–4 months hence the manifestations of folic acid deficiency appear in about 3–4 months.

Causes of Folic Acid Deficiency

1. Dietary deficiency: Most common.
2. Decreased absorption (malabsorption, tropical sprue), coeliac disease.
3. Diminished storage (hepatic disease, vitamin C deficiency).
4. Decreased utilization (due to drugs, *e.g.*, phenytoin, phenobarbitone, chronic alcoholics).
5. Increased demand (pregnancy, lactation, hemolytic anaemias).
6. Drug induced (anti folates, *e.g.*, methotrexate, trimethoprim, pyrimethamine).

Preparations: It is availbale as folic acid and folinic acid (Oral and IM).

Uses

1. *Megaloblastic anaemias.*
2. *Pernicious anaemia:* Give a combination of B_{12} and folic acid. Avoid use of folic acid alone.
3. *Prophylactic therapy:* During pregnancy, routine prophylactically folic acid 5 mg/day orally given from the first trimester to prevent neural tube defects.

4. *Methotrexate toxicity.*
5. Malabsorption syndrome 2–5 mg/day (therapeutic dose), 0.5 mg/day (prophylactic).

Oral folic acid is safe, but injections may rarely cause hypersensitivity reactions.

Erythropoietin

Erythropoietin is a glycoprotein produced by peritubular interstitial cells of the kidney in response to anaemia and myelosuppression. Commercially, erythropoietin is produced by recombinant DNA technology.

Erythropoietin stimulates erythropoiesis by acting on the erythropoietic stem cells. It is administered by I.V./SC route.

Uses

Anaemia associated with chronic renal failure and cancer, due to anti-cancer drugs and zidovudine therapy in HIV infected patients.

Adverse effects include rise in blood pressure, hemtocrit and thromboembolic complications. Rarely allergic reactions also may occur.

Fat Soluble Vitamins (A, D, E And K)

Vitamin D and K are already discussed.

Vitamin A (Retinol)

Source: Green leafy vegetables, carrots, mango, papaya, eggs, milk, butter, cheese, liver and fish liver oils. It is essential nutrient required for normal reproduction, vision and immune competence (antioxidant) and integrity of epithelial cells.

Signs and symptoms of deficiency: Xerophthalmia, Bitot's spots in the conjunctiva, night blindness, diarrhoea, dry and rough skin are seen in early stages. In the later stages, keratomalacia, perforation of the cornea, necrosis and blindness can occur. There is increased susceptibility for urinary calculus and faulty moulding of bones.

Dose: 3000-5000 IU/day is used for prophylaxis.

50000-100000 IU/IM used for 3 days followed by supplement doses in night blindness.

Retinoic acid or synthetic analogs of vitamin A like tretinoin or isotretinoin are used in the treatment of acne.

Vitamin E (Alpha Tocopherol)

Source: Wheat germ oil, rice germ oil and soyabean oil. Vitamin E is essential for normal structure and function of the nervous system and is an anti-sterility agent. Vitamin E deficiency in human beings usually does not occur. **Deficiency** may cause peripheral neuropathy with spinocerebellar degeneration, sterility, muscular dystrophy, haemolytic anaemia.

Daily requirement is 10–15 mg.

It can be used as antioxidant in menopausal syndrome, scleroderma and in various skin disorders.

Liquid paraffin emulsifies fat soluble vitamins and leads to their deficiency.

Water Soluble Vitamins

Vitamin B Complex

Thiamine (Vitamin B_1)

Source: Outer layer of cereals, pulses, peanuts, organ meat, yeast.

Thiamine is converted to thiamine pyrophosphate which acts as a coenzyme in carbohydrate metabolism. Daily requirement is 1.5–2 mg. Thiamine deficiency produces beriberi. It can be:

Dry beriberi, which is characterized by peripheral neuritis and muscular atrophy and treated by 5–10 mg/day.

Wet beriberi, which is characterized by dependent edema and high output cardiac failure. Wernicke's encephalopathy and Korsakoff's psychosis are also thought to be due to thiamine deficiency and treated by 100 mg/day IV/IM.

Riboflavin (Vitamin B_2)

Source: Milk, egg, liver, meat, grains, green leafy vegetables and sprouted pulses.

Flavin mononucleotide (FMN) and flavin adenine dinucleotide (FAD) containing the active form of riboflavin, which are coenzymes in various oxidation reduction reactions of carbohydrates and in the transfer of hydrogen in amino acid.

Symptoms of deficiency: Stomatitis, glossitis, seborrhoeic keratosis of the nose, ulcers in the mouth, dry skin, burning sensation in the plantar surface of the feet, vascularization of the cornea and alopecia, retard growth and development of fetus (if mother is having deficiency). Dose 1–5 mg/day (prophylaxis).

Nicotinic Acid and Nicotinamide (Vitamin B_3)

Nicotinic acid and nicotinamide are together known as niacin.

Source: Rice (polish), liver, fish, milk, eggs, nuts and pulses.

Nicotinic acid is converted to nicotinamide. Nicotinamide adenine dinucleoticle (NAD) and its phosphate (NADP) are coenzymes involved in several oxidation reduction reactions. Niacin deficiency results in pellagra characterized by dermatitis, diarrhoea and dementia (3Ds). It occurs commonly in alcoholics. It is used in:

1. Prophylaxis and treatment of pellagra (50–500 mg).
2. Nicotinic acid is used in hyperlipoproteinaemia.

Pyridoxine (Vitamin B_6)

Source: Cereals, legumes, liver, milk, meat, eggs and soyabean.

Pyridoxal phosphate is a coenzyme involved in the synthesis of several amino acids, biogenic amines and other compounds (like GABA) and decarboxylation and transamination reactions.

Symptoms of deficiency: Glossitis, peripheral neuritis, anaemia, dermatitis, low seizure threshold due to decreased GABA levels in the brain, hyperirritability, growth retardation, diarrhea and vomiting. It is used in:

1. Anaemia due to pyridoxine deficiency.
2. INH induced peripheral neuropathy used both for prophylaxis and treatment.
3. Convulsions in infants due to pyridoxine deficiency.
4. Morning sickness in pregnancy, pyridoxine may reduce vomiting by an unknown mechanism.

Pantothenic Acid (Vitamin B_5)

Source: Wheat, cereals, milk, peanuts, liver, egg yolk, vegetables and meat.

Pantothenic acid is converted into coenzyme A which is involved in several metabolic reactions. Calcium pantothenate is a component of multivitamin preparations. Deficiency of vitamin B_5 may cause symptoms of neuromuscular degeneration and adrenocortical insufficiency.

Biotin (Vitamin B_7)

Biotin is an organic acid found in liver, nuts, egg yolk and other foods. Biotin deficiency in humans is not known.

Vitamin C (Ascorbic Acid)

Source: Citrus fruits, tomatoes, goose berry, green vegetables and potatoes are rich in vitamin C.

Ascorbic acid is involved in several metabolic reactions including oxidation reduction reactions and in cellular respiration. It is essential for the integrity of connective tissue, for the development of cartilage, bone and teeth and for wound healing.

Vitamin C deficiency results in scurvy characterized by connective tissue defects resulting in hemorrhages in subcutaneous tissues, petechiae, echymoses, impaired wound healing, tender bleeding gums, deformed teeth, brittle bones, anaemia and growth retardation in infants.

Uses

1. Scurvy (prophylaxis and treatment).
2. *Common cold:* Large doses of vitamin C has been tried as prophylactic against common cold with controversial benefits.
3. To acidify urine.
4. Anaemia due to vitamin deficiency.

   Dose: 50-500 mg/day for prophylaxis.
   1-1.5 gm/day for scurvy.

IMMUNOSUPPRESSANTS AND IMMUNOMODULATORS

Immunosuppressants

Immunosuppressants are drugs which inhibit immunity. They may suppress cell mediated or humoral immunity or both. They are useful in various auto immune disease and organ transplantation.

Classification

1. *T cell inhibitors:* Cyclosporine, Tacrolimus, Sirolimus, Mycophenolate mofetil.
2. *Cytotoxic drugs:* Azathioprine, Methotrexate, Cyclophosphamide, Chlorambucil.
3. *Glucocorticoids.*

4. *Antibodies against immune cells molecules:* Muromonab CD3, Alemtuzumab, Efalizumab, Anti-thymocyte globulin (ATG), Anti-pymphocytic globulin (ALG).
5. *Tolerogenes:* Anti-CD80 and Anti-CD86.
6. *TNF_{alpha} inhibitor:* Etanercept.
7. *IL- antagonist:* Anakinra, Rilonacept, Daclizumab, Basiliximab.

T Cell Inhibitors

Cyclosporine acts at an early stage, selectively inhibits T cell proliferation and suppresses cell mediated immunity. It can be given orally and intravenously. Cyclosporine binds to cyclophilin, an immunophilin and this complex binds to and inhibits the enzyme calcineurin phosphatase. This results in inhibition of T cell activation and IL-2 production.

Sirolimus acts by inhibiting calcineurin like cyclosporine.

Tacrolimus / Rapamycin binds to another immunophilin and then the complex inhibits calcineurin. It does not interfere with process of maturation of stem cells.

Adverse effects include nephrotoxicity, hepatotoxicity, anorexia, gum hypertrophy, increased susceptibility to infections, hypertension, hyperkalemia, hyperglycemia, hyperlipidaemia and hirsutism.

It is used in:

- Organ transplantation (for prophylaxis and treatment) to reduce graft rejection in organ transplantation.
- Autoimmune disorders, *e.g.*, rheumatoid arthritis, severe psoriasis, atopic dermatitis, inflammatory bowel disease and nephrotic syndrome.
- Sirolimus may be used in combination with other drugs for the prophylaxis to reduce organ transplant rejection, in psoriasis, uveoretinitis and for coronary angioplasty.

Mycophenolate mofetil a prodrug, is converted to mycophenolic acid, which inhibits guanine nucleotide synthesis and inhibits the proliferation and functions of lymphocytes. It is indicated as an adjunct to other immunosuppressive drugs in the prophylaxis of transplant rejection. It also reduces replication of HIV virus.

Cytotoxic Drugs

Cytotoxic drugs inhibit cell mediated immunity. They are used in the prevention of graft rejection and in autoinumme disorders.

Glucocorticoids are used for prevention of transplant rejection, in the treatment of RA,SLE, and other auto immune disorders.

Antibody Agents

Muromonab D_3 is a monoclonal antibody to D_3 antigens on T lymphocytes. On intravenous administration, T cells disappear from the circulation within minutes. It is used with other immunosuppressant in organ transplantation.

Antithymocyte globulin (ATG) and anti-lymphocytic globulin (ALG) binds to T lymphocytes and depletes them thereby suppressing immune response. They are antigenic, causes serum sickness and nephritis. ALG binds with a protein on the lymphocyte surface. They are used in renal transplant and bone marrow transplant.

Infliximab is a monoclonal antibody and **Etanercept and Anakinra** are proteins that blocks TNF alpha. They are useful in rheumatoid arthritis and Crohn's disease.

Rilonacept: Under trial for use in gout.

Immunostimulants (Immunomodulators)

Immunostimulating and immunomodulating agents are drugs that modulate the immune response and can be used to increase the immune responsiveness of patients with immunodeficiency as in AIDS, chronic illness and cancers. The drugs currently used for this purpose are BCG and levamisole. BCG has been tried in cancers. Levamisole used as anthelmintic is also found to enhance cell-mediated immunity in humans. It has been tried in some cancers.

Interferons are cytokines with antiviral and immunomodulatory properties. Recombinant interferons (alpha, beta and gamma) are available for clinical use. They bind to specific receptors and bring about immune activation and increase host defense. Interferons are indicated in several tumors including malignant melanoma, hairy cell leukaemia lymphomas, Kasposi's sarcoma, condylomata acuminata and in viral infections.

Various peptides (*e.g.*, Neuropeptides, Tuftsin) cytokines (IL, interferon, immunoglobulins) also have immune stimulatory properties.

Gene Therapy

Gene therapy is the replacement of defective gene by the insertion of a normal, functional gene. It is the genetic modification of cells for the prevention or treatment of a disease and correcting the defect in the affected part of the body. Gene therapy can confer new functions to the cell.

Gene transfer requires the use of vectors to deliver the DNA material. An ideal vector should be safe and effective. Vector may be:

- *Physical vectors:* DNA is complexes with substances like lipids and then administered.
- *Chemical vectors:* Lipósomes are used to carry genes into the cells.
- *Biological vectors:* Most important biological vectors are viral vectors. Viruses invade cells and use the metabolic processes of these host cells for replication.

  The principal applications of gene therapy are in single gene defects like thalassemia, cystic fibrosis, hemoglobinopathies, in the treatment of cancer, cardiovascular diseases, atherosclerosis, immunodeficiency disorders–particularly AIDS, anaemia, Alzheimer's disease and many infectious diseases.

CHELATING AGENTS

Heavy metals bind to and inactivate the functional groups (ligands) of essential tissue enzymes and interfere with normal cell functions. Heavy metals cannot be metabolized in the body.

Chelating agents or heavy metal antagonists bind the heavy metal ions and make them nontoxic. The chemical complex formed is called chelate (Chele = claw). The complex so formed is water soluble and is eliminated by the kidneys.

The clinically useful chelating agents are calcium disodium edetate ($CaNa_2$ EDTA), dimercaprol, d-penicillamine and desferrioxamine. Chelating agents are more effective when they are given earlier, as they prevent the utilization of ligands rather than reactivating them. Adverse effects include nephrotoxicity, fatigue, fever, myalgia and dermatitis.

Calcium disodium edetate ($CaNa_2$ EDTA) is mainly used in lead poisoning. It can also be used in zinc, manganese and iron poisoning. It is nephrotoxic, may cause vitamin B_6 deficiency.

Dimercaprol: British anti-lewisite (BAL) is a colorless, oily liquid. Dimercaprol chelates arsenic, mercury, lead and other heavy metals, used in lead encephalopathy as it rapidly crosses BBB. It may cause hemolysis in patients with G6 PD deficiency.

Unithiol is a water soluble analogue of dimercaprol that can be given both orally and parenterally. It enhances the excretion of mercury, arsenic and lead.

The incidence of side effects is low. It may cause Stevens-Johnson's syndrome.

Succimer is another water soluble analogue of dimercaprol. It is used in acute arsenic poisoning and it is also effective in lead and mercury poisoning. It is effective orally. It is used in lead poisoning and reverses many of the biochemical indication of toxicity.

D-penicillamine: It chelates copper, mercury, zinc and lead. It is used for the treatment of Wilson's disease and cystinuria. It is also used orally. Bone marrow depression and allergic reaction are common with it. Pyridoxine should be administered with it.

Desferrioxamine is used in the treatment of iron poisoning. It is poorly absorbed through GIT, so given parenterally. It is contraindicated in renal insufficiency, anuria and during pregnancy.

DRUGS USED IN THE TREATMENT OF MIGRAINE

Migraine is a common disorder characterized by severe, throbbing, unilateral, headache often associated with nausea, vomiting and fatigue, lasting for several hours. An attack is triggered by factors like stress, anxiety, excitement, food etc. These triggering factors stimulate the release of vasoactive substances from nerve endings which are responsible for the events that follow.

Drugs Used in Acute Attack are:

- Aspirin, paracetamol or other NSAIDs.
- Metoclopramide can be combined with aspirin as it is an antiemetic and also speeds up absorption of aspirin.
- Sumatriptan is very effective but short acting.

Drugs Used for Prophylaxis

When the attacks are frequent and severe, prophylaxis is needed.

- *Beta adrenergic blockers:* Propranolol reduces frequency and severity of attacks. The mechanism of action is not exactly known.
- *Calcium channel blocker:* Flunarizine may be useful.
- Pizotifen and cyproheptadine block 5-HT and H_1 histamine receptors. They may be used as alternatives.
- *Tricyclic antidepressants:* Amitriptyline may be tried but it is associated with many adverse effects.

Serotonin Agonists and Antagonists Used in the Treatment of Migraine

Drugs	Receptor	Uses	Comments
Sumatriptan	5-HT1$_D$	Acute migraine, cluster headache	Short acting
Ergot alkaloids			
Ergotamine	5-HT$_1$ partial agonist/ antagonist	Acute attack of migraine	
Methysergide	5-HT$_2$ partial agonist/ antagonist	Prophylaxis of migraine	Not preferred due to risk of retroperitoneal and mediastinal fibrosis

DRUGS ACTING ON UTERUS

Uterine Stimulants (Oxytocics)

Oxytocics are the drugs that cause uterine contraction. They include

A. **Oxytocin.**
B. **Ergot derivatives:** Ergometrine, Methylergometrine, Ergonovine
C. **Prostaglandins:** PGE_2, PGF_2 alpha, 15-methyl PGF_{2alpha}, Misoprostol.

A. Oxytocin

It is a peptide hormone synthesized in the hypothalamus along with ADH and stored and secreted from posterior pituitary.

Mechanism of Action

Oxytocin binds to specific G protein coupled receptors on myometrium. This leads to generation of IP_3 (inositol triphosphate), release of Ca^{2+} from intracellular stores and increased production of PGs by endometrium. This leads to contraction of the pregnant uterus.

Pharmacological Actions

1. **Uterus:** Non-pregnant uterus is not sensitive to oxytocin.
   During parturition: Uterus is highly sensitive to oxytocin. It increases both force and frequency of uterine contractions. This results in expulsion of the fetus from the uterus.
   With I.V. infusion of low dose of oxytocin, there is a period of complete relaxation between two successive uterine contractions that allows refilling of the placental blood vessels by the maternal

arterial blood and thus prevents fetal asphyxia. Higher doses of oxytocin cause sustained uterine contractions that interfere with blood flow through the placenta and cause fetal distress, which leads to asphyxial injury to the baby.

2. **Breast:** Oxytocin contracts the myoepithelial cells of the female breast and causes milk ejection.
3. **CVS:** Small doses have no effect but high doses causes vasodilatation and transient hypotension, reflex tachycardia and flushing. Umbilical vessels are contracted.
4. **Kidney:** It has ADH like action and decreases urine output, renal plasma flow and causes sodium and water retention.

Uses

a. *Therapeutic*
   1. Induction of labour: Oxytocin is the drug of choice for induction of labour because:
      a. It has short plasma half life and causes complete relaxation between the uterine contractions that allow refilling of the placental blood vessels by the maternal arterial blood and thus prevents fetal asphyxia.
      b. Lower uterine segment is not contracted, so the fetal descent is not compromised.
   2. Uterine inertia.
   3. Postpartum hemorrhage: Oxytocin may be used for the prevention as well as treatment of postpartum hemorrhage (PPH) (but ergometrine is preferred).
   4. Breast engorgement.
   5. In veterinary practice to increase production of milk.

b. *Diagnostic oxytocin challenge test:* It is an invasive method, which is preferred in selected cases to assess the uteroplacental adequacy.

Averse Effects

1. Hyperstimulation of uterus: Over dosage can cause strong uterine contractions and even rupture of uterus.
2. Prolonged or large doses may cause fetal hypoxia or even fetal death.
3. Prolonged IV infusion can cause water intoxication due to ADH like action.

B. Ergot Derivatives

Pharmacological Actions

1. *Uterus:* They stimulate uterine contractions involving both upper and lower segments. At low doses, contractions are rhythmic with a period of relaxation in between. But at higher doses, the contractions become more powerful and raise the resting tone, and the uterus passes into a state of sustained tonic contractions called uterine tetany.
2. *GIT:* In high doses, they can increase the peristaltic movements.
3. *CVS:* In therapeutic doses, they can increase the BP, but it is not significant.

Therapeutic Uses

1. Postpartum hemorrhage (PPH).
2. After caesarean section to prevent uterine atony and thus control bleeding.
3. To hasten the involution of the uterus when it is delayed.
4. Migraine.

Adverse Effects

Nausea, vomiting and rise in BP especially in hypertensive patients. Prolonged use may cause gangrene of fingers and toes due to vasoconstrictor effect. They may interfere with lactation, so used with caution.

Contraindications

1. Hypertension and other cardiac diseases.
2. Preeclampsia and eclampsia.
3. Rh negative mother.

C. Prostaglandins

They inhibit the spontaneous activity of isolated non-pregnant human uterus. They stimulate myometrial smooth muscle, hasten the process of softening and dilatation of cervix (cervical ripening) and act as leuteolytic agent by inhibiting the secretion of progesterone by corpus luteum. They are more effective in 2nd trimester of pregnancy. In 3rd trimester they are less effective than oxytocin.

Advers effects are nausea, vomiting, headache, diarrhoea. They should be used with caution in presence of increased IOP, hypertension, diabetes mellitus, epilepsy and angina. They are contraindicated in renal, cardiac, pulmonary and hepatic diseases.

Uses

1. Therapeutic abortion.
2. Cervical priming (Dinoprostone is used).
3. Postpartal bleeding (ergometrine is preferred).
4. Induction of term labour (when oxytocin is contraindicated).

Uterine Relaxants (Tocolytics)

Tocolytics are drugs that inhibit uterine contractions.

a. Beta Adrenergic Agonists

The selective $beta_2$ agonists used as uterine relaxants are isoxsuprine, orciprenaline, salbutamol, terbutaline and ritodrine.

b. Magnesium Sulphate

It has a depressant action on uterine smooth muscle, central nervous system and myocardium. It is used to control convulsions and BP in toxemia of pregnancy. It is useful when $beta_2$ agonists are contraindicated.

c. Calcium Channel Blockers

Nifedipine acts by inhibiting the influx of Ca^{2+} ions into the myometrial cells. It is used orally as tocolytic.

d. Prostaglandin Synthesis Inhibitors

NSAIDs like indomethacin, ibuprofen, mefenamic acid, aspirin etc. have tocolytic effect by inhibiting prostaglandin synthesis. But they are not used because of adverse effects such as premature closure of ductus arteriosus with subsequent development of pulmonary hypertension.

e. Progesterone

Progestins are used in the treatment of threatened abortion. They may cause masculinization of female fetus.

f. Atosiban (Oxytocin Receptor Antagonist)

It competitively blocks the oxytocin receptors of the uterus and induces uterine relaxation. Side effects are nausea, vomiting, hypotension, headache and skin rashes.

Uses

1. To delay preterm labour.
2. Threatened abortion.
3. Dysmenorrhoea.

MULTIPLE CHOICE QUESTIONS

Q. 1 In the treatment of pernicious anaemia Vitamin B_{12} and folic acid should be given together because:

(A) Vitamin B_{12} acts as a cofactor for dihydrofolate reductase
(B) Folic acid alone causes improvement of anemic symptoms but not neurological dysfunction
(C) Vitamin B_{12} deficiency may result in methyl folate trap
(D) Folic acid is required for conversion of methyl malonyl-CoA to succenyl CoA

Q. 2 Which drug do not produce methemoglobinemia?

(A) Nitroglycerine (B) Prilocaine
(C) Phenytoin (D) Dapsone

Q. 3 Which of the following side effect of oral iron therapy limits compliance by the patient?

(A) Epigastric pain and bowel alteration
(B) Fever
(C) Joint pain
(D) Lymphadenopathy

Q. 4 Chelating agents are the group of drugs primarily used for:

(A) Gout (B) Barbiturate poisoning
(C) Cyanide poisoning (D) Heavy metal poisoning

Q. 5 Which of the following is true regarding infliximab?

(A) It is a recombinant antibody to TNF-alpha
(B) It is a humanized antibody to TNF-alpha
(C) It is a recombinant proteins resembling IL-1
(D) It is recombinant protein composed of a portion of LFA-3

Q. 6 Regarding correction of iron deficiency anaemia which of the following statement is most appropriate?

(A) Parenteral iron corrects the deficiency more rapidly
(B) Sustained release preparations are more suited as they provide continuous release
(C) Oral ion in the form of desiccated ferrous sulphate is the preparation of choice
(D) Oral iron corrects the deficiency just as rapidly as parenteral iron in most cases

---

1 (B) 2 (C) 3 (A) 4 (D) 5 (A) 6 (D)

Q. 7 Which statement is true regarding the treatment of migraine?

(A) Simple analgesics like paracetamol are ineffective in migraine
(B) Ergot alkaloids are used for the prophylaxis
(C) Use of ergot alkaloids is restricted to severe or resistant cases
(D) Ergot alkaloids should be given till 24 hours after an attack has subsided

Q. 8 Ergotamine relieves migraine by which of the following mechanism:

(A) Blocking vascular 5-HT_2 receptors
(B) Constricting cranial vessels and reducing perivascular neurogenic inflammation
(C) Blocking vascular alpha-adrenergic receptors
(D) Constrict the dilated cranial arteriovenous shunt channels

Q. 9 Which of the following is true for the sumatriptan?

(A) It activates all types of serotonergic neurons
(B) It tends to suppress vomiting accompanying migraine
(C) It does not carry risk of precipitating coronary vasospasm
(D) It is combined with ergotamine for treatment of severe migraine

Q. 10 Which of the following drug is most commonly used for prophylaxis of migraine?

(A) Ergotamine (B) Propranolol
(C) Methesergide (D) Sumatriptan

Q. 11 Oxytocin is preferred over ergometrine for augmenting labour because:

(A) It has brief and titrable action
(B) It is less likely to cause fetal anoxia (asphyxia)
(C) It is less likely to impede fetal descent
(D) All of the above

Q. 12 Ergometrine is used in all of the following *except:*

(A) Post partum hemorrhage (PPH)
(B) Inadequate uterine involution
(C) Uterine inertia during labour
(D) Uterine atony after cesarean section

---

7 (C) 8 (D) 9 (B) 10 (B) 11 (D) 12 (C)

Q. 13 Ergonovine is having following mechanism to control PPH:

(A) It causes vasoconstriction of uterine arteries
(B) It increases tone of uterine muscles
(C) It prompt coagulation
(D) It induces platelet aggregation

Q. 14 Which of the following drugs is preferred to suppress labour?

(A) Atropine
(B) Ritodrine
(C) PGE_2
(D) Progesterone

Q. 15 Which of the following preparation has highest elemental iron content?

(A) Ferrous sulfate
(B) Ferrous gluconate
(C) Ferrous fumarate
(D) Ferric hydroxide polymaltose complex

Q. 16 Deficiency of which vitamin can result in CNS effect?

(A) Vitamin B_1
(B) Vitamin B_6
(C) Vitamin B_3
(D) Vitamin B_2

Q. 17 In therapeutic doses Vitamin E is useful in:

(A) Recurrent abortion
(B) Male sterility
(C) Retrolental fibroplasias
(D) Progressive muscular dystrophy

Q. 18 A patient with Wilson's disease allergic to penicillamine can be treated with:

(A) Calcium edetate (B) Dimercaprol
(C) Tetracycline (D) Desferrioxamine

Q. 19 Cyanide poisoning is treated by:

(A) Desferrioxamine (B) Penicillamine
(C) Sodium nitrite (D) Acetonitrite

---

13 (B) 14 (B) 15 (D) 16 (A) 17 (C) 18 (B) 19 (C)

ANSWERS

Ans. 1 (B) Folic acid does not help in conversion of methyl malonyl CoA to succenyl CoA. So deficiency of Vitamin B_{12} leads to accumulation of methyl malonyl CoA which may worsen the neurological symptoms.

Ans. 2 (C) Prilocaine's metabolite ortho-toluidine causes methemoglobinemia. Nitroglycerine converts hemoglobin to methemoglobinemia, so can be used in the treatment of cyanide poisoning. Dapsone causes non-hemolytic anaemia and methemoglobinemia in patients with G-6 PD deficiency. Phenytoin does not cause methemoglobinemia.

Ans. 3 (A) Oral iron therapy may cause epigastric pain, heartburn, nausea, vomiting, staining of teeth, metallic taste, blotting and bowel alteration (diarrhea or constipation). All other effects, *e.g.*, fever; joint pain and lymphadenopathy are the adverse effects of parenteral iron therapy.

Ans. 4 (D) Chelating agents are used in the treatment of heavy metal poisoning, *e.g.*, As, Hg, Au, Bi etc. They form stable non-toxic and easily excreted complexes with toxic metals Dimercaprol, Desferrioxamine, Penicillamine, Calcium disodium edetate are some useful chelating agents. In case of cyanide poisoning, nitrates are used while no antidote is there for barbiturate poisoning.

Ans. 5 (A) Infliximab is a recombinant antibody to TNF-alpha. It has been successfully used in the treatment of Crohn's disease, rheumatoid arthritis and some other auto immune conditions. For RA, it is given in a dose of 3-5 mg/kg IV infusion at 0, 2 and 6 weeks interval over a period of not less than 2 hours.

Ans. 6 (D) Response to oral or parenteral iron preparation is essentially similar with average daily hemoglobin rise of about 0.2 gm%. Hence parenteral therapy is used only under special circumstances.

Ans. 7 (C) In all case of migraine NSAIDs, *e.g.*, aspirin, paracetamol etc. with or without antiemetic should be tried. Ergot alkaloids are also effective in acute attack of migraine but due to availability of better drug (sumatriptan etc.), and due to toxic effect, it is not preferred nowadays. NSAIDs should be taken till the attack subsides.

Ans. 8 (D) Ergotamine is very effective drug to abort acute attack of migraine. It is a partial agonist of 5-HT_{1D} and 5-HT_{1B} receptors. It is used with or without caffeine to potentiate its effect. They constrict dilated cranial vessels and suppress neurogenic inflammation. They are not effective for prophylaxis.

Ans. 9 (B) Sumatriptan and its congeners are selective agonist at 5-HT_{1D} receptors. They cause constriction of dilated extracranial vessels and suppress inflammation. It causes coronary vasospasm, paraesthesia and muscle weakness. It suppresses nausea and vomiting. It should not be combined with ergot alkaloid (not given until 24 hours after the last dose).

Ans. 10 (B) Propranolol is most commonly used for prophylaxis of migraine. Other drugs are CCB (flunarizine), clonidine, pizotifen (5-HT antagonist), TCADs (amitriptyline).

Ans. 11 (D) Oxytocin is a peptide hormone secreted from the posterior pituitary. It increases the magnitude as well as rate of contractions of the upper segment of the uterus (fundus). This facilitates the relaxation of cervix. Uterine contractions occur in the benefit of childbirth.

Ans. 12 (C) Ergometrine and it synthetic derivative methyl ergonovine, increases myometrial contractions involving the fundus, the body and the cervical segment of the uterus. In therapeutic doses, intermittent relaxation is there in between the contractions. But in higher doses there is no relaxation in between the tonic contractions. Therapeutic uses include management of third stage of labour, to treat PPH and for normal involution of uterus. It is not given during labour.

Ans. 13 (B) Ergonovine causes contraction of myometrial meshwork compress the bleeding arteries, which stops the bleeding.

Ans. 14 (B) The primary use of uterine relaxant is in the prevention of premature labour. Tocolytic agents act either directly or act indirectly by inhibiting synthesis/release of PG or oxytocin. $Beta_2$ agonist, *e.g.*, salbutamol, terbutaline, ritodrine, isoxsuprine, magnesium sulfate and CCB, *e.g.*, nifedipine can be used to prevent premature labour.

Ans. 15 (D) The most common oral preparation of iron are ferrous salts, *e.g.*, ferrous sulfate, ferrous fumerate, ferrous gluconoate, which provide 20%, 33% and 19% of elemental iron respectively. Iron polysaccharide complex, carbony-iron complex and ferric hydroxide polymaltose complex have 100% iron content, carry least risk of overdose toxicity and have better GI tolerance.

Ans. 16 (A) Vitamin B_1 (thiamine) deficiency leads to failure of glucose metabolism and lactic acidosis. It causes dry beriberi which affects CNS and PNS, causing peripheral neuropathy, numbness, cramps and muscle weakness.

Ans. 17 (C) Vitamin E is used in nocturnal muscle cramps, to reduce risk of retrolental fibroplasias, fibrocystic breast disease, intermittent claudication, acenthocytosis, to increase survival time of erythrocyte and as anti-oxidant.

Ans. 18 (B) Dimercaprol can be used in patients allergic to penicillamine.

Ans. 19 (C) Cyanide chelate iron of cytochrome oxidase. This causes tissue anoxia, coma and death. Amyl nitrite or sodium nitrite converts hemoglobin into methemoglobin, which traps CN^- and converts it into an unstable cyanmethemoglobin. Subsequent administration of sodium thiosulfate reacts with it and from sodium thiocyanate which get excreted.

